Essential
Evidence-Based
Psychopharmacology

Second Edition

Essential Evidence-Based Psychopharmacology

Second Edition

Edited by

Dan J. Stein
Professor and Chair, Department of Psychiatry, University of Cape Town, Cape Town, South Africa

Bernard Lerer
Professor of Psychiatry and Director, Biological Psychiatry Laboratory, Hadassah-Hebrew University Medical Center, Jerusalem, Israel

Stephen M. Stahl
Adjunct Professor of Psychiatry, University of San Diego, San Diego, California, USA;
Honorary Visiting Senior Fellow in Psychiatry, University of Cambridge, Cambridge, UK

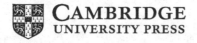

CAMBRIDGE
UNIVERSITY PRESS

CAMBRIDGE
UNIVERSITY PRESS

University Printing House, Cambridge CB2 8BS, United Kingdom

Cambridge University Press is part of the University of Cambridge.

It furthers the University's mission by disseminating knowledge in the pursuit of
education, learning and research at the highest international levels of excellence.

www.cambridge.org
Information on this title: www.cambridge.org/9781107400108

First edition first published 2005
Second edition first published 2012

A catalogue record for this publication is available from the British Library

Library of Congress Cataloguing in Publication data
Essential evidence-based psychopharmacology / edited by
Dan J. Stein, Bernard Lerer, Stephen M. Stahl. – 2nd ed.
    p.   cm.
Rev. ed. of: Evidence-based phamacology.
Includes index.
ISBN 978-1-107-00795-6 (hardback)
1. Mental illness – Chemotherapy.   2. Psychotropic drugs.
3. Psychopharmacology.   4. Evidence-based medicine.
I. Stein, Dan J.   II. Lerer, Bernard.   III. Stahl, S. M.
IV. Evidence-based pharmacology.
RC483.E95   2012
616.89'18 – dc23   2011053165

ISBN 978-1-107-00795-6 Hardback
ISBN 978-1-107-40010-8 Paperback

Contents

Contributors

Christer Allgulander
Karolinska Institutet, Stockholm, Sweden

David S. Baldwin
Clinical Neuroscience Division, School of
Medicine, University of Southampton, UK

Neeltje M. Batelaan
Department of Psychiatry and EMGO
institute, VU University Medical Center
and GGZ inGeest, Amsterdam, the
Netherlands

Hany Bissada
The Ottawa Hospital, Ottawa, ON, Canada

Carlos Blanco
Department of Psychiatry, Columbia
College of Physicians and Surgeons, and
the New York State Psychiatric Institute,
New York, NY, USA

Laura B. Bragdon
Department of Psychiatry, Columbia
College of Physicians and Surgeons, and
the New York State Psychiatric Institute,
New York, NY, USA

Angus Brown
Hertfordshire NHS Trust, UK

Martin Brown
Hampshire Partnership NHS Trust,
Dunsbury Way Clinic, Havant,
Hampshire, UK

Darren Cotterell
Solent Healthcare NHS Trust, St James
Hospital, Portsmouth, Hampshire, UK

John M. Davis
Department of Psychiatry, University of
Illinois at Chicago, IL, USA

Jamie M. Dupuy
Department of Psychiatry, Massachusetts
General Hospital and Harvard Medical
School, Boston, MA, USA

Naomi A. Fineberg
University of Hertfordshire and Queen
Elizabeth II Hospital, Welwyn Garden
City, UK

Martine F. Flament
University of Ottawa Institute of Mental
Health Research, Ottawa, ON, Canada

John R. Geddes
University Department of Psychiatry,
Warneford Hospital, Oxford UK

Stephan Heres
Department of Psychiatry and
Psychotherapy, Technische Universität
München, Klinikum rechts der Isar,
München, Germany

Jeffrey Huffman
Department of Psychiatry, Massachusetts
General Hospital and Harvard Medical
School, Boston, MA, USA

Jonathan C. Ipser
Mailman School of Public Health,
Department of Epidemiology, Columbia
University, New York, NY, USA

Werner Kissling
Department of Psychiatry and
Psychotherapy, Technische Universität
München, Klinikum rechts der Isar,
München, Germany

Christopher J. Kratochvil
University of Nebraska Medical Center,
Omaha, NE, USA

Stefan Leucht
Department of Psychiatry and
Psychotherapy, Technische Universität
München, Klinikum rechts der Isar,
München, Germany

Michael R. Liebowitz
Department of Psychiatry, Columbia
College of Physicians and Surgeons, and
the New York State Psychiatric Institute,
New York, NY, USA

John S. March
Duke University Medical Center, Durham,
NC, USA

Andrew A. Nierenberg
Department of Psychiatry, Massachusetts
General Hospital and Harvard Medical
School, Boston, MA, USA

Michael J. Ostacher
Department of Psychiatry and Behavioral
Sciences, Stanford University School of
Medicine, Stanford, CA, USA

Ilenia Pampaloni
Surrey and Borders Partnership NHS
Trust, UK

Roy H. Perlis
Department of Psychiatry, Massachusetts
General Hospital and Harvard Medical
School, Boston, MA, USA

Luis H. Ripoll
Mental Illness Research Education and
Clinical Center, James J. Peters VA Medical
Center, Bronx, NY, USA

Franklin R. Schneier
Department of Psychiatry, Columbia
College of Physicians and Surgeons, and
the New York State Psychiatric Institute,
New York, NY, USA

Larry J. Siever
Mental Illness Research Education and
Clinical Center, James J. Peters VA Medical
Center, Bronx, NY, USA

Wendy Spettigue
Children's Hospital of Eastern Ontario,
Ottawa, ON, Canada

Dan J. Stein
Department of Psychiatry, University of
Cape Town, Cape Town, South Africa.

Matthew J. Taylor
Institute of Psychiatry, King's College
London, UK

Joseph Triebwasser
Mental Illness Research Education and
Clinical Center, James J. Peters VA Medical
Center, Bronx, NY, USA

Anton J. L. M. Van Balkom
Department of Psychiatry and EMGO
Institute, VU University Medical Center
and GGZ inGeest, Amsterdam, the
Netherlands

Wim van den Brink
Academic Medical Center of the University
of Amsterdam, Department of Psychiatry,
Amsterdam Institute for Addiction
Research (AIAR), Amsterdam, The
Netherlands

Brigette S. Vaughan
University of Nebraska Medical Center,
Omaha, NE, USA

Sarah Waldman
Mood and Anxiety Disorders Service,
Hampshire Partnership NHS Foundation
Trust, UK

Preface

The pioneers of modern psychopharmacology prided themselves on the empirical nature of their work, and the rigor of their clinical data. Evidence-based medicine emphasizes the importance of searching for relevant studies and making decisions in the light of the data, and therefore has immediate appeal for psychopharmacology. This volume attempts to summarize recent advances in evidence-based medication treatment of psychiatric disorders.

Clinical decisions are only as good as the existing evidence, and critics have rightly pointed out the necessity for good clinical judgment and for further research when the data is poor. Nevertheless, there has been a steady growth in methods for systematically reviewing the literature, assessing the clinical trials database, and optimizing clinical decision-making, as well as an ongoing expansion of the evidence-base. We therefore felt that it was timely to update our previous collection of evidence-based chapters on psychopharmacology.

This volume comprises chapters on each of the major psychiatric disorders, and addresses questions such as (1) what is the best first-line psychopharmacological intervention for a particular disorder; (2) how long should such an intervention be continued, and (3) what is the next best strategy should the first-line psychopharmacological agent fail? These questions lie at the heart of clinical psychopharmacology, and we are hopeful that the volume will therefore appeal to practicing clinicians, whether they work in a primary or specialty setting.

Dan J. Stein
Beni Lerer
Stephen Stahl

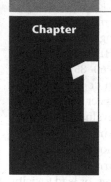

Chapter

1

Evidence-based pharmacotherapy of attention deficit hyperactivity disorder

Brigette S. Vaughan, John S. March, and Christopher J. Kratochvil

Introduction

Attention deficit hyperactivity disorder (ADHD) is a neurobiological disorder, affecting significant numbers of children, adolescents, and adults worldwide. Research throughout the past century has established a strong scientific foundation for our current understanding of the etiology, epidemiology, and treatment of ADHD. The American Medical Association's Council on Scientific Affairs in 1998 stated, "Overall, ADHD is one of the best-researched disorders in medicine, and the overall data on its validity are far more compelling than for many medical conditions" (Goldman et al., 1998). The American Academy of Child & Adolescent Psychiatry (AACAP), in their 2007 ADHD Practice Parameters concluded, "Although scientists and clinicians debate the best way to diagnose and treat ADHD, there is no debate among competent and well-informed healthcare professionals that ADHD is a valid neurobiological condition that causes significant impairment in those whom it afflicts" (Pliszka, 2007).

Neuropsychological, neuroimaging, and genetic studies have demonstrated the biological underpinnings of ADHD. These studies have correlated deficits in executive functioning, response inhibition, delay aversion, vigilance, working memory, and planning with specific regions of the brain (Willcutt et al., 2005). Structural imaging studies have demonstrated that children with ADHD have significantly smaller brain volumes, on average, than same-aged comparison children (Castellanos & Tannock, 2002; Durston et al., 2004; Mostofsky et al., 2002), with smaller cerebellar and total cerebral volumes noted (Castellanos et al., 2002). In addition, functional imaging has revealed discrete variations in brain activation, specifically in the frontal-striatal cerebellar circuits (Krain & Castellanos, 2006). Family, twin, and more recently, genotyping studies provide further support for the biological basis of ADHD. There is considerable evidence that the principal cause of ADHD is genetic, with an estimated heritability of 76% (Faraone et al., 2005). Parents of children with ADHD are 2–8 times more likely to have the disorder themselves, and the risk is similar for siblings of affected children (Faraone & Biederman, 2000).

ADHD has been conservatively estimated to occur in 3–7% of children (APA, 2000), with other estimates as high as 7–12% (CDC, 2005; Woodruff et al., 2004). While most commonly diagnosed between ages 7 and 10 years, symptom presentation and impairment can often be seen in children as young as age 3 years (Lavigne *et al.*, 1996). Epidemiological studies have shown that 2–6% of preschool children meet diagnostic criteria for ADHD (Angold *et al.*, 2000; Lavigne *et al.*, 1996). Of those diagnosed with ADHD as children, 60–85% continue to meet criteria for the disorder as adolescents, and as many as 60% continue to experience symptoms as adults (Barkley *et al.*, 1990, 2002; Biederman *et al.*, 1996; Kessler *et al.*, 2005).

A comprehensive differential diagnosis is essential for an accurate evaluation. Behaviors which are characteristic of normal childhood development may be misinterpreted as ADHD if not considered in an age-appropriate context. In addition, developmental disabilities, learning disorders, mental retardation, and hearing or vision impairments, as well as general medical problems such as hyperthyroidism, partial complex seizures, or lead toxicity may mimic ADHD. Several aspects of the core symptoms of inattention, hyperactivity, and impulsivity, can also be indicative of depressive and anxiety disorders, substance abuse, or pediatric bipolar disorder.

The diagnostic criteria for ADHD require the presence of at least 6/9 inattentive symptoms, and/or 6/9 hyperactive-impulsive symptoms, with onset prior to age 7 years. Symptoms must be developmentally inappropriate and result in clinically significant impairment in social, academic, and/or occupational functioning (APA, 2000). Even preschool children with ADHD are at high risk for academic, social, behavioral, and family dysfunction due to the disorder (DuPaul *et al.*, 2001), and are more likely to be placed in specialized educational settings (Lahey *et al.*, 1998, 2004). These children also have increased rates of accidents and injuries (Lahey *et al.*, 1998), aggression (Connor *et al.*, 2003), and internalizing symptoms (Cunningham & Boyle, 2002). School-aged children with ADHD as a group have more difficulties with peer interactions, academic tasks, and conflicts with parents than do same-aged peers without ADHD. In addition to ongoing difficulties common to younger children, adolescents have elevated rates of substance use and abuse, motor vehicle accidents, academic and occupational impairments, teen pregnancy, and sexually transmitted diseases (Barkley, 2006).

Nearly two-thirds of children diagnosed with ADHD also have at least one co-occurring psychiatric condition. The Multimodal Treatment Study of Children with ADHD (MTA) consisted of one of the largest and best characterized ADHD populations to date ($n = 579$ children aged 7–9.9 years), and demonstrated that only 31% of participants had ADHD alone, while 40% also met criteria for oppositional defiant disorder, 38% for anxiety/mood disorders, 14% for conduct disorder, and 11% for tic disorders (MTA Cooperative Group, 1999).

The National Initiative for Children's Healthcare Quality (NICHQ) recommends that children with ADHD and their families receive individualized treatment with ongoing support and education (Bodenheimer *et al.*, 2002a, 2002b). They recommend that an effective ADHD management plan for children should generally include parent training, behavioral modification and social-skills training, and school-based interventions. In preschool children, or those with mild symptoms, the AACAP (Pliszka, 2007) and American Academy of Pediatrics (AAP, 2001) recommend a trial of behavioral interventions prior to starting medication. Unfortunately, studies have shown that while behavioral therapies offer some benefit, they may have limited effectiveness as a monotherapy for treating moderate to severe ADHD. In the majority of cases, behavioral interventions may be only one component of a more extensive treatment plan.

Table 1.1. Treatment recommendations from the AACAP Practice Parameters for the assessment and treatment of attention deficit hyperactivity disorder (Pliszka, 2007).

Treatment	Monitoring
• The treatment plan for the patient with ADHD should be well thought out and comprehensive.	• Patients receiving pharmacotherapy for ADHD should have their height and weight monitored throughout treatment.
• Pharmacological treatment should begin with an agent approved by the FDA for the treatment of ADHD.	• The patient should be monitored for treatment-emergent side-effects during pharmacotherapy.
• If a patient responds robustly to pharmacotherapy, medication treatment of their ADHD alone may be sufficient.	• If a patient has a suboptimal response to medication, a comorbid diagnosis, or psychosocial stressors, adjunctive psychosocial intervention is often beneficial.
• If none of the FDA-approved medications result in satisfactory treatment, the clinician should review the diagnosis and consider behavioral therapy and/or the use of medications not approved by the FDA for the treatment of ADHD.	• Treatment should continue as long as symptoms remain present and cause impairment. The need for treatment should be periodically reassessed.

The MTA study randomized participants to intensive behavioral therapy, pharmacotherapy with systematically delivered methylphenidate, a combination of the two, or standard community care. The pharmacotherapy and combined treatment groups demonstrated significant improvement, and both were superior to behavioral therapy alone. Interestingly, however, the combined treatment group's response was not significantly better than pharmacotherapy alone for the treatment of core ADHD symptoms. Medication, therefore, appears to have the most significant acute impact on the treatment of ADHD (MTA Cooperative Group, 1999). The addition of behavioral interventions to pharmacotherapy did, however, increase parent and teacher satisfaction with treatment, improved children's interpersonal relationships, and on average, children receiving behavioral interventions required lower medication doses (MTA Cooperative Group, 1999). A later study of children aged 3–5.5 years with moderate to severe ADHD, the Preschool ADHD Treatment Study (PATS), demonstrated limited response to behavioral therapy alone, resulting in the majority of children warranting the initiation of pharmacotherapy following treatment with only behavioral intervention (Greenhill *et al.*, 2006).

Practice parameters

The AACAP Practice Parameters for ADHD published in 2007 combine short- and long-term empirical evidence with expert opinion from pediatric mental health researchers and clinicians. They offer specific recommendations (Table 1.1) for a comprehensive treatment plan, potentially consisting of pharmacological and behavioral interventions, and that if pharmacotherapy is indicated, the initial agent selected should be one with US Food and Drug Administration (FDA) approval for ADHD. The AACAP further states that if the response to an FDA-approved treatment is robust and normalizes the patient's functioning, medication alone may be sufficient (Pliszka, 2007).

In their 2001 clinical practice guideline for treating ADHD in children, the AAP recommended that the first intervention for the young child with ADHD be behavioral (AAP, 2001).

Table 1.2. Treatment algorithm for preschool children with attention deficit hyperactivity disorder (Gleason *et al.*, 2007).

General principles
• Assessment and diagnosis should be comprehensive, developmentally appropriate and contextually sensitive.
• An adequate trial of psychotherapy should precede pharmacotherapy, and should continue even if medication is used.
• Pharmacotherapy should be considered in the context of the clinical diagnosis and degree of functional impairment.
• Referral of the parent for treatment may optimize family mental health.
• Medication discontinuation trials are recommended following 6 months of treatment.
• The use of additional medication to manage side-effects of medication is discouraged.

Stage 0: Diagnostic assessment and psychotherapeutic intervention.
Stage 1: Methylphenidate trial.
Stage 2: Amphetamine trial.
Stage 3: a-adrenergic or atomoxetine trial.

The 2007 AACAP (Pliszka, 2007) parameters indicate that behavioral therapy alone may be appropriate in mild cases of ADHD and should be considered for young children. Additionally, Gleason and colleagues made specific recommendations regarding treatment algorithms for pharmacotherapy in preschool-aged children (Table 1.2) (Gleason *et al.*, 2007). Gleason and colleagues went on to specifically address treatment of preschool-aged patients with ADHD and referenced the PATS study when providing guidance for treating young children with a psychostimulant. The AACAP does note that subjects in PATS were only randomized to pharmacotherapy if they did not demonstrate significant or satisfactory improvement following 10 weeks of parent training (Greenhill *et al.*, 2006).

What is the first-line treatment for ADHD?

The role of pharmacotherapy (Table 1.3) as a first-line treatment of ADHD is strongly supported in the literature (Biederman & Spencer, 2008). The stimulant medications have decades of efficacy data from hundreds of controlled trials, beginning as early as the 1930s, and were well-established as effective treatments for ADHD by the 1970s. The pediatric safety and efficacy database on acute and long-term use of these agents has continued to grow and includes data not only on school-aged children, but more recently has expanded into preschool children and adolescents (AAP, 2001; Biederman & Spencer, 2008; Brown *et al.*, 2005; Greenhill *et al.*, 2002; Pliszka *et al.*, 2007). There has also been a significant increase in data supporting the utility of non-stimulant agents for ADHD in the past 10 years (AAP, 2001; Biederman & Spencer, 2008; Brown *et al.*, 2005; Greenhill *et al.*, 2002; Madaan *et al.*, 2006; Pliszka *et al.*, 2007). A meta-analysis of atomoxetine and stimulant studies revealed a robust effect size for atomoxetine and the stimulants, both of which are currently approved by the FDA for the treatment of ADHD. Atomoxetine demonstrated an effect size of 0.62, which would be considered a medium effect size, compared with 0.91 and 0.95, considered large effect sizes, for immediate- and extended-release stimulants, respectively (Faraone, 2003). A more recent FDA-approved agent, the a_2 agonist guanfacine XR, demonstrated effect sizes of 0.43–0.86 in two double-blind, placebo-controlled (DBPC) trials (Biederman *et al.*, 2008b; Sallee *et al.*, 2009b).

Table 1.3. Medications with FDA approval for the treatment of attention deficit hyperactivity disorder.

Name	Delivery system	Duration of effect (Daughton & Kratochvil, 2009)	Trade name
Methylphenidate	Solution	4 h	Methylin
	Chewable tablet	4 h	Methylin
	Tablet	4 h	Ritalin
	Sustained release tablet	Up to 8 h	Ritalin SR
	Beaded capsule	7–8 h	Metadate ER, Methylin ER, Ritalin LA
	Beaded capsule	8–9 h	Metadate CD
	OROS capsule	Up to 12 h	Concerta
	Transdermal patch	12 h	Daytrana
d-Methylphenidate	Tablet	4 h	Focalin
	Beaded capsule	Up to 12 h	Focalin XR
Amphetamine	Tablet	6 h	Adderall
	Beaded capsule	10 h	Adderall XR
d-Amphetamine	Tablet	4 h	Dexedrine, Dextrostat
	Spansule capsule	10 h	Dexedrine Spansule
Lisdexamfetamine	Capsule	10 h	Vyvanse
Atomoxetine	Capsule	24 h	Strattera
Guanfacine extended-release	Tablet	8–12 h	Intuniv
Clonidine extended release	Tablet	12 h	Kapvay

Stimulants

Stimulants have historically been considered a first-line treatment for ADHD, with approximately 75% of children responding to the first agent selected, and 80–90% eventually responding if two different stimulants are tried consecutively (Pliszka, 2003). Although the MTA study examined the use of immediate-release methylphenidate, extended-release preparations are now commonly used to improve adherence to the treatment schedule, thus providing less opportunity for gaps in coverage. A combination of immediate- and extended-release preparations, selected and titrated according to tolerability and response, may ultimately be required to optimally manage the child's individual pharmacotherapy needs. All stimulant medications currently approved for the treatment of ADHD are derivatives of either methylphenidate or amphetamine, both of which act by enhancing the neurotransmission of dopamine, and to a lesser extent, norepinephrine (Biederman & Spencer, 2008). DBPC studies in children, adolescents, and adults have demonstrated that 65–75% of subjects typically respond to stimulant treatment, compared with 4–30% of those on placebo (Greenhill et al., 2002; Pliszka, 2007). Recent research has focused on improving the delivery mechanisms of the stimulant medications in order to extend the duration of action. With multiple formulations of these medications (short-, intermediate-, and long-acting) as well as a variety of administration options available (e.g. capsules, sprinkleable capsules, tablets, chewable tablets, oral solution, transdermal patches), treatment can be tailored to individual patient needs.

The MTA study demonstrated the tolerability and efficacy of t.i.d. immediate-release methylphenidate in a randomized trial of 579 children aged 7–9.9 years with the combined subtype of ADHD. Dose titration was based on effect as reported by parent and teacher rating scales, and tolerability. Children in the manualized pharmacotherapy arm of the study had mean final doses of 32.1 ± 15.4 mg/day, and those assigned to manualized pharmacotherapy plus behavioral intervention had mean final doses of 28.9 ± 13.7 mg/day. The MTA study allowed children weighing <25 kg to have methylphenidate doses of up to 35 mg/day, and allowed doses up to 50 mg/day for children who weighed more. Average doses in the smaller children were 0.95 ± 0.40 mg/kg, and 1.13 ± 0.55 mg/kg in those that were heavier (MTA Cooperative Group, 1999).

Prior to the NIMH-funded PATS there were fewer than a dozen small placebo-controlled trials of psychostimulants in preschool children, and all utilized immediate-release methylphenidate (Kratochvil et al., 2004). Doses in these studies did not exceed 0.6 mg/kg, a narrower range than the 0.3–1.0 mg/kg used in older children (Kratochvil et al., 2004), and were administered q.i.d. or b.i.d., rather than the t.i.d. schedule often required for optimal effect. Efficacy of methylphenidate in the preschool age group varies from older children (Connor, 2002), as does the adverse effect profile (Firestone et al., 1998). PATS, which used a titration model similar to the MTA's, included 165 children aged 3.5–5 years initially randomized to either placebo or immediate-release methylphenidate (1.25 mg, 2.5 mg, 5 mg, or 7.5 mg t.i.d.). Subjects received a week of treatment with each dose during the double-blind cross-over titration phase. Twenty-two percent of subjects were identified as best responding to 7.5 mg t.i.d. The mean final best dose in PATS was 14.22 ± 8.1 mg/day, or 0.7 ± 0.4 mg/kg.day (Greenhill et al., 2006).

When PATS data were compared with MTA data, it was noted that the younger children had lower optimal doses, by weight, of immediate-release methylphenidate (0.7 mg/kg.day compared with 1.0 mg/kg.day). Pharmacokinetic data also demonstrated a slower clearance of a single dose of methylphenidate in 4- and 5-year-old children compared with school-aged children (Wigal et al., 2007). Tolerability seems to have age-related variability, with younger children demonstrating more emotional adverse events (e.g. crabbiness, irritability, and proneness to crying) than school-aged children. Thus, slower titration, closer monitoring and smaller doses of stimulants are advised when treating preschool children (Pliszka, 2007).

Adverse effects

All formulations of the stimulant medications have similar adverse-event profiles (Greenhill et al., 2002). Delayed sleep-onset, decreased appetite, weight loss, headache, stomach upset and increased heart rate and blood pressure are common. Emotional outbursts and irritability have also been frequently reported in younger children (Wigal et al., 2006).

Concerns with cardiovascular safety of ADHD pharmacotherapies have led to specific recommendations for pre-treatment evaluation, treatment selection, and monitoring. Much scrutiny is given to the risks present for children with structural cardiac abnormalities, but potentially medication-related changes in heart rate and blood pressure are also observed in healthy children with ADHD. In a study of 10 years of Florida Medicaid claims, stimulant use in patients with ADHD was associated with 20% more emergency-room visits, and 21% more office visits for cardiac symptoms (Winterstein et al., 2007).

Gould et al. (2009) reported that the rate of sudden death in pediatric patients taking a psychostimulant was the same as that seen in the general population, with 11 sudden deaths reported between 1992 and 2005. However, in a matched case-control study, a significant association of stimulant use with sudden death was seen when comparing data for 564 reports of sudden death in 7- to 19-year-olds with the deaths of 564 same-aged patients who died in motor vehicle accidents (odds ratio 7.4, 95% confidence interval (CI) 1.4–74.9) (Gould et al., 2009).

The AAP (Perrin et al., 2008) recommends that a targeted cardiac history and physical examination be part of the assessment of a child prior to initiating ADHD treatment. Questions regarding a prior patient history of heart disease, palpitations, syncope or seizures, or a family history of sudden death in children or young adults, cardiomyopathy or long-QT syndrome should be asked. If these are present, an ECG and/or referral to a cardiologist may be warranted prior to initiating treatment. These cardiovascular risks may become more of an issue in the treatment of adults who may have concurrent hypertension and/or cardiovascular disease.

Atomoxetine

Atomoxetine, which selectively blocks re-uptake at the noradrenergic neuron, was the first non-stimulant medication approved by the FDA for the treatment of ADHD. Two large, DBPC efficacy studies demonstrated significant improvement in ADHD symptoms with atomoxetine compared with placebo, with 64.1% and 58.7% of atomoxetine subjects responding (Spencer et al., 2002). More than a dozen DBPC trials have provided evidence supporting the safety and efficacy of atomoxetine dosed both once- and twice-daily for the treatment of ADHD in children, adolescents, and adults (Kelsey et al., 2004; Michelson et al., 2001, 2002, 2003; Spencer et al., 2002; Weiss et al., 2005).

The FDA-approved target therapeutic dose of 1.2 mg/kg.day was selected following a dose-finding study which observed a graded dose-response to atomoxetine 0.5 mg/kg.day and 1.2 mg/kg.day, but no significant difference between 1.2 mg/kg.day and 1.8 mg/kg.day for reduction of core ADHD symptoms. Improvements in psychosocial functioning, however, were seen when the dose was increased to 1.8 mg/kg.day without any significant difference in adverse events (Michelson et al., 2001).

Atomoxetine is not approved for use in children aged < 6 years. However, there has been one DBPC trial $(n = 101)$, examining the use of atomoxetine in 5- and 6-year-olds. Improvements were noted on parent and teacher ADHD–IV ratings for children assigned to atomoxetine compared with those on placebo $(p < 0.05)$. Three subjects withdrew from the study due to adverse events (atomoxetine = 0, placebo = 3). The mean final daily dose of atomoxetine was 1.38 mg/kg.day. Despite statistically significant improvements in ADHD symptoms, and the fact that the parents received concomitant education on ADHD and behavioral interventions as a part of the study, the children continued to have ADHD–IV (parent) scores above the 86th percentile for age and gender at study completion (Kratochvil et al., 2008b).

Adverse effects

Common acute adverse effects of atomoxetine include sedation, loss of appetite, nausea, vomiting, irritability, and headaches. In an analysis of the efficacy and tolerability of atomoxetine in young vs. older children, no significant differences were noted in the adverse event profile or response to atomoxetine (Kratochvil et al., 2008a).

Atomoxetine carries additional warnings for hepatotoxicity and suicidality risk. An analysis of laboratory data from 7961 adult and pediatric subjects in atomoxetine clinical trials revealed 41 instances of elevations in AST and ALT. There were 351 spontaneous reports of hepatic events in the first 4 years atomoxetine was on the market. Of these, three suggested atomoxetine as a probable cause, and 1/3 had a positive re-challenge. In all three cases, symptoms resolved following discontinuation of atomoxetine. These data resulted in recommendation that atomoxetine be discontinued if jaundice or elevations in hepatic enzymes are present (Bangs *et al.*, 2008*a*). A 2008 analysis of data from 14 studies of atomoxetine by Bangs and colleagues demonstrated that suicide ideation was more common in subjects receiving atomoxetine (0.37%, 5/1357 subjects) compared with those receiving placebo (0%, 0/851 subjects). To place the risk of suicidality in context, the number needed to harm (NNH) was 227, whereas the number needed to treat (NNT) to achieve remission of ADHD symptoms was five. No suicides occurred in any of the trials in the analysis (Bangs *et al.*, 2008*b*).

Stimulant and atomoxetine comparator trials

Atomoxetine and osmotic release oral system (OROS) methylphenidate

In a comparator trial in 516 children and adolescents aged 6–16 with ADHD, subjects were randomized to 6 weeks of treatment with either atomoxetine up to 1.8 mg/kg.day ($n = 222$), OROS methylphenidate up to 54 mg/day ($n = 220$) or placebo ($n = 74$). Atomoxetine and OROS methylphenidate were both superior to placebo, with 45% ($p < 0.003$) and 56% ($p < 0.001$) responding, respectively. Effect sizes were 0.6 for atomoxetine and 0.8 for OROS methylphenidate. Decreased appetite was the only adverse event separating from placebo for both active treatments ($p < 0.05$). Subjects receiving OROS methylphenidate reported experiencing insomnia, while those assigned to atomoxetine had more frequent complaints of somnolence. Weight loss and increased diastolic blood pressure ($p < 0.05$) were noted to be significant for both drugs compared with placebo, and an increased pulse rate was significant in the atomoxetine group compared with OROS methylphenidate and placebo ($p < 0.05$) (Newcorn *et al.*, 2008).

For the stimulant-naive patients ($n = 191$) participating in this trial, response rates to atomoxetine (57%, $p = 0.004$) and methylphenidate (64%, $p < 0.001$) were comparable ($p = 0.43$), but those subjects with prior exposure to stimulants ($n = 301$), had better responses to methylphenidate (51%, $p = 0.002$) than to atomoxetine (37%, $p = 0.09$) ($p = 0.03$) (Newcorn *et al.*, 2008). The effect size for atomoxetine was greater in stimulant-naive patients (0.9), compared with patients previously treated with stimulants (0.5), while the effect-sizes for OROS methylphenidate in patients not previously treated with a stimulant and with prior exposure were 1.0 and 0.8, respectively (Newcorn *et al.*, 2008).

Subjects initially assigned to OROS methylphenidate were then switched to atomoxetine at the end of the 6-week acute treatment phase of the study. Forty-two percent (29/69 subjects) who did not respond to atomoxetine in the second phase of the study had previously responded to OROS methylphenidate during acute treatment, while 43% of subjects who did not respond acutely to OROS methylphenidate (30/70 subjects) went on to respond to atomoxetine. This may indicate a differential response to treatment for some patients (Newcorn *et al.*, 2008).

Atomoxetine and mixed-amphetamine salts

In a 3-week laboratory school comparison of atomoxetine and extended-release mixed amphetamine salts in 6- to 12-year-olds with either combined or hyperactive-impulsive type ADHD, improved attention and academic performance were noted with both treatments. Mixed amphetamine salts-treated subjects had greater improvements than those who received atomoxetine ($p < 0.001$). The difference at end-point was statistically and clinically significant; however, the relatively short 3-week duration of the study may not have been sufficient to demonstrate the full effect of atomoxetine treatment. The mixed amphetamine salts group reported experiencing insomnia, decreased appetite, upper abdominal pain, anorexia and headache, while the most common adverse events reported in the atomoxetine group were somnolence, appetite decrease, upper abdominal pain, vomiting, and headache. Vital sign changes were similar for both groups and were not statistically significant (Wigal et al., 2005).

a_2 agonists

The a_2 adrenergic agents, clonidine (Catapres) and immediate-release guanfacine (Tenex), have been used relatively commonly over the past decade as second-line or adjunctive treatments in the USA. International comparisons (Winterstein et al., 2008), however, show very different co-medication patterns between the USA and European countries where a_2 adrenergic agents are rarely used. Clonidine has been shown to reduce ADHD symptoms in patients with comorbid tics, aggression and conduct disorder. Immediate-release clonidine is short-acting and requires multiple divided doses throughout the day (Brown et al., 2005). In the USA clonidine is also available as a transdermal patch, allowing for once-weekly application. An extended-release formulation (Kapvay™) was approved by the FDA in September 2010, for the treatment of ADHD in children and adolescents aged 6–17 years. Kapvay received approval as both monotherapy and in combination with a stimulant.

Guanfacine is a more selective a_2-adrenergic agonist with less sedation and a longer duration of action (Biederman & Spencer, 2008). A small open-label study of immediate-release guanfacine showed improvements in hyperactivity and inattention, with transient sedation as the most common adverse event (Hunt et al., 1995), and additional studies have demonstrated its utility and good tolerability in treating ADHD with co-occurring tic disorders and Tourette's (Chappell et al., 1995; Scahill et al., 2001). An extended-release form of guanfacine was given FDA approval in 2009 as monotherapy for pediatric ADHD following two controlled trials (study 1: $n = 345$, ages 6–17 years; study 2: $n = 324$, ages 6–17 years). Adverse events were largely dose-dependent. Both studies had similar tolerability data, with the most common treatment-emergent adverse events being headache, somnolence, fatigue, sedation, and upper abdominal pain. No clinically significant vital sign or ECG changes were seen (Biederman et al., 2008b; Sallee et al., 2009b). Dose-based effect sizes ranged from 0.43 to 0.86, and response rates were 43% for the 3-mg dose and 62% for the 4-mg dose.

Guanfacine's most common acute adverse effects include somnolence, headache, fatigue, upper abdominal pain, and sedation. Bradycardia was reported in long-term studies (Biederman et al., 2008a; Sallee et al., 2009a).

What is the impact of ADHD pharmacotherapy?

The benefits of pharmacotherapy are most evident in reduction of the core symptoms of ADHD. By reducing inattention, hyperactivity, and impulsivity, patients with ADHD are better able to perform academically and socially. Studies have demonstrated that children treated with stimulants have improved attention to school work, decreased disruptive behaviors, and decreased non-compliance. Short-term data also show improvements in academic performance and productivity (Barkley, 1998). Some data suggest that children with ADHD treated with psychostimulants demonstrate better academic outcomes as evidenced by WIAT-II subtests and high school grade point average (GPA) than children with ADHD who were not treated. However, the treated children did not do as well as non-ADHD controls. It is unclear if pharmacotherapy alone translates to long-term academic success (Powers *et al.*, 2008).

Social interactions between affected children and their parents, teachers, and peers are significantly improved with stimulant treatment. Treated children are more compliant with commands and more appropriately responsive to interactions with others, with less negative and off-task behavior. As a result, adult redirections and supervision needs decrease, and praise and positive attention to the child increase. ADHD children treated with stimulants also appear to be better accepted by peers, probably as a result of reduced negative and aggressive behavior (Barkley, 1998). Health-related quality-of-life outcomes measured by the Child Health Questionnaire (CHQ) were improved along with ADHD symptoms in children treated with atomoxetine in a DBPC dosimetry study in children and adolescents aged 8–18 years (Michelson *et al.*, 2001).

Early treatment with methylphenidate does not appear to increase risk for negative outcomes, and may have beneficial long-term effects (Mannuzza *et al.*, 2008). However, long-term data from the MTA study notes that benefits of pharmacotherapy are sustainable up to 2 years for the majority of subjects followed, but by the third year of follow-up, only about one third of subjects demonstrated ongoing benefit with medication treatment (Swanson *et al.*, 2008). Despite decreases in ADHD symptoms, the MTA subjects as a group still had relatively poorer ratings of behavior, academic, and overall functioning compared with normal controls at 6- and 8-year follow-ups.

How long should treatment last?

Epidemiological surveys of community samples indicate that 2–6% of preschool children meet diagnostic criteria for ADHD (Angold *et al.*, 2000; Lavigne *et al.*, 1996), with prevalence rates in school-aged children conservatively estimated to be between 3% and 7% (APA, 2000). As children grow into adolescence and adulthood the prevalence of ADHD decreases, yet still persists in significant numbers, estimated at approximately 3–4% in adults (Fayyad *et al.*, 2007). Even though the presentation may vary from early childhood to adulthood, the impairment there is no less significant (Kessler *et al.*, 2006). A multitude of studies have demonstrated a correlation between ADHD in adults and global impairment in functioning, including: smoking and substance abuse, diminished rates of college graduation, occupational/vocational difficulties, motor vehicle accidents, legal problems, unplanned pregnancies, and relationship problems (Barkley, 2006).

In a 10-year case-controlled follow-up study of 112 male adults with ADHD, potential protective factors of stimulant treatment for ADHD were assessed. Biederman *et al.* (2008c, 2009) found no evidence that stimulant treatment in childhood or adolescence either increased or decreased the risk for development of substance use disorders in young adulthood, but that ADHD patients treated with stimulants were at significantly less risk of developing depressive and anxiety disorders, disruptive behavior, and repeating a grade in school than the ADHD patients who were not treated. Daviss *et al.* also demonstrated a similar finding of ADHD pharmacotherapy reducing the risk of later major depression (Daviss *et al.*, 2008).

With the longitudinal course of ADHD documented, the AACAP Practice Parameter recommendations serve as a reminder to periodically evaluate the need for ongoing treatment of ADHD with pharmacotherapy. Follow-up clinic visits ensure that medication remains effective, dosing is optimal, and adverse events are minimized. The AACAP recommends that ADHD treatment be individualized, and that the duration of treatment should continue as long as impairing symptoms are present (Pliszka, 2007).

Considerable evidence demonstrating the efficacy of psychostimulants in treating adults with ADHD (Asherson, 2005) led to FDA approval of both methylphenidate (extended-release methylphenidate and d-methylphenidate) and amphetamine (extended-release mixed amphetamine salts). Atomoxetine has also received FDA approval for adults with ADHD based on two DBPC studies (Buitelaar *et al.*, 2007).

Adverse effects

A specific concern with long-term pharmacotherapy is impact on growth, so much so that the AACAP Practice Parameter for ADHD treatment includes a specific recommendation regarding regular height and weight monitoring, including serial plotting of growth parameters. The AACAP advises that a change in height or weight crossing two percentile lines is suggestive of abnormal growth and warrants a medication holiday, dose adjustment, or change. Reductions in growth must be balanced with benefits of treatment (Pliszka, 2007).

Swanson *et al.* (2005) demonstrated that children treated with stimulants grew more slowly and appeared to gain less weight than expected; however, they also theorized that, in general, children with ADHD may have different growth trajectories than their 'normal' peers. Statistically significant delays in height and weight were also seen with stimulant treatment in a meta-analysis of 22 studies by Faraone *et al.* (2008). The pooled data showed that the weight deficits were more significant than the deficits seen in height ($p = 0.002$), although both appeared to normalize over time (Faraone *et al.*, 2008).

Based upon a qualitative meta-analysis, Faraone *et al.* suggested that the effects on weight and height may be dose-dependent. There was no apparent difference, however, in the growth effects between methylphenidate and amphetamine, and cessation of treatment appeared to normalize growth (Faraone *et al.*, 2008). This normalization of growth with breaks over the summer or with drug discontinuation has been demonstrated in additional studies (Gittelman *et al.*, 1988; Kaffman *et al.*, 1979; Klein & Mannuzza, 1988; Safer *et al.*, 1975); although analysis of data from the MTA study (MTA Cooperative Group, 2004) showed that while discontinuation of methylphenidate treatment did not reverse losses in expected height, it did have a beneficial effect on weight gain.

Atomoxetine has also been clearly linked with changes in height and weight trajectories, which for the group appeared to dissipate over time, despite continued treatment (Spencer *et al.*, 2005, 2007). These data appear to indicate that for most children growth suppression, if present, will be transient and not clinically significant over time. Nonetheless, there is clearly an effect of these medications on growth. Therefore, while group averages over time may not be overly concerning, close monitoring of individual children taking ADHD medication is clearly indicated.

What is the management of treatment-resistant cases?

The vast majority of patients with ADHD will respond to one of the FDA-approved pharmacotherapies for the treatment of ADHD. If a patient does not respond adequately to appropriate trials (adequate duration and optimal dose) of these agents, a re-assessment of the diagnosis is warranted both to confirm the diagnosis of ADHD and to re-examine for missed co-occurring disorders (AACAP recommendation). Co-occurrence of learning disorders, developmental disorders, and other psychiatric conditions can affect response to treatment and/or complicate treatment planning, and the addition of behavioral therapy to a medication regimen may be required. Non-FDA-approved pharmacotherapies (e.g. bupropion or tricyclic antidepressants) may be tried if interventions with a greater evidence base are either ineffective or contraindicated. Finally, combination therapy with FDA-approved agents and/or non-approved agents might be clinically indicated. Use of medications not approved for the treatment of ADHD, and treatment with more than one medication simultaneously elevates potential risks, however, and these risks as well as other treatment options must be discussed with the patient and caregivers, and if employed monitored closely (Pliszka, 2007).

Conclusion

ADHD is one of the best-studied disorders in psychiatry. Reliable diagnosis at a young age is possible, and recognition of ADHD as a potentially life-long impairing disorder is increasing. As data emerge which describe the physiological evidence behind the historically "behavioral" diagnosis, acceptance of the role of pharmacotherapy has increased for preschool children through adults. Guidelines such as those from the AACAP provide clear recommendations to the practising clinician for diagnosing, treating and monitoring patients with ADHD, in a manner which maximizes effectiveness, tolerability, and ultimately, functionality of the patient. As improvements are made in the delivery systems and durations of effect of the various psychostimulant agents, clinicians and patients will still be faced with what to do for those who do not respond. Research is expanding into non-stimulant agents, and the specific role these may have. Further examination of a potential "differential response," as suggested in the comparator trial of atomoxetine and OROS methylphenidate, may ultimately better inform clinicians as to the selection of a specific pharmacotherapy for a specific individual. In the interim, appropriate diagnosis, informed prescribing, clinical monitoring, and collaborative treatment planning can all help to optimize outcomes in ADHD management.

Statement of interest

Dr. Kratochvil was supported by NIMH Grant 5K23MH06612701; received grant support from Eli Lilly, McNeil, Shire, Abbott, Somerset and Cephalon; was a consultant for Eli Lilly, AstraZeneca, Abbott Quintiles Seaside, and Pfizer. He is Editor of the *Brown University Child & Adolescent Psychopharmacology Update*, member of the REACH Institute Primary Pediatric Psychopharmacology Steering Committee, member of the American Professional Society for ADHD & Related Disorders Board of Directors, and received study drug for a NIMH-funded study from Eli Lilly and Abbott. Dr. Kratochvil receives royalties from Oxford University Press.

Ms. Vaughan has received salary support from NIMH Grant 5K23MH06612701, Eli Lilly, and Bristol-Myers Squibb.

Dr. March has served as a consultant or scientific advisor to Pfizer, Eli Lilly, Wyeth, Glaxo-SmithKline, BMS, Johnson and Johnson, Psymetrix, Scion, Transition Therapeutics and MedAvante; has received research support from Eli Lilly and Pfizer; has received study drug for a NIMH-funded study from Eli Lilly and from Pfizer; is an equity holder in MedAvante; receives royalties from Guilford Press, Oxford University Press and MultiHealth Systems; and receives research support from NARSAD, NIMH, and NIDA.

References

American Academy of Pediatrics (AAP) (2001). Clinical practice guideline: treatment of the school-aged child with attention-deficit/hyperactivity disorder. *Pediatrics* **108**, 1033–1044.

American Psychiatric Association (APA) (2000). *Diagnostic and Statistical Manual of Mental Disorders (4th edn) – Text Revision*. Washington, DC: American Psychiatric Association.

Angold A, Erkanli A, Egger HL, Costello EJ (2000). Stimulant treatment for children: a community perspective. *Journal of the American Academy of Child and Adolescent Psychiatry* **39**, 975–984; discussion 984–994.

Asherson P (2005). Clinical assessment and treatment of attention deficit hyperactivity disorder in adults. *Expert Review of Neurotherapeutics* **5**, 525–539.

Bangs ME, Jin L, Zhang S et al. (2008a). Hepatic events associated with atomoxetine treatment for attention-deficit hyperactivity disorder. *Drug Safety* **31**, 345–354.

Bangs ME, Tauscher-Wisniewski S, Polzer J et al. (2008b). Meta-analysis of suicide-related behavior events in patients treated with atomoxetine. *Journal of the American Academy of Child and Adolescent Psychiatry* **47**, 209–218.

Barkley RA (1998). *Attention-Deficit Hyperactivity Disorder. A Handbook for Diagnosis and Treatment*, 2nd edn. New York: The Guilford Press.

Barkley RA (2006). *Attention-Deficit Hyperactivity Disorder: A Handbook for Diagnosis and Treatment*, 3rd edn. New York: Guilford Press.

Barkley RA, Fischer M, Edelbrock CS, Smallish L (1990). The adolescent outcome of hyperactive children diagnosed by research criteria: I. An 8-year prospective follow-up study. *Journal of the American Academy of Child and Adolescent Psychiatry* **29**, 546–557.

Barkley RA, Fischer M, Smallish L, Fletcher K (2002). The persistence of attention-deficit/hyperactivity disorder into young adulthood as a function of reporting source and definition of disorder. *Journal of Abnormal Psychology* **111**, 279–289.

Biederman J, Faraone S, Milberger S et al. (1996). A prospective 4-year follow-up study of attention-deficit hyperactivity and related disorders. *Archives of General Psychiatry* **53**, 437–446.

Biederman J, Melmed RD, Patel A et al. (2008a). Long-term, open-label extension study of guanfacine extended release in children and adolescents with ADHD. *CNS Spectrums* **13**, 1047–1055.

Biederman J, Melmed RD, Patel A et al. (2008b). A randomized, double-blind, placebo-controlled study of guanfacine extended release in children and adolescents with attention-deficit/hyperactivity disorder. *Pediatrics* **121**, e73–e84.

Biederman J, Monuteaux MC, Spencer T et al. (2008c). Stimulant therapy and risk for subsequent substance use disorders in male adults with ADHD: a naturalistic controlled 10-year follow-up study. *American Journal of Psychiatry* **165**, 597–603.

Biederman J, Monuteaux MC, Spencer T et al. (2009). Do stimulants protect against psychiatric disorders in youth with ADHD? A 10-year follow-up study. *Pediatrics* **124**, 71–78.

Biederman J, Spencer TJ (2008). Psychopharmacological interventions. *Child and Adolescent Psychiatric Clinics of North America* **17**, 439–458, xi.

Bodenheimer T, Wagner EH, Grumbach K (2002a). Improving primary care for patients with chronic illness. *Journal of the American Medical Association* **288**, 1775–1779.

Bodenheimer T, Wagner EH, Grumbach K (2002b). Improving primary care for patients with chronic illness: the chronic care model, part 2. *Journal of the American Medical Association* **288**, 1909–1914.

Brown RT, Amler RW, Freeman WS et al. (2005). Treatment of attention-deficit/hyperactivity disorder: overview of the evidence. *Pediatrics* **115**, e749–e757.

Buitelaar JK, Michelson D, Danckaerts M et al. (2007). A randomized, double-blind study of continuation treatment for attention-deficit/hyperactivity disorder after 1 year. *Biological Psychiatry* **61**, 694–699.

CDC (2005). Mental health in the United States. Prevalence of diagnosis and medication treatment for attention-deficit/hyperactivity disorder – United States, 2003. *Morbidity and Mortality Weekly Report* **54**, 842–847.

Castellanos FX, Lee PP, Sharp W et al. (2002). Developmental trajectories of brain volume abnormalities in children and adolescents with attention-deficit/hyperactivity disorder. *Journal of the American Medical Association* **288**, 1740–1748.

Castellanos FX, Tannock R (2002). Neuroscience of attention-deficit/hyperactivity disorder: the search for endophenotypes. *Nature Reviews Neuroscience* **3**, 617–628.

Chappell PB, Riddle MA, Scahill L et al. (1995). Guanfacine treatment of comorbid attention-deficit hyperactivity disorder and Tourette's syndrome: preliminary clinical experience. *Journal of the American Academy of Child and Adolescent Psychiatry* **34**, 1140–1146.

Connor DF (2002). Preschool attention deficit hyperactivity disorder: a review of prevalence, diagnosis, neurobiology, and stimulant treatment. *Journal of Developmental and Behavioral Pediatrics* **23** (Suppl. 1), S1–S9.

Connor DF, Edwards G, Fletcher KE et al. (2003). Correlates of comorbid psychopathology in children with ADHD. *Journal of the American Academy of Child and Adolescent Psychiatry* **42**, 193–200.

Cunningham CE, Boyle MH (2002). Preschoolers at risk for attention-deficit hyperactivity disorder and oppositional defiant disorder: family, parenting, and behavioral correlates. *Journal of Abnormal Child Psychology* **30**, 555–569.

Daughton JM, Kratochvil CJ (2009). Review of ADHD pharmacotherapies: advantages,

disadvantages, and clinical pearls. *Journal of the American Academy of Child and Adolescent Psychiatry* **48**, 240–248.

Daviss WB, Birmaher B, Diler RS, Mintz J (2008). Does pharmacotherapy for attention-deficit/hyperactivity disorder predict risk of later major depression? *Journal of Child and Adolescent Psychopharmacology* **18**, 257–264.

DuPaul GJ, McGoey KE, Eckert TL, VanBrakle J (2001). Preschool children with attention-deficit/hyperactivity disorder: impairments in behavioral, social, and school functioning. *Journal of the American Academy of Child and Adolescent Psychiatry* **40**, 508–515.

Durston S, Hulshoff Pol HE, Schnack HG et al. (2004). Magnetic resonance imaging of boys with attention-deficit/hyperactivity disorder and their unaffected siblings. *Journal of the American Academy of Child and Adolescent Psychiatry* **43**, 332–340.

Faraone S (2003). Understanding the effect size of ADHD medications: implications for clinical care. *Medscape Psychiatry & Mental Health* **8**, 1–7.

Faraone SV, Biederman J (2000). Nature, nurture, and attention deficit hyperactivity disorder. *Child Development Review* **20**, 568–581.

Faraone SV, Biederman J, Morley CP, Spencer TJ (2008). Effect of stimulants on height and weight: a review of the literature. *Journal of the American Academy of Child and Adolescent Psychiatry* **47**, 994–1009.

Faraone SV, Perlis RH, Doyle AE et al. (2005). Molecular genetics of attention-deficit/hyperactivity disorder. *Biological Psychiatry* **57**, 1313–1323.

Fayyad J, De Graaf R, Kessler R et al. (2007). Cross-national prevalence and correlates of adult attention-deficit hyperactivity disorder. *British Journal of Psychiatry* **190**, 402–409.

Firestone P, Musten LM, Pisterman S et al. (1998). Short-term side effects of stimulant medication are increased in preschool children with attention-deficit/hyperactivity disorder: a double-blind placebo-controlled study. *Journal of Child and Adolescent Psychopharmacology* **8**, 13–25.

Gittelman R, Landa B, Mattes J, Klein D (1988). Methylphenidate and growth in hyperactive children: a controlled withdrawal study. *Archives of General Psychiatry* **45**, 1127–1130.

Gleason MM, Egger HL, Emslie GJ et al. (2007). Psychopharmacological treatment for very young children: contexts and guidelines. *Journal of the American Academy of Child and Adolescent Psychiatry* **46**, 1532–1572.

Goldman LS, Genel M, Bezman RJ, Slanetz PJ (1998). Diagnosis and treatment of attention-deficit/hyperactivity disorder in children and adolescents. Council on Scientific Affairs, American Medical Association. *Journal of the American Medical Association* **279**, 1100–1107.

Gould MS, Walsh BT, Munfakh JL et al. (2009). Sudden death and use of stimulant medications in youths. *American Journal of Psychiatry* **166**, 992–1001.

Greenhill L, Kollins S, Abikoff H et al. (2006). Efficacy and safety of immediate-release methylphenidate treatment for preschoolers with ADHD. *Journal of the American Academy of Child and Adolescent Psychiatry* **45**, 1284–1293.

Greenhill LL, Pliszka S, Dulcan MK et al. (2002). Practice parameter for the use of stimulant medications in the treatment of children, adolescents, and adults. *Journal of the American Academy of Child and Adolescent Psychiatry* **41** (Suppl. 2), 26S–49S.

Hunt RD, Arnsten AF, Asbell MD (1995). An open trial of guanfacine in the treatment of attention deficit hyperactivity disorder. *Journal of the American Academy of Child and Adolescent Psychiatry* **34**, 50–54.

Kaffman M, Sher A, Bar-Sinai N (1979). MBD children – variability in developmental patterns or growth inhibitory effects of stimulants? *Israeli Annals of Psychiatry and Related Disciplines* **17**, 58–66.

Kelsey DK, Sumner CR, Casat CD et al. (2004). Once-daily atomoxetine treatment for children with attention-deficit/hyperactivity disorder, including an assessment of evening and morning behavior: a double-blind, placebo-controlled trial. *Pediatrics* **114**, e1–e8.

Kessler RC, Adler L, Barkley R et al. (2006). The prevalence and correlates of adult ADHD in the United States: results from the national comorbidity survey replication. *American Journal of Psychiatry* **163**, 716–723.

Kessler RC, Adler LA, Barkley R et al. (2005). Patterns and predictors of attention-deficit/ hyperactivity disorder persistence into adulthood: results from the national comorbidity survey replication. *Biological Psychiatry* **57**, 1442–1451.

Klein RG, Mannuzza S (1988). Hyperactive boys almost grown up. III. Methylphenidate effects on ultimate height. *Archives of General Psychiatry* **45**, 1131–1134.

Krain AL, Castellanos FX (2006). Brain development and ADHD. *Clinical Psychology Review* **26**, 433–444.

Kratochvil CJ, Greenhill LL, March JS et al. (2004). The role of stimulants in the treatment of preschool children with attention-deficit hyperactivity disorder. *CNS Drugs* **18**, 957–966.

Kratochvil CJ, Milton DR, Vaughan BS, Greenhill LL (2008a). Acute atomoxetine treatment of younger and older children with ADHD: a meta-analysis of tolerability and efficacy. *Child and Adolescent Psychiatry and Mental Health* **2**, 25.

Kratochvil CJ, Vaughan BS, Daughton JM et al. (2008b). Atomoxetine vs. placebo for the treatment of ADHD in 5- and 6- year-old children. Paper presented at the Annual Meeting of the American Academy of Child and Adolescent Psychiatry, Chicago, IL, October 27–31, 2008.

Lahey BB, Pelham WE, Loney J et al. (2004). Three-year predictive validity of DSM-IV attention deficit hyperactivity disorder in children diagnosed at 4–6 years of age. *American Journal of Psychiatry* **161**, 2014–2020.

Lahey BB, Pelham WE, Stein MA et al. (1998). Validity of DSM-IV attention-deficit/ hyperactivity disorder for younger children. *Journal of the American Academy of Child and Adolescent Psychiatry* **37**, 695–702.

Lavigne JV, Gibbons RD, Christoffel KK et al. (1996). Prevalence rates and correlates of psychiatric disorders among preschool children. *Journal of the American Academy of Child and Adolescent Psychiatry* **35**, 204–214.

Madaan V, Kinnan S, Daughton J, Kratochvil CJ (2006). Innovations and recent trends in the treatment of ADHD. *Expert Review of Neurotherapeutics* **6**, 1375–1385.

Mannuzza S, Klein RG, Truong NL et al. (2008). Age of methylphenidate treatment initiation in children with ADHD and later substance abuse: prospective follow-up into adulthood. *American Journal of Psychiatry* **165**, 604–609.

Michelson D, Adler L, Spencer T et al. (2003). Atomoxetine in adults with ADHD: two randomized, placebo-controlled studies. Biological Psychiatry 53, 112–120.

Michelson D, Allen AJ, Busner J et al. (2002). Once-daily atomoxetine treatment for children and adolescents with attention deficit hyperactivity disorder: a randomized, placebo-controlled study. American Journal of Psychiatry 159, 1896–1901.

Michelson D, Faries D, Wernicke J et al. (2001). Atomoxetine in the treatment of children and adolescents with attention-deficit/hyperactivity disorder: a randomized, placebo-controlled, dose-response study. Pediatrics 108, E83.

Mostofsky SH, Cooper KL, Kates WR et al. (2002). Smaller prefrontal and premotor volumes in boys with attention-deficit/hyperactivity disorder. Biological Psychiatry 52, 785–794.

MTA Cooperative Group (1999). A 14-month randomized clinical trial of treatment strategies for attention-deficit/hyperactivity disorder. Multimodal treatment study of children with ADHD. Archives of General Psychiatry 56, 1073–1086.

MTA Cooperative Group (2004). National Institute of Mental Health multimodal treatment study of ADHD follow-up: changes in effectiveness and growth after the end of treatment. Pediatrics 113, 762–769.

Newcorn JH, Kratochvil CJ, Allen AJ et al. (2008). Atomoxetine and osmotically released methylphenidate for the treatment of attention deficit hyperactivity disorder: acute comparison and differential response. American Journal of Psychiatry 165, 721–730.

Perrin JM, Friedman RA, Knilans TK (2008). Cardiovascular monitoring and stimulant drugs for attention-deficit/ hyperactivity disorder. Pediatrics 122, 451–453.

Pliszka S (2007). Practice parameter for the assessment and treatment of children and adolescents with attention-deficit/ hyperactivity disorder. Journal of the American Academy of Child and Adolescent Psychiatry 46, 894–921.

Pliszka SR (2003). Non-stimulant treatment of attention-deficit/hyperactivity disorder. CNS Spectrums 8, 253–258.

Pliszka SR, Liotti M, Bailey BY et al. (2007). Electrophysiological effects of stimulant treatment on inhibitory control in children with attention-deficit/hyperactivity disorder. Journal of Child and Adolescent Psychopharmacology 17, 356–366.

Powers RL, Marks DJ, Miller CJ et al. (2008). Stimulant treatment in children with attention-deficit/hyperactivity disorder moderates adolescent academic outcome. Journal of Child and Adolescent Psychopharmacology 18, 449–459.

Safer D, Allen R, Barr E (1975). Growth rebound after termination of stimulant drugs. Pediatrics 86, 113–116.

Sallee FR, Lyne A, Wigal T, McGough JJ (2009a). Long-term safety and efficacy of guanfacine extended release in children and adolescents with attention-deficit/ hyperactivity disorder. Journal of Child and Adolescent Psychopharmacology 19, 215–226.

Sallee FR, McGough J, Wigal T et al. (2009b). Guanfacine extended release in children and adolescents with attention deficit/ hyperactivity disorder: a placebo-controlled trial. Journal of the American Academy of Child and Adolescent Psychiatry 48, 155–165.

Scahill L, Chappell PB, Kim YS et al. (2001). A placebo-controlled study of guanfacine in the treatment of children with tic disorders and attention deficit hyperactivity disorder. American Journal of Psychiatry 158, 1067–1074.

Spencer T, Heiligenstein JH, Biederman J et al. (2002). Results from two proof-of-concept, placebo-controlled studies of atomoxetine in children with attention-deficit/hyperactivity disorder. Journal of Clinical Psychiatry 63, 1140–1147.

Spencer TJ, Kratochvil CJ, Sangal RB et al. (2007). Effects of atomoxetine on growth in children with attention-deficit/hyperactivity disorder following up to five years of treatment. Journal of Child and Adolescent Psychopharmacology 17, 689–700.

Spencer TJ, Newcorn JH, Kratochvil CJ et al. (2005). Effects of atomoxetine on growth after 2-year treatment among pediatric patients with attention-deficit/hyperactivity disorder. Pediatrics 116, e74–e80.

Swanson J, Arnold LE, Kraemer H et al. (2008). Evidence, interpretation, and qualification from multiple reports of long-term outcomes in the multimodal treatment study of children with ADHD (MTA): Part II:

supporting details. *Journal of Attention Disorders* **12**, 15–43.

Swanson JM, Ruff DD, Feldman PD *et al.* (2005). *Characterization of Growth in Children with ADHD*. Paper presented at the Annual Meeting of the American Academy of Child and Adolescent Psychiatry, Toronto, Canada, October 18–23, 2005.

Weiss M, Tannock R, Kratochvil C *et al.* (2005). A randomized, placebo-controlled study of once-daily atomoxetine in the school setting in children with ADHD. *Journal of the American Academy of Child and Adolescent Psychiatry* **44**, 647–655.

Wigal SB, Gupta S, Greenhill L *et al.* (2007). Pharmacokinetics of methylphenidate in preschoolers with attention-deficit/ hyperactivity disorder. *Journal of Child and Adolescent Psychopharmacology* **17**, 153–164.

Wigal SB, McGough JJ, McCracken JT *et al.* (2005). A laboratory school comparison of mixed amphetamine salts extended release (Adderall XR) and atomoxetine (Strattera) in school-aged children with attention deficit/hyperactivity disorder. *Journal of Attention Disorders* **9**, 275–289.

Wigal T, Greenhill L, Chuang S *et al.* (2006). Safety and tolerability of methylphenidate in preschool children with ADHD. *Journal of the American Academy of Child and Adolescent Psychiatry* **45**, 1294–1303.

Willcutt EG, Doyle AE, Nigg JT *et al.* (2005). Validity of the executive function theory of attention-deficit/hyperactivity disorder: a meta-analytic review. *Biological Psychiatry* **57**, 1336–1346.

Winterstein AG, Gerhard T, Shuster J *et al.* (2007). Cardiac safety of central nervous system stimulants in children and adolescents with attention-deficit/ hyperactivity disorder. *Pediatrics* **120**, e494–e501.

Winterstein AG, Gerhard T, Shuster J *et al.* (2008). Utilization of pharmacologic treatment in youths with attention deficit/hyperactivity disorder in Medicaid database. *Annals of Pharmacotherapy* **42**, 24–31.

Woodruff TJ, Axelrad DA, Kyle AD *et al.* (2004). Trends in environmentally related childhood illnesses. *Pediatrics* **113** (Suppl. 4), 1133–1140.

Evidence-based pharmacotherapy of schizophrenia

2

Stefan Leucht, Stephan Heres, Werner Kissling, and John M. Davis

Introduction

Enormous scientific efforts have been made since the development of chlorpromazine in 1953 to improve the drug treatment of schizophrenia leading to more than 10 000 controlled trials currently summarized in the Cochrane Schizophrenia Group's register (Adams *et al.*, 2008). In this context, the current article presents our personal interpretation of the core evidence about the pharmacological treatment of schizophrenia. Other interpretations exist and the article cannot compete with national treatment guidelines that have been methodologically developed (e.g. Lehman *et al.*, 2004). But what makes our article different is that it attempts to follow the logical steps of clinical care. Arranged as a simple algorithm it starts from the choice of an antipsychotic for acutely ill patients and ends with the most important questions about maintenance treatment.

Method

The report is based on published systematic reviews or relevant key articles on topics not yet covered by a systematic review. We did not perform a literature search for this review but the first author (S.L.) regularly runs MEDLINE searches with the key words 'antipsychotic* OR schizophreni*'.

Treatment of an acute episode (see Fig. 2.1 for outline)

Choice of antipsychotic drug and what is the first-line pharmacotherapy

More than 50 years of psychopharmacological research on antipsychotics have yielded little evidence-based data for the choice among the at least 50 antipsychotic drugs available worldwide (Gaebel & Awad, 1994). Much hope has been placed in pharmacogenetics, but this field is still in its infancy (Stone *et al.*, 2010). As all drugs have advantages and disadvantages, it is impossible to define a single first-line compound. In this context we briefly summarize our interpretation of the discussion about second-generation antipsychotics (SGAs) *vs.* first-generation antipsychotics (FGAs), and which is the best SGA, mainly based on recent systematic reviews (Leucht *et al.*, 2008*b*, 2009*a*, 2009*b*) and effectiveness studies CATIE (Lieberman *et al.*, 2005) and EUFEST (Kahn *et al.*, 2008). We did not include the most recent

Essential Evidence-Based Psychopharmacology, Second Edition, ed. Dan J. Stein, Bernard Lerer, and Stephen M. Stahl. Published by Cambridge University Press. © Cambridge University Press.

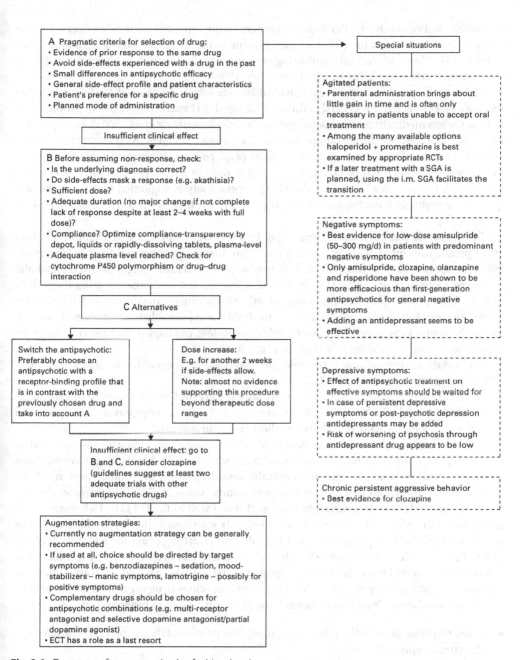

A Pragmatic criteria for selection of drug:
• Evidence of prior response to the same drug
• Avoid side-effects experienced with a drug in the past
• Small differences in antipsychotic efficacy
• General side-effect profile and patient characteristics
• Patient's preference for a specific drug
• Planned mode of administration

Special situations

Insufficient clinical effect

B Before assuming non-response, check:
• Is the underlying diagnosis correct?
• Do side-effects mask a response (e.g. akathisia)?
• Sufficient dose?
• Adequate duration (no major change if not complete lack of response despite at least 2–4 weeks with full dose)?
• Compliance? Optimize compliance-transparency by depot, liquids or rapidly-dissolving tablets, plasma-level
• Adequate plasma level reached? Check for cytochrome P450 polymorphism or drug–drug interaction

C Alternatives

Switch the antipsychotic:
Preferably choose an antipsychotic with a receptor-binding profile that is in contrast with the previously chosen drug and take into account A

Dose increase:
E.g. for another 2 weeks if side-effects allow. Note: almost no evidence supporting this procedure beyond therapeutic dose ranges

Insufficient clinical effect: go to B and C, consider clozapine (guidelines suggest at least two adequate trials with other antipsychotic drugs)

Augmentation strategies:
• Currently no augmentation strategy can be generally recommended
• If used at all, choice should be directed by target symptoms (e.g. benzodiazepines – sedation, mood-stabilizers – manic symptoms, lamotrigine – possibly for positive symptoms)
• Complementary drugs should be chosen for antipsychotic combinations (e.g. multi-receptor antagonist and selective dopamine antagonist/partial dopamine agonist)
• ECT has a role as a last resort

Agitated patients:
• Parenteral administration brings about little gain in time and is often only necessary in patients unable to accept oral treatment
• Among the many available options haloperidol + promethazine is best examined by appropriate RCTs
• If a later treatment with a SGA is planned, using the i.m. SGA facilitates the transition

Negative symptoms:
• Best evidence for low-dose amisulpride (50–300 mg/d) in patients with predominant negative symptoms
• Only amisulpride, clozapine, olanzapine and risperidone have been shown to be more efficacious than first-generation antipsychotics for general negative symptoms
• Adding an antidepressant seems to be effective

Depressive symptoms:
• Effect of antipsychotic treatment on affective symptoms should be waited for
• In case of persistent depressive symptoms or post-psychotic depression antidepressants may be added
• Risk of worsening of psychosis through antidepressant drug appears to be low

Chronic persistent aggressive behavior
• Best evidence for clozapine

Fig. 2.1. Treatment of an acute episode of schizophrenia.

antipsychotic drugs (paliperidone, asenapine, iloperidone) except for listing their optimum dose ranges as comparative data are still sparse.

We interpret the meta-analyses such that overall clozapine, amisulpride, olanzapine and risperidone may be somewhat more efficacious than FGAs and other SGAs (Davis *et al.*, 2003; Geddes *et al.*, 2000; Leucht *et al.*, 2009*a*, 2009*b*). The magnitude of the efficacy superiority was small, and certainly smaller than differences in the most frequent side-effects. The use of clozapine is restricted to refractory patients due to the increased risk of agranulocytosis (Alvir, 1994). However, careful monitoring of changes in the blood count has almost eliminated agranuloctyosis-induced death (Lieberman, 1998).

Haloperidol produced more extrapyramidal side-effects (EPS) and tardive dyskinesia than SGAs, even when it was used at doses < 7.5 mg/day (Leucht *et al.*, 2009a). Prophylactic antiparkinson medication reduces haloperidol's EPS (Rosenheck *et al.*, 2003). Low-potency FGAs produce fewer EPS than haloperidol, and not more than all SGAs (Leucht *et al.*, 2003b, 2009a). The risk of mid-potency FGAs such as perphenazine, is between that of high- and low-potency FGAs (Klein & Davis, 1969), and it was similar to risperidone according to Hoyberg & Fensbo (1993). Among the SGAs a meta-analysis suggested that clozapine and quetiapine probably have the lowest and risperidone the highest EPS risk (Rummel-Kluge *et al.*, 2010).

In contrast to this partial amelioration of EPS with SGAs there is also a shift in the side-effect profile with most SGAs increasing the risk of metabolic abnormalities (de Hert *et al.*, 2009; Newcomer, 2005). Clozapine and olanzapine produced most weight gain and metabolic problems (Allison *et al.*, 1999) (the PORT guideline recommends against using them first-line in first-episode patients; Buchanan *et al.*, 2010), while ziprasidone and haloperidol caused the least followed by aripiprazole, amisulpride, and probably mid-potency FGAs such as perphenazine. Low-potency FGAs, zotepine, sertindole, quetiapine, and risperidone probably lie somewhere in the middle (Leucht *et al.*, 2009a).

Thioridazine, ziprasidone, sertindole, and pimozide are probably associated with most QTc prolongation (Buchanan *et al.*, 2010).

Risperidone and amisulpride seem to produce the greatest prolactin increase, even more so than haloperidol (Bushe *et al.*, 2008; Kleinberg *et al.*, 1999). Aripiprazole, clozapine, and quetiapine may be associated with the smallest prolactin increase.

Any creation of a clear hierarchy is difficult. Ideally, studies including all agents would be necessary, but for obvious reasons such studies are not available. Many drugs have not been compared head-to-head and methodologically sound dose-finding studies have not been conducted for almost all first-generation compounds (Davis, 1974). For example, the evidence on sulpiride and perphenazine – drugs that did well in the CATIE (Lieberman *et al.*, 2005) and CUtLASS studies (Jones *et al.*, 2006) – is scarce and their optimum doses have not been established in appropriate fixed-dose designs (Hartung *et al.*, 2005; Omori & Wang, 2009). Furthermore, it is difficult to weigh all these differences in efficacy and side-effects. For many patients weight gain may be unacceptable, while for other patients EPS are undesired. Again other patients may want to receive the most efficacious drug regardless of side-effects.

Recommendation: Drug choice needs to be primarily based on pragmatic criteria:

- Prior response to an antipsychotic assuming that previous efficacy predicts efficacy in the current episode.
- The avoidance of an antipsychotic that produced side-effects in an earlier episode.
- General side-effect profile of the substances (see above) and patient characteristics (e.g. in a patient with diabetes, substances causing weight gain should be avoided).
- Slight differences in efficacy.
- The intended long-term administration. If it is clear that a depot substance is to be administered for maintenance therapy, the choice of an oral antipsychotic that is available as a depot can facilitate the later change.

• If possible, patients' preferences should be taken into account in a shared decision-making process. This may improve compliance and in the end it is the patient who must take the medication. Therefore patients should be involved (Hamann et al., 2003).

Sedation strategies in agitated patients

There are many strategies for the treatment of agitated patients such as monotherapy with an antipsychotic (high or low potency, oral or parenteral), monotherapy with a benzodiazepine, combining both, adding a sedating low-potency FGA, rapidly dissolving tablets, liquid formulations, etc. Due to a lack of RCTs a definite recommendation is not possible and probably most options work in some way. Liquid and rapidly dissolving tablets are options for safeguarding drug intake. Parenteral administrations do not lead to a much faster onset of action (Moller et al., 1982). A review found no significant difference between intramuscular formulations of haloperidol and chlorpromazine (Leucht et al., 2008a). The combination of haloperidol and lorazepam seems to be more efficacious than their monotherapy (Alexander et al., 2004; Battaglia et al., 1997). The SGAs aripiprazole, olanzapine and ziprasidone are available as intramuscular formulations (Citrome, 2007). Their advantage includes fewer EPS than haloperidol. A general problem is that the SGA studies were conducted for registrational purposes and all participants had to give informed consent. These are not the patients for whom intramuscular medication is indicated (often violent patients who are not willing to take medication). From a methodological perspective four large (200–300 participants), real-world pragmatic trials with intramuscular medication need to be highlighted (Alexander et al., 2004; Huf et al., 2003, 2007; Raveendran et al., 2007). In these the combination of haloperidol and promethazine produced more rapid tranquillization with fewer dystonic reactions than haloperidol alone (Huf et al., 2007) and no more EPS than lorazepam alone (Alexander et al., 2004). It did outperform olanzapine in secondary outcomes (number of additional injections) with no difference in EPS, probably due to the anticholinergic properties of promethazine (Raveendran, 2007). Only intramuscular midazolam, a highly sedating benzodiazepine, was more efficacious than haloperidol plus promethazine (Huf et al., 2003) but the mean dose of haloperidol in this study was lower compared with the other listed trials and so a dosing effect leading to the favorable outcome for the benzodiazepine compound cannot be completely ruled out. In the case of chronic, persistent aggressive behavior clozapine was superior to haloperidol and olanzapine (Krakowski et al., 2006). The evidence for other SGAs or mood stabilizers is indirect at best (e.g. derived from non-schizophrenic populations), because RCTs in this specific group of patients have not been conducted.

Recommendation: Parenteral administration should usually only be applied in emergency situations when patients refuse medication. Among the many available options the best evidence is available for haloperidol combined with promethazine. If the subsequent oral treatment is planned to be an SGA it can be reasonable to choose its intramuscular formulation for sedation.

Treatment of patients with depressive symptoms

Depressive symptoms are frequently present in acutely ill patients with schizophrenia (Barnes & McPhillips, 1995) and may first improve with antipsychotics alone. Based on limited data some SGAs have shown superior antidepressant properties (Leucht et al., 2009a). A Cochrane review found some evidence that antidepressants are effective for post-psychotic depression (Whitehead *et al.*, 2003). The risk that an adjunctive antidepressant may provoke psychosis has been judged to be small (Siris, 1991; Whitehead *et al.*, 2003).

Recommendation: Depressive symptoms associated with an acute episode should not be automatically treated with an antidepressant. Neuroleptic-induced depressive symptoms might be ruled out by anti-parkinson medication or switching to a drug with fewer EPS. Post-psychotic depression may be treated with an antidepressant.

Treatment of patients with negative symptoms

All SGAs and haloperidol improved negative symptoms more than placebo (Leucht *et al.*, 2008*b*). In Leucht *et al.* (2009*a*), only four SGAs (amisulpride, clozapine, olanzapine, risperidone) were more efficacious than FGAs for negative symptoms. However, almost all relevant studies were conducted in patients suffering predominantly from positive symptoms. In such patients it is unclear whether it is a superiority for negative symptoms related to primary, or only to secondary, negative symptoms which can stem from positive symptoms, depression or EPS. Only studies in patients with primary/predominant negative symptoms could clarify whether SGAs are truly more efficacious. Here, the best evidence is available for low-dose amisulpride (50–300 mg/day) which proved superior compared with placebo in several trials (Leucht *et al.*, 2002*b*). However, comparing SGAs to FGAs only a few RCTs in predominant negative symptoms are available and among these only a single small trial showed superiority of olanzapine compared with haloperidol (Lindenmayer *et al.*, 2007). Three meta-analyses showed that adding an antidepressant can be effective for predominant negative symptoms (Rummel *et al.*, 2006) or in chronic patients with schizophrenia (Sepehry *et al.*, 2007; Singh *et al.*, 2010).

Recommendation: Secondary negative symptoms due to EPS should be ruled out (e.g. by antiparkinson medication or changing the antipsychotic). Low-dose amisulpride is the best-examined drug in patients with predominant negative symptoms. Adding an antidepressant can be tried.

Factors that need to be ruled out before non-response is assumed

Before assuming non-response and introducing a major change in treatment, a number of items need to be ruled out.

Is the diagnosis of schizophrenia correct? A psychotic depression/mania or severe personality disturbances can be difficult to distinguish from schizophrenia.

Do side-effects mask a response? Akathisia can resemble psychotic agitation and parkinsonism can mimic negative symptoms.

Sufficient dose? There is better information about the therapeutic dose ranges of SGAs than FGAs because dose-finding studies have been conducted during their registration processes. There is some variability between guidelines, but we present the recommendations of the PORT guideline (Buchanan *et al.*, 2010), supplemented by Falkai *et al.* (2005) or our own evaluation if necessary: amisulpride 400–800 mg/day for predominant positive symptoms and 50–300 mg/day for predominant negative symptoms, aripiprazole 10–30 mg/day, asenapine 10–20 mg/day, clozapine 300–800 mg/day (in treatment-resistant patients), iloperidone 12–24 mg/day, olanzapine 10–20 mg/day, quetiapine 300–800 mg/day, paliperidone 3–15 mg/day, risperidone 2–8 mg/day, sertindole 12–20(24) mg/day, ziprasidone 80–160 mg/day, zotepine 150–250 mg/day. Regarding FGAs, an influential review concluded that very high doses (>700 mg/day chlorpromazine) are generally no more efficacious than

moderate doses (Baldessarini *et al.*, 1988). A Cochrane review suggested that in uncomplicated patients higher doses than 7.5 mg/day haloperidol do not bring about more efficacy
(Waraich *et al.*, 2002) and in single RCTs, 4 mg/day (Zimbroff *et al.*, 1997) or neuroleptic
threshold doses (average 3.3 mg/day) were as effective as higher doses (McEvoy *et al.*, 1991).
Much less is known about the doses of other FGAs and dose-equivalence tables are problematic among others since they assume linear relationships. We orient the interested reader to
recent publications on dose equivalence (Andreasen *et al.*, 2010; Davis & Chen, 2004; Gardner *et al.*, 2010; Kane *et al.*, 2003). First-episode and elderly patients often need lower doses.
The latter are also more sensitive to side-effects due to reduced metabolism and one-third of
the dose in younger patients has been suggested as a rule of thumb (Jeste *et al.*, 1993).

Was the patient compliant? Compliance problems are so frequent that they should always
be addressed by switching to liquid medication or rapidly dissolving tablets in inpatients; or
considering depot medication in outpatients (Leucht & Heres, 2006). Plasma levels and the
determination of a patient's cytochrome P450 status can also be useful.

Sufficient plasma level? There is not sufficient evidence to allow the exact titration of
antipsychotics guided by therapeutic drug monitoring except for clozapine, where it can be
useful. Therefore, plasma-level measurements are only indicated in the following situations
(for review of therapeutic ranges see Baumann *et al.*, 2004):

- Suspicion of non-compliance.
- Lack of response in spite of taking usually sufficient doses to rule out ultra-rapid
  excessive metabolization of the antipsychotic due to a polymorphism of the cytochrome
  P450 enzyme system.
- Pronounced side-effects despite the administration of a usual dose to rule out 'poor
  metabolizers' due to too little production of cytochrome P450 enzymes.
- Medication interactions, smoking, etc., which can also lead to elevated or lowered
  plasma levels via effects on the cytochrome P450 system.

Has the patient been treated sufficiently long? The onset of response to treatment of individual patients is highly variable and recent analyses attempted to resolve some of the heterogeneity by identifying different trajectories (Levine & Leucht, 2010; Levine & Rabinowitz,
2010). Nevertheless, recent meta-analyses rejected the long-held hypothesis that there is a
general 'delay of onset of action' of several weeks for antipsychotic drugs. The largest part
of the drug effect occurred in the first week and became consistently smaller thereafter
(Agid *et al.*, 2003; Leucht *et al.*, 2005a). Two further studies demonstrated that the antipsychotic drug effect can be disentangled from placebo as early as 24 h (Agid *et al.*, 2008;
Kapur *et al.*, 2005).

These findings call into question guidelines that a drug should not be considered ineffective and switched before 3–6 weeks (Gaebel *et al.*, 2006; Lehman *et al.*, 2004; McGorry, 2005;
NICE, 2003). Indeed, several studies have now suggested that non-responders might be identified as soon as after 2 weeks. Very roughly, those patients who did not have an improvement
of at least 20–25% in PANSS or BPRS total score reduction (corresponding to less than mini-
mally improved on the Clinical Global Impressions Scale; Leucht *et al.*, 2005b, 2005c, 2006) at
2 weeks were unlikely to respond later (Ascher-Svanum *et al.*, 2008; Chang *et al.*, 2006; Correll
et al., 2003; Jager *et al.*, 2009; Kinon *et al.*, 2008a, Leucht *et al.*, 2007a, 2008c; Lin *et al.*, 2007).
In one analysis, however, only improvement at 4 weeks but not at 2 weeks predicted later
response (Lambert *et al.*, 2009). Although only little evidence is available that early switching of medication is effective (see below), keeping the patient on the original drug is likely

to lead to a poor outcome. Therefore, changing treatment earlier than the usually proposed 4–6 weeks could be justified.

Recommendation: Before non-response is assumed, the diagnosis should be confirmed, and side-effects masking response, non-compliance, insufficient dose, and too-fast drug metabolism should be ruled out (e.g. by plasma levels). Any major change in treatment should not be considered before absolute non-response to at least 2–4 weeks of treatment with a full antipsychotic dose.

Switching the drug or increasing the dose in initial non-responders

Surprisingly few RCTs have examined the effectiveness of switching medication or of a major dose increase.

(*a*) *Switching to a different antipsychotic*. To date only one trial examined switching after only 2 weeks of virtually no improvement. It found that switching from risperidone to olanzapine was more effective than keeping patients on risperidone, but the superiority was small (Kinon *et al.*, 2010).

Kinon *et al.* (1993) treated 115 participants with 20 mg/day fluphenazine for 4 weeks. The 47 non-responders were randomized to double-blind treatment with (*a*) continuation with 20 mg/day fluphenazine (control group), (*b*) 80 mg/day fluphenazine (dose increase group) or 20 mg/day haloperidol (switching group). Regardless of the strategy, only four (9%) of these patients responded.

Shalev *et al.* (1993) randomized 60 patients with acute schizophrenia to haloperidol, perphenazine, or chlorpromazine. Non-responders after 4 weeks of treatment were randomized twice to open treatment with one of the other two antipsychotics. At the end of the study, the majority of the participants had responded with an overall higher number of patients responding to perphenazine or chlorpromazine than to haloperidol.

Suzuki *et al.* (2007) randomized 78 patients with schizophrenia to olanzapine, quetiapine or risperidone. After up to 8 weeks treatment, the non-responders were twice re-randomized to the remaining compounds. Only 16 patients did not respond to any of the three antipsychotic drugs with olanzapine and risperidone showing comparable efficacy while quetiapine was less effective. As in Shalev *et al.* (1993) the major limitation of the study was the lack of a control group of patients who stayed on the initial drug to rule out that the improvement was not simply an effect of time.

Stroup *et al.* (2007) post-hoc analyzed those 114 participants who had received perphenazine in CATIE phase I, but discontinued it. Those participants who were randomized to quetiapine or olanzapine in phase II did better than those randomized to risperidone. This was explained by the similar profile of perphenazine and risperidone. Thus, if the antipsychotic drug is changed, it is reasonable to choose a compound with a different receptor-binding profile.

(*b*) *Substantially increasing the dose*. The aforementioned study by Kinon *et al.* (1993) showed no incremental efficacy of increasing fluphenazine from 20 mg/day to 80 mg/day. McEvoy *et al.* (1991) randomized patients who did not respond to neuroleptic threshold doses of haloperidol (mean 2.3 mg/day) to either continuation of threshold doses or doses up to 10 times greater. The dose increase was not associated with better efficacy. In Kinon *et al.* (2008*b*) there was no efficacy difference between 10 mg/day, 20 mg/day, and 40 mg/day olanzapine in patients with suboptimal response to previous treatment. Olanzapine (40 mg/day) was, however, slightly better in a severely ill subgroup.

Recommendation: More evidence may be available for switching a drug rather than a massive dose increase beyond the official ranges, although even for the former strategy the evidence is scarce. Individual patients respond only to very high doses and such a history should be considered, but we would not recommend this as a general strategy. If a dose increase beyond the optimum doses was not effective, the dose should be reduced to previous levels. An antipsychotic with a different receptor-binding profile should be chosen in case of a switch. There is no randomized evidence whether patients should be started on a loading dose, a medium dose, or titrated slowly upwards. This decision needs to be adapted to the situation (e.g. the acuteness of the symptoms) and the antipsychotic (some require titration or have clearly dose-related side-effects).

Clozapine and other SGAs for treatment resistance

Clozapine had been continuously prescribed in several European countries in the 1970s and 1980s (Naber & Hippius, 1990). It was reintroduced in the USA and other countries after the landmark study of Kane *et al.* (1988) reporting clozapine to be superior to chlorpromazine in refractory patients. This finding was confirmed by subsequent studies (Kane *et al.*, 2001; Rosenheck *et al.*, 1997) and meta-analyses (Chakos *et al.*, 2001; Essali *et al.*, 2009; Wahlbeck *et al.*, 1999). Clozapine was superior to other SGAs in CATIE phase II but it was the only open-label arm (McEvoy *et al.*, 2006). In the CUtLASS study clozapine was more effective than other SGAs as a group (Lewis *et al.*, 2006). A meta-analysis of 28 blinded RCTs did not find significant superiority of clozapine compared with other SGAs (Leucht *et al.*, 2009b). We suggested that too-low clozapine doses explained this unexpected finding. Nevertheless, we believe that a conclusive clozapine *vs.* other SGAs trial is still needed.

Concerning the efficacy of other SGAs compared to FGAs in treatment-resistant patients a meta-analysis published in 2001 concluded that in contrast to clozapine none was convincingly superior (Chakos *et al.*, 2001). The evidence base has not substantially changed since. We briefly summarize the studies in treatment-resistant participants in Leucht *et al.* (2009a). There was no RCT comparing amisulpride, sertindole, or zotepine with FGAs in treatment-resistant schizophrenia. Kane *et al.* (2007) found no difference between aripiprazole and perphenazine in 300 participants who had not responded to olanzapine or risperidone. Olanzapine was superior to haloperidol in a post-hoc analysis of treatment-resistant patients from a large pivotal trial (Breier & Hamilton, 1999; Tollefson *et al.*, 1997). It was also found superior to haloperidol in patients having poorly responded to FGAs in Volavka *et al.* (2002). Four smaller studies did not find olanzapine clearly superior (Altamura *et al.*, 2002; Buchanan *et al.*, 2005; Conley *et al.*, 1998; Smith *et al.*, 2001). Conley *et al.* (2005) found no difference between quetiapine, risperidone and fluphenazine, while in Emsley *et al.* (2000) partial non-responders to fluphenazine did better when they were randomized to quetiapine instead of haloperidol. Wirshing *et al.* (1999) found a superiority of risperidone compared with haloperidol in the first 4 weeks of an 8-week study, while Conley *et al.* (2005), See *et al.* (1999) and Volavka *et al.* (2002) did not find any clear superiority. Kane *et al.* (2006) found superiority of ziprasidone compared with chlorpromazine in terms of negative symptoms but not overall symptoms. In our opinion none of these findings are robust enough to generally recommend another SGA than clozapine for refractory patients.

Recommendation: Clozapine remains the gold standard for treatment-refractory patients while for none of the other SGAs is there sufficient evidence available. By most guidelines clozapine is recommended after at least two adequate trials with different antipsychotic drugs.

Augmentation strategies

Among the many augmentation strategies that have been examined, there was no clear effect of benzodiazepines (apart from sedation; Volz et al., 2007), beta-blockers (Cheine et al., 2001), lithium (Leucht et al., 2007b), carbamazepine (Leucht et al., 2002a) and valproate (Basan et al., 2004). The largest valproate study (249 participants) showed a more rapid onset of improvement in the augmentation group at 2 weeks (Casey et al., 2003), but even this effect was not replicated in a recent trial with 402 participants (Casey et al., 2009). Lamotrigine is a promising adjunct according to a Cochrane review (Premkumar & Pick, 2006) and a meta-analysis focusing on clozapine non-responders (Tiihonen et al., 2009). However, the latter meta-analyses were relatively small and possibly not robust (Trikalinos et al., 2004). Attempts to add acetylcholinesterase inhibitors to improve cognitive deficits have not proven effective (Stip et al., 2007). The effects of other augmentation strategies such as polyunsaturated fatty acids (omega-3 and omega-6 fatty acids; Joy et al., 2006), glutamatergic agents (Tuominen et al., 2006), estrogens (Chua et al., 2005), dehydroepiandrosterone (DHEA; Elias & Kumar, 2007), amphetamines (Nolte et al., 2004), cyclooxygenase-2 (COX-2) inhibitors such as celecoxib (Akhondzadeh et al., 2007; Muller et al., 2002), and erythropoietin (Ehrenreich et al., 2007) are either still in the experimental stage or inconclusive.

Recommendation: Monotherapy should be the aim, because combinations of medications increase the risk of side-effects and drug–drug interactions. In drug combinations it is often not clear which compound has led to success and which should be discontinued. Compliance with several agents is difficult. Most importantly, there is no convincing evidence for any combination strategy. It might at best be tried for target symptoms (e.g. benzodiazepines for anxiety) and quickly discontinued if ineffective.

Combinations of antipsychotic drugs

Although antipsychotic drugs are frequently combined in clinical practice, several recent systematic reviews did not show a clear benefit. Correll et al. (2009) suggested a better response in the combination group compared with monotherapy, but it remained unclear which of the many combinations were effective, the positive results were mainly based on Chinese studies in which antipsychotics were combined right from the start rather than after non-response (which is current practice), if clozapine was part of the combination treatment, and if the trials lasted > 10 weeks (confirmed by Paton et al., 2007; but not by Taylor & Smith, 2009). Furthermore, there was a possibility of publication bias. Barbui et al. (2009) included only studies in clozapine non-responders and found a positive effect only in randomized open studies, but not in double-blind studies. Recent RCTs suggested some benefits of adding aripiprazole to risperidone for reducing prolactin (Kane et al., 2009) and to clozapine for reducing weight (Fleischhacker et al., 2008). Another study suggested possible efficacy for aripiprazole augmentation for negative symptoms (Chang et al., 2008).

Recommendation: Due to lack of convincing evidence, combining antipsychotic drugs cannot be generally recommended (Goodwin et al., 2009). If used, drugs with different receptor-binding profiles should be combined. For example, clozapine, which has relatively few antidopaminergic properties, may be combined with selective dopamine receptor antagonists such as amisulpride, sulpiride, aripiprazole, or low-dose haloperidol, while, for example, combining olanzapine and quetiapine makes less sense.

Electroconvulsive therapy (ECT) and repetitive transcranial magnetic stimulation (rTMS)

In a Cochrane review, ECT monotherapy was more effective than sham ECT, but less effective than anti-psychotic drugs (Tharyan & Adams, 2005). Very limited evidence supported the combination of ECT with antipsychotics. Meta-analyses found medium effect sizes for rTMS for positive symptoms (Aleman *et al.*, 2007; Tranulis *et al.*, 2008). Fewer studies examined the effect of rTMS applied over frontal areas in order to influence negative symptoms with more equivocal results (Hajak *et al.*, 2004; Klein *et al.*, 1999). Guidelines consider rTMS to be still in the experimental stage (Gaebel *et al.*, 2006; Lehman *et al.*, 2004).

Recommendation: ECT is recommended only as a last resort (except for special indications such as severe catatonia), but advantageously compared with the other augmentation strategies, it is effective as monotherapy and has a different mechanism of action than antipsychotics.

Maintenance treatment (see Fig. 2.2 for outline)

Indication

In naturalistic studies, only ~20% of patients with a first episode did not experience another episode within 5 years (Robinson *et al.*, 1999; Shepherd *et al.*, 1989). We assume that in multiple-episode patients this proportion is even smaller. Maintenance treatment with antipsychotic drugs clearly reduced relapse rates from 53% to 16% within 9.7 months (Gilbert *et al.*, 1995). Intermittent treatment (tapering medication once a patient is in remission and only re-starting it when there are early warning signs) was less efficacious than continuous treatment (Carpenter *et al.*, 1990; Herz *et al.*, 1991; Jolley & Hirsch, 1990; Pietzcker *et al.*, 1993; Schooler *et al.*, 1997), even in first-episode patients (Gaebel *et al.*, 2010).

Recommendation: As there are no valid indicators that could predict who will not relapse, we follow an early guideline (Kissling *et al.*, 1991) that suggested continuous maintenance treatment with antipsychotic drugs for all patients, except for those in whom side-effects outweigh the benefits, those with very mild episodes, and unclear diagnoses.

Choice of the antipsychotic drug in maintenance treatment

In Leucht *et al.* (2003*a*), SGAs as a group reduced relapse rates compared with FGAs from 23% to 15%. In an update the various SGAs were not pooled because we felt that they were too different to form a class. Among the single SGAs, only olanzapine, risperidone and, based on a single trial, sertindole were superior to FGAs (Leucht *et al.*, 2009*a*). A clearer advantage includes lower incidence of tardive dyskinesia, which occurred with an annual incidence of 3.0% in SGAs *vs.* 7.7% with FGAs (see Correll & Schenk, 2008, an update of Correll *et al.*, 2004).

Recommendation: For pragmatic reasons, maintenance treatment can be carried out with the antipsychotic drug to which the patient responded in the acute episode as long as there are no important side-effects. However, the higher risk of FGAs for tardive dyskinesia or weight gain-related risks associated with several SGAs should be considered.

Depot medication

Depot formulations are not more efficacious per se, but they could have advantages in terms of improved compliance, although the randomized evidence is limited. A summary of Cochrane reviews found little supportive evidence but included short-term studies and

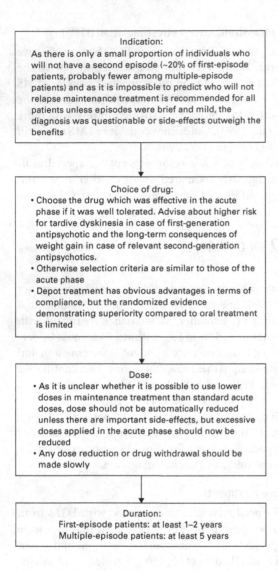

Fig. 2.2. Maintenance treatment of schizophrenia.

Indication:
As there is only a small proportion of individuals who will not have a second episode (~20% of first-episode patients, probably fewer among multiple-episode patients) and as it is impossible to predict who will not relapse maintenance treatment is recommended for all patients unless episodes were brief and mild, the diagnosis was questionable or side-effects outweigh the benefits

Choice of drug:
• Choose the drug which was effective in the acute phase if it was well tolerated. Advise about higher risk for tardive dyskinesia in case of first-generation antipsychotic and the long-term consequences of weight gain in case of relevant second-generation antipsychotics.
• Otherwise selection criteria are similar to those of the acute phase
• Depot treatment has obvious advantages in terms of compliance, but the randomized evidence demonstrating superiority compared to oral treatment is limited

Dose:
• As it is unclear whether it is possible to use lower doses in maintenance treatment than standard acute doses, dose should not be automatically reduced unless there are important side-effects, but excessive doses applied in the acute phase should now be reduced
• Any dose reduction or drug withdrawal should be made slowly

Duration:
First-episode patients: at least 1–2 years
Multiple-episode patients: at least 5 years

studies in inpatients – both factors that may have limited the compliance-improving effect (Adams *et al.*, 2000). Indeed, a recent meta-analysis including only long-term RCTs in outpatients found a superiority of depot compared with oral treatment, but there were limitations (Leucht *et al.*, 2011). Interested readers might refer to a comprehensive supplement on treatment with depot in the *British Journal of Psychiatry* (Patel *et al.*, 2009).

Recommendation: Despite the currently limited evidence, we believe that depot medication has obvious advantages such as assured medication and the awareness of when a patient stopped treatment (Kane *et al.*, 2003).

Duration of relapse prevention with antipsychotic drugs

There is little evidence to guide us about the ideal duration of antipsychotic relapse prevention. An early consensus conference suggested keeping first-episode patients on maintenance medication for at least 1–2 years and multiple-episode patients for at least 5 years. In severe cases the prophylaxis might even be indefinite (Kissling *et al.*, 1991). This recommendation was based on a few, small, controlled (but not all randomized), withdrawal trials. Multiple-episode patients who had been stable for up to 5 years had significantly higher relapse rates when their medication was withdrawn compared with those staying on drugs (Cheung, 1981; Johnson, 1976, 1979; Odejide & Aderounmu, 1982). A later study found the same result in patients who had been stable for 6 years (Sampath *et al.*, 1992). In first-episode patients the duration was restricted to 2 years, because this was the longest study duration here (Chen *et al.*, 2010, Crow *et al.*, 1986; Hogarty & Ulrich, 1998; Kane, 1982). In the last 20 years we have gained little new evidence and this remains a gap. But even a gradual symptom-guided tapering (and discontinuation if feasible) of antipsychotic treatment after 6 months of symptom absence led to doubled relapse rates compared with maintenance treatment in first-episode patients in a recent trial (Wunderink *et al.*, 2007). It should also be noted that lack of evidence beyond 6 years (or 2 years for first-episode patients) does not mean that the risk for relapse goes down. Empirically, multiple-episode patients stable for 2 years relapsed at the same rates as patients newly entered into a relapse study (Hogarty *et al.*, 1976). Many national guidelines have adopted the early suggestions. Their recommendations range between 1 and 2 years for first-episode patients, and between 2 and 5 years for multiple-episode patients (Gaebel *et al.*, 2005).

Recommendation: First-episode patients should usually be kept on maintenance medication for at least 1–2 years and multiple-episode patients for at least 5 years.

The optimal dosage in maintenance treatment

It is unclear whether lower doses than those usually applied in the acute phase are sufficient for maintenance treatment. Studies in the 1980s and 1990s attempted to identify doses of depot FGAs that were high enough to prevent relapses, but low enough to minimize side-effects. Unfortunately, the definition of an ideal dose was not clear-cut and the lowest doses led to the highest relapse rates, although the differences were not always statistically significant (Hogarty & McEvoy, 1988; Johnson *et al.*, 1987; Kane *et al.*, 1983, 2002; Marder *et al.*, 1984; Schooler *et al.*, 1997). In a systematic review, higher dosages of conventional antipsychotics than 375 mg/day chlorpromazine equivalent did not produce additional effectiveness in maintenance therapy (Bollini, 1994). In another review, dosages between 50 mg/day and 100 mg/day chlorpromazine equivalents led to more relapses than doses between 200 and 500 chlorpromazine equivalents (Barbui *et al.*, 1996). Only a few dose-finding studies on relapse prevention with SGAs are available. Arato *et al.* (2002) found no difference between 40 mg/day ziprasidone and higher doses. Simpson *et al.* (2006) reported a trend superiority of risperidone 50 mg bi-weekly compared with 25 mg bi-weekly, and Wang *et al.* (2010) found the lowest relapse rate when the risperidone dose that was effective in the acute phase was maintained compared with 50% and 25% reductions. In a systematic review including SGAs and FGAs, standard doses were clearly more effective than "very low" doses, while the comparisons of relapses with "low" doses was only of borderline statistical significance (Uchida *et al.*, 2009). On the other hand, it may not be so important to lower the dose of SGAs, since within their official dose ranges many side-effects are not very dose related.

Recommendation: Given the uncertainty whether lower doses are as effective as standard doses, we recommend keeping the dose of the acute phase as long as there are no important side-effects. Nevertheless, due to various pressures, psychiatrists sometimes tend to give very high doses or combination treatments in the acute phase. The maintenance phase should definitely be used for reducing such excessive dosing. Any dose reduction should be performed very slowly to avoid withdrawal effects and rebound psychoses.

Statement of Interest

Stefan Leucht has received speaker/consultancy/advisory board honoraria from Sanofi-Aventis, Bristol-Myers Squibb, Eli Lilly, Essex Pharma, GlaxoSmithKline, Janssen/Johnson and Johnson, Lundbeck and Pfizer including the fees and travel expenses for attending these functions; he has received funding for research projects from Eli Lilly and Sanofi-Aventis. Stephan Heres has received honoraria from Janssen-Cilag, Sanofi-Aventis, Pharmastar, and Johnson & Johnson; he has accepted travel or hospitality payment from Janssen-Cilag, Sanofi-Aventis, Johnson & Johnson, Pfizer, Bristol-Myers Squibb, AstraZeneca, Lundbeck, Novartis, and Eli Lilly and Company. Werner Kissling has received speaker and/or advisory board/consultancy honoraria from Janssen, Sanofi-Aventis, Johnson & Johnson, Pfizer, Bayer, Bristol-Myers Squibb, AstraZeneca, Lundbeck, Novartis, and Eli Lilly.

References

Adams CE, Coutinho E, Davis JM *et al.* (2008). *Cochrane Schizophrenia Group.* The Cochrane Library. Chichester: John Wiley & Sons.

Adams CE, Fenton MKP, Quraishi S, David AS (2000). Systematic meta-review of depot antipsychotic drugs for people with schizophrenia. *British Journal of Psychiatry* **179**, 190–199.

Agid O, Kapur S, Arenovich T, Zipursky RB (2003). Delayed-onset hypothesis of antipsychotic action – a hypothesis tested and rejected. *Archives of General Psychiatry* **60**, 1228–1235.

Agid O, Kapur S, Warrington L *et al.* (2008). Early onset of antipsychotic response in the treatment of acutely agitated patients with psychotic disorders. *Schizophrenia Research* **102**, 241–248.

Akhondzadeh S, Tabatbaee M, Amini H *et al.* (2007). Celecoxib as adjunctive therapy in schizophrenia: a double-blind, randomized and placebo-controlled trial. *Schizophrenia Research* **90**, 179–185.

Aleman A, Sommer IE, Kahn RS (2007). Efficacy of slow repetitive transcranial magnetic stimulation in the treatment of resistant auditory hallucinations in schizophrenia: a meta-analysis. *Journal of Clinical Psychiatry* **68**, 416–421.

Alexander J, Tharyan P, Adams C *et al.* (2004). Rapid tranquillisation of violent or agitated patients in a psychiatric emergency setting –

pragmatic randomised trial of intramuscular lorazepam v. haloperidol plus promethazine. *British Journal of Psychiatry* **185**, 63–69.

Allison DB, Mentore JL, Heo M *et al.* (1999). Antipsychotic-induced weight gain: a comprehensive research synthesis. *American Journal of Psychiatry* **156**, 1686–1696.

Altamura AC, Velona I, Curreli R *et al.* (2002). Is olanzapine better than haloperidol in resistant schizophrenia? A double-blind study in partial responders. *International Journal of Psychiatry in Clinical Practice* **6**, 107–111.

Alvir JMJ (1994). Agranulocytosis: incidence and risk factors. *Journal of Clinical Psychiatry* **55**, 137–138.

Andreasen NC, Pressler M, Nopoulos P *et al.* (2010). Antipsychotic dose equivalents and dose-years: a standardized method for comparing exposure to different drugs. *Biological Psychiatry* **67**, 255–262.

Arato M, O'Connor R, Meltzer H, Zeus Study Group (2002). Ziprasidone in the long-term treatment of negative symptoms and the prevention of exacerbation of schizophrenia. *International Clinical Psychopharmacology* **17**, 207–215.

Ascher-Svanum H, Nyhuis AW, Faries DE *et al.* (2008). Clinical, functional, and economic ramifications of early nonresponse to antipsychotics in the naturalistic treatment of schizophrenia. *Schizophrenia Bulletin* **34**, 1163–1171.

Baldessarini RJ, Cohen BM, Teicher MH (1988). Significance of neuroleptic dose and plasma level in the pharmacological treatment of psychoses. *Archives of General Psychiatry* **45**, 79–91.

Barbui C, Saraceno B, Liberati A, Garattini S (1996). Low-dose neuroleptic therapy and relapse in schizophrenia: meta-analysis of randomized controlled trials. *European Psychiatry* **11**, 306–311.

Barbui C, Signoretti A, Mule S *et al.* (2009). Does the addition of a second antipsychotic drug improve clozapine treatment? *Schizophrenia Bulletin* **35**, 458–468.

Barnes TR, McPhillips MA (1995). How to distinguish between the neuroleptic-induced deficit syndrome, depression and disease-related negative symptoms in schizophrenia. *International Clinical Psychopharmacology* **10** (Suppl. 3), 115–121.

Basan A, Kissling W, Leucht S (2004). Valproate as an adjunct to antipsychotics for schizophrenia: a systematic review of randomized trials. *Schizophrenia Research* **70**, 33–37.

Battaglia J, Moss S, Rush J *et al.* (1997). Haloperidol, lorazepam, or both for psychotic agitation: a multicenter, prospective, double blind, emergency department study. *American Journal of Emergency Medicine* **15**, 335–340.

Baumann P, Hiemke C, Ulrich S *et al.* (2004). The AGNP-TDM expert group consensus guidelines: therapeutic drug monitoring in psychiatry. *Pharmacopsychiatry* **37**, 243–265.

Bollini P (1994). Antipsychotic drugs: is more worse? A meta analysis of the published randomized controlled trials. *Psychological Medicine* **24**, 307–316.

Breier A, Hamilton SH (1999). Comparative efficacy of olanzapine and haloperidol for patients with treatment-resistant schizophrenia. *Biological Psychiatry* **45**, 403–411.

Buchanan RW, Ball MP, Weiner E *et al.* (2005). Olanzapine treatment of residual positive and negative symptoms. *American Journal of Psychiatry* **162**, 124–129.

Buchanan RW, Kreyenbuhl J, Kelly DL *et al.* (2010). The 2009 schizophrenia PORT psychopharmacological treatment recommendations and summary statements. *Schizophrenia Bulletin* **36**, 71–93.

Bushe C, Shaw M, Peveler RC (2008). A review of the association between antipsychotic use and hyperprolactinaemia. *Journal of Psychopharmacology* **22**, 46–55.

Carpenter WT, Hanlon TE, Heinrichs DW *et al.* (1990). Continuous *vs.* targeted medication in schizophrenic outpatients: outcome results. *American Journal of Psychiatry* **147**, 1138–1163.

Casey DE, Daniel DG, Tamminga C *et al.* (2009). Divalproex ER combined with olanzapine or risperidone for treatment of acute exacerbations of schizophrenia. *Neuropsychopharmacology* **34**, 1330–1338.

Casey DE, Daniel DG, Wassef AA *et al.* (2003). Effect of divalproex combined with olanzapine or risperidone in patients with an acute exacerbation of schizophrenia. *Neuropsychopharmacology* **28**, 182–192.

Chakos M, Lieberman J, Hoffman E *et al.* (2001). Effectiveness of second generation antipsychotics for treatment-resistant schizophrenia: a review and meta-analysis of randomized trials. *American Journal of Psychiatry* **158**, 518–526.

Chang JS, Ahn YM, Park HJ *et al.* (2008). Aripiprazole augmentation in clozapine-treated patients with refractory schizophrenia: an 8-week, randomized, double-blind, placebo-controlled trial. *Journal of Clinical Psychiatry* **69**, 720–731.

Chang YC, Lane HY, Yang KH, Huang CL (2006). Optimizing early prediction for antipsychotic response in schizophrenia. *Journal of Clinical Psychopharmacology* **26**, 554–559.

Cheine M, Ahonen J, Wahlbeck K (2001). Beta-blocker supplementation of standard drug treatment for schizophrenia. *Cochrane Database of Systematic Reviews* **3**, CD000234.

Chen EYH, Hui CLM, Lam MML *et al.* (2010). Maintenance treatment with quetiapine *vs.* discontinuation after one year of treatment in patients with remitted first episode psychosis: randomised controlled trial. *British Medical Journal* **341**, c4024.

Cheung HK (1981). Schizophrenics fully remitted on neuroleptics for 3–5 years – to stop or continue drugs? *British Journal of Psychiatry* **138**, 490–494.

Chua WL, Santiago AD, Kulkarni J, Mortimer A (2005). Estrogen for schizophrenia. *Cochrane Database of Systematic Reviews* **4**, CD004719.

Citrome L (2007). Comparison of intramuscular ziprasidone, olanzapine, or aripiprazole for agitation: a quantitative review of efficacy and safety. *Journal of Clinical Psychiatry* **68**, 1876–1885.

Conley RR, Kelly DL, Nelson MW *et al.* (2005). Risperidone, quetiapine, and fluphenazine in the treatment of patients with therapy-refractory schizophrenia. *Clinical Neuropharmacology* **28**, 163–168.

Conley RR, Tamminga CA, Bartko JJ *et al.* (1998). Olanzapine compared with chlorpromazine in treatment-resistant schizophrenia. *American Journal of Psychiatry* **155**, 914–920.

Correll CU, Leucht S, Kane JM (2004). Lower risk for tardive dyskinesia associated with second-generation antipsychotics: a systematic review of one-year studies. *American Journal of Psychiatry* **161**, 414–415.

Correll CU, Malhotra AK, Kaushik S *et al.* (2003). Early prediction of antipsychotic response in schizophrenia. *American Journal of Psychiatry* **160**, 2063–2065.

Correll CU, Rummel-Kluge C, Corves C *et al.* (2009). Antipsychotic combinations *vs.* monotherapy in schizophrenia: a meta-analysis of randomized controlled trials. *Schizophrenia Bulletin* **35**, 443–457.

Correll CU, Schenk EM (2008). Tardive dyskinesia and new antipsychotics. *Current Opinion in Psychiatry* **21**, 151–156.

Crow TJ, MacMillan JF, Johnson AL, Johnstone EC (1986). A randomised controlled trial of prophylactic neuroleptic treatment. *British Journal of Psychiatry* **148**, 120–127.

Davis JM (1974). Dose equivalence of the antipsychotic drugs. *Journal of Psychiatric Research* **11**, 65–69.

Davis JM, Chen N (2004). Dose-response and dose equivalence of antipsychotics. *Journal of Clinical Psychopharmacology* **24**, 192–208.

Davis JM, Chen N, Glick ID (2003). A meta-analysis of the efficacy of second-generation antipsychotics. *Archives of General Psychiatry* **60**, 553–564.

De Hert M, Dekker JM, Wood D *et al.* (2009). Cardiovascular disease and diabetes in people with severe mental illness position statement from the European Psychiatric Association (EPA), supported by the European Association for the Study of Diabetes (EASD) and the European Society of Cardiology (ESC). *European Psychiatry* **24**, 412–424.

Ehrenreich H, Hinze-Selch D, Stawicki S *et al.* (2007). Improvement of cognitive functions in chronic schizophrenic patients by recombinant human erythropoietin. *Molecular Psychiatry* **12**, 206–220.

Elias A, Kumar A (2007). Testosterone for schizophrenia. *Cochrane Database of Systematic Reviews* **3**, CD006197.

Emsley RA, Raniwalla J, Bailey PJ, Jones AM (2000). A comparison of the effects of quetiapine ('Seroquel') and haloperidol in schizophrenic patients with a history of and a demonstrated, partial response to conventional antipsychotic treatment. *International Clinical Psychopharmacology* **15**, 121–131.

Essali A, Al-Haj HN, Li C, Rathbone J (2009). Clozapine *vs.* typical neuroleptic medication for schizophrenia. *Cochrane Database of Systematic Reviews* **1**, CD000059.

Falkai P, Wobrock T, Lieberman J *et al.* (2005). World Federation of Societies of Biological Psychiatry (WFSBP) – Guidelines for biological treatment of schizophrenia, part 1: Acute treatment of schizophrenia. *World Journal of Biological Psychiatry* **6**, 132–191.

Fleischhacker WW, Heikkinen ME, Olie JP *et al.* (2008). Weight change on aripiprazole-clozapine combination in schizophrenic patients with weight gain and suboptimal response on clozapine: 16-week double-blind study. *European Psychiatry* **23**, S114–S115.

Gaebel W, Awad AG (1994). *Prediction of Neuroleptic Treatment Outcome in Schizophrenia. Concepts and Methods.* Vienna: Springer Verlag.

Gaebel W, Falkai P, Weinmann S, Wobrock T (2006). *Behandlungsleitlinie Schizophrenic.* Darmstadt: Steinkopff.

Gaebel W, Riesbeck M, Wölwer W *et al.* (2010). Relapse prevention in first episode schizophrenia. Maintenance *vs.* intermittent drug treatment with a prodrome based early intervention: Results of a randomised controlled trial within the German research network on schizophrenia. *Journal of Clinical Psychiatry.* Published online: 29 June 2010. doi:10.4088/JCP.09m05459yel.

Gaebel W, Weinmann S, Sartorius N *et al.* (2005). Schizophrenia practice guidelines:

international survey and comparison. *British Journal of Psychiatry* 187, 248–255.

Gardner DM, Murphy AL, O'Donnell H *et al.* (2010). International consensus study of antipsychotic dosing. *American Journal of Psychiatry* 167, 686–693.

Geddes J, Freemantle N, Harrison P, Bebbington P (2000). Atypical antipsychotics in the treatment of schizophrenia: systematic overview and meta-regression analysis. *British Medical Journal* 321, 1371–1376.

Gilbert P, Harris J, McAdams LA, Jeste DV (1995). Neuroleptic withdrawal in schizophrenia. Review of the literature. *Archives of General Psychiatry* 52, 173–188.

Goodwin G, Fleischhacker W, Arango C *et al.* (2009). Advantages and disadvantages of combination treatment with antipsychotics ECNP Consensus Meeting, March 2008, Nice. *European Neuropsychopharmacology* 19, 520–532.

Hajak G, Marienhagen J, Langguth B *et al.* (2004). High-frequency repetitive transcranial magnetic stimulation in schizophrenia: a combined treatment and neuroimaging study. *Psychological Medicine* 34, 1157–1163.

Hamann J, Leucht S, Kissling W (2003). Shared decision making in psychiatry. *Acta Psychiatrica Scandinavica* 107, 403–409.

Hartung B, Wada M, Laux G, Leucht S (2005). Perphenazine for schizophrenia. *Cochrane Database of Systematic Reviews* 1, CD003443.

Herz MI, Glazer WM, Mostert MA *et al.* (1991). Intermittent *vs.* maintenance medication in schizophrenia. Two-year results. *Archives of General Psychiatry* 48, 333–339.

Hogarty GE, McEvoy JP (1988). Dose of fluphenazine, familial expressed emotions and outcome in schizophrenia. *Archives of General Psychiatry* 45, 797–805.

Hogarty GE, Ulrich RF (1998). The limitations of antipsychotic medication on schizophrenia relapse and adjustment and the contributions of psychosocial treatment. *Journal of Psychiatric Research* 32, 243–250.

Hogarty GE, Ulrich RF, Mussare F, Aristigueta N (1976). Drug discontinuation among long term, successfully maintained schizophrenic outpatients. *Diseases of the Nervous System* 37, 494–500.

Hoyberg OJ, Fensbo C (1993). Risperidone *vs.* perphenazine in the treatment of chronic schizophrenic patients with acute exacerbation. *Acta Psychiatrica Scandinavica* 88, 396–402.

Huf G, Coutinho ES, Adams CE (2007). Rapid tranquillisation in psychiatric emergency settings in Brazil: pragmatic randomised controlled trial of intramuscular haloperidol *vs.* intramuscular haloperidol plus promethazine. *British Medical Journal* 335, 869.

Huf G, Coutinho ESF, Adams CE *et al.* (2003). Rapid tranquillisation for agitated patients in emergency psychiatric rooms: a randomised trial of midazolam *vs.* haloperidol plus promethazine. *British Medical Journal* 327, 708–711.

Jager M, Schmauss M, Laux G *et al.* (2009). Early improvement as a predictor of remission and response in schizophrenia: results from a naturalistic study 3. *European Psychiatry* 24, 501–506.

Jeste DV, Lacro JP, Gilbert PL *et al.* (1993). Treatment of late-life schizophrenia with neuroleptics. *Schizophrenia Bulletin* 19, 817–830.

Johnson DA (1976). The duration of maintenance therapy in chronic schizophrenia. *Acta Psychiatrica Scandinavica* 53, 298–301.

Johnson DA, Ludlow JM, Street K, Taylor RD (1987). Double-blind comparison of half-dose and standard-dose flupenthixol decanoate in the maintenance treatment of stabilised out-patients with schizophrenia. *British Journal of Psychiatry* 151, 634–638.

Johnson DAW (1979). Further observation on the duration of depot neuroleptic maintenance therapy in schizophrenia. *British Journal of Psychiatry* 135, 524–530.

Jolley AG, Hirsch SR (1990). Trial of brief intermittent neuroleptic prophylaxis for selected schizophrenic outpatients: clinical and social outcome at two years. *British Medical Journal* 301, 837–842.

Jones PB, Barnes TRE, Davies L *et al.* (2006). Randomized controlled trial of the effect on quality of life of second- *vs.* first-generation antipsychotic drugs in schizophrenia – cost utility of the latest antipsychotic drugs in schizophrenia study (CUtLASS 1). *Archives of General Psychiatry* 63, 1079–1086.

Joy CB, Mumby-Croft R, Joy LA (2006). Polyunsaturated fatty acid supplementation for schizophrenia. *Cochrane Database of Systematic Reviews* **3**, CD001257.

Kahn RS, Fleischhacker WW, Boter H *et al.* (2008). Effectiveness of antipsychotic drugs in first-episode schizophrenia and schizophreniform disorder: an open randomised clinical trial. *Lancet* **371**, 1085–1097.

Kane JM (1982). Fluphenazine *vs.* placebo in patients with remitted, acute first-episode schizophrenia. *Archives of General Psychiatry* **39**, 70–73.

Kane JM, Correll CU, Goff DC *et al.* (2009). A multicenter, randomized, double-blind, placebo-controlled, 16-week study of adjunctive aripiprazole for schizophrenia or schizoaffective disorder inadequately treated with quetiapine or risperidone monotherapy. *Journal of Clinical Psychiatry* **70**, 1348–1357.

Kane JM, Davis JM, Schooler N *et al.* (2002). A multidose study of haloperidol decanoate in the maintenance treatment of schizophrenia. *American Journal of Psychiatry* **159**, 554–560.

Kane JM, Honigfeld G, Singer J *et al.* (1988). Clozapine for the treatment-resistant schizophrenic. A double-blind comparison with chlorpromazine. *Archives of General Psychiatry* **45**, 789–796.

Kane JM, Khanna S, Rajadhyaksha S, Giller E (2006). Efficacy and tolerability of ziprasidone in patients with treatment-resistant schizophrenia. *International Clinical Psychopharmacology* **21**, 21–28.

Kane JM, Leucht S, Carpenter D, Docherty JP (2003). Optimising pharmacologic treatment of psychotic disorders. *Journal of Clinical Psychiatry* **64** (Suppl. 12), 1–100.

Kane JM, Marder SR, Schooler NR *et al.* (2001). Clozapine and haloperidol in moderately refractory schizophrenia – a 6-month randomized and double-blind comparison. *Archives of General Psychiatry* **58**, 965–972.

Kane JM, Meltzer HY, Carson WH *et al.* (2007). Aripiprazole for treatment-resistant schizophrenia: results of a multicenter, randomized, double-blind, comparison study *vs.* perphenazine. *Journal of Clinical Psychiatry* **68**, 213–223.

Kane JM, Rifkin A, Woerner M *et al.* (1983). Low-dose neuroleptic treatment of outpatient schizophrenics. I. Preliminary results for relapse rates. *Archives of General Psychiatry* **40**, 893–896.

Kapur S, Arenovich T, Agid O *et al.* (2005). Evidence for onset of antipsychotic effects within the first 24 h of treatment. *American Journal of Psychiatry* **162**, 939–946.

Kinon BJ, Chen L, Ascher-Svanum H *et al.* (2008a). Predicting response to atypical antipsychotics based on early response in the treatment of schizophrenia. *Schizophrenia Research* **102**, 230–240.

Kinon BJ, Chen L, Ascher-Svanum H *et al.* (2010). Early response to antipsychotic drug therapy as a clinical marker of subsequent response in the treatment of schizophrenia. *Neuropsychopharmacology* **35**, 581–590.

Kinon BJ, Kane JM, Johns C *et al.* (1993). Treatment of neuroleptic-resistant schizophrenic relapse. *Psychopharmacology Bulletin* **29**, 309–314.

Kinon BJ, Volavka J, Stauffer V *et al.* (2008b). Standard and higher dose of olanzapine in patients with schizophrenia or schizoaffective disorder: a randomized, double-blind, fixed-dose study. *Journal of Clinical Psychopharmacology* **28**, 392–400.

Kissling W, Kane JM, Barnes TR *et al.* (1991). Guidelines for neuroleptic relapse prevention in schizophrenia: towards consensus view. In Kissling W (Ed.), *Guidelines for Neuroleptic Relapse Prevention in Schizophrenia* (pp. 155–163). Heidelberg: Springer.

Klein DF, Davis JM (1969). *Diagnosis and Drug Treatment of Psychiatric Disorders.* Baltimore, MD: Williams and Wilkins.

Klein E, Kolsky Y, Puyerovsky M *et al.* (1999). Right prefrontal slow repetitive transcranial magnetic stimulation in schizophrenia: a double-blind sham-controlled pilot study. *Biological Psychiatry* **46**, 1451–1454.

Kleinberg DL, Davis JM, de Coster R *et al.* (1999). Prolactin levels and adverse events in patients treated with risperidone. *Journal of Clinical Psychopharmacology* **19**, 57–61.

Krakowski MI, Czobor P, Citrome L, Bark N, Cooper TB (2006). Atypical antipsychotic agents in the treatment of violent patients with schizophrenia and schizoaffective disorder. *Archives of General Psychiatry* **63**, 622–629.

Lambert M, Schimmelmann BG, Naber D, Eich FX *et al.* (2009). Early- and delayed antipsychotic response and prediction of outcome in 528 severely impaired patients with schizophrenia treated with amisulpride. *Pharmacopsychiatry* 42, 277–283.

Lehman AF, Lieberman JA, Dixon LB et al. (2004). Practice guideline for the treatment of patients with schizophrenia, second edition. *American Journal of Psychiatry* 161, 1–56.

Leucht C, Heres S, Kane JM et al. (2011). Oral versus depot antipsychotic drugs for schizophrenia – a critical systematic review and meta-analysis of randomised long-term trials. *Schizophrenia Research* 127, 83–92.

Leucht C, Kitzmantel M, Chua L et al. (2008a). Haloperidol *vs.* chlorpromazine for schizophrenia. *Cochrane Database of Systematic Reviews* 1, CD004278.

Leucht S, Arbter D, Engel RR et al. (2008b). How effective are second-generation antipsychotic drugs? A meta-analysis of placebo-controlled trials. *Molecular Psychiatry.* Published online: 8 January 2008. doi:10.1038/sj.mp .4002136.

Leucht S, Barnes TRE, Kissling W et al. (2003a). Relapse prevention in schizophrenia with new-generation antipsychotics: a systematic review and exploratory meta-analysis of randomized, controlled trials. *American Journal of Psychiatry* 160, 1209–1222.

Leucht S, Busch R, Hamann J et al. (2005a). Early onset of antipsychotic drug action: a hypothesis tested, confirmed and extended. *Biological Psychiatry* 57, 1543–1549.

Leucht S, Busch R, Kissling W, Kane JM (2007a). Early prediction of antipsychotic non-response. *Journal of Clinical Psychiatry* 68, 352–360.

Leucht S, Corves C, Arbter D et al. (2009a). Second-generation *vs.* first-generation antipsychotic drugs for schizophrenia: a meta-analysis. *Lancet* 373, 31–41.

Leucht S, Heres S (2006). Epidemiology, clinical consequences, and psychosocial treatment of nonadherence in schizophrenia. *Journal of Clinical Psychiatry* 67, 3–8.

Leucht S, Kane JM, Etschel E et al. (2006). Linking the PANSS, BPRS, and CGI: clinical implications. *Neuropsychopharmacology* 31, 2318–2325.

Leucht S, Kane JM, Kissling W et al. (2005b). Clinical implications of BPRS scores. *British Journal of Psychiatry* 187, 363–371.

Leucht S, Kane JM, Kissling W et al. (2005c). What does the PANSS mean? *Schizophrenia Research* 79, 231–238.

Leucht S, Kissling W, McGrath J (2007b). Lithium for schizophrenia. *Cochrane Database of Systematic Reviews* 3, CD003834.

Leucht S, Komossa K, Rummel-Kluge C et al. (2009b). A meta-analysis of head to head comparisons of second generation antipsychotics in the treatment of schizophrenia. *American Journal of Psychiatry* 166, 152–163.

Leucht S, McGrath J, White P, Kissling W (2002a). Carbamazepine augmentation for schizophrenia: how good is the evidence? *Journal of Clinical Psychiatry* 63, 218–224.

Leucht S, Pitschel-Walz G, Engel R, Kissling W (2002b). Amisulpride – an unusual atypical antipsychotic. A meta-analysis of randomized controlled trials. *American Journal of Psychiatry* 159, 180–190.

Leucht S, Shamsi AS, Busch R et al. (2008c). Early prediction of antipsychotic response – replication and six weeks extension. *Schizophrenia Research* 101, 312–319.

Leucht S, Wahlbeck K, Hamann J, Kissling W (2003b). New generation antipsychotics *vs.* low-potency conventional antipsychotics: a systematic review and meta-analysis. *Lancet* 361, 1581–1589.

Levine SZ, Leucht S (2010). Elaboration on the early-onset hypothesis of antipsychotic drug action: treatment response trajectories. *Biological Psychiatry* 68, 86–92.

Levine SZ, Rabinowitz J (2010). Trajectories and antecedents of treatment response over time in early-episode psychosis. *Schizophrenia Bulletin* 36, 624–632.

Lewis SW, Barnes TR, Davies L et al. (2006). Randomized controlled trial of effect of prescription of clozapine *vs.* other second-generation antipsychotic drugs in resistant schizophrenia. *Schizophrenia Bulletin* 32, 715–723.

Lieberman JA (1998). Maximizing clozapine therapy: managing side effects. *Journal of Clinical Psychiatry* 59, 38–43.

Lieberman JA, Stroup TS, McEvoy JP et al. (2005). Effectiveness of antipsychotic drugs in patients with chronic schizophrenia. *New England Journal of Medicine* 353, 1209–1223.

Lin CH, Chou LS, Lin CH et al. (2007). Early prediction of clinical response in schizophrenia patients receiving the atypical antipsychotic zotepine. *Journal of Clinical Psychiatry* **68**, 1522–1527.

Lindenmayer JP, Khan A, Iskander A *et al.* (2007). A randomized controlled trial of olanzapine *vs.* haloperidol in the treatment of primary negative symptoms and neurocognitive deficits in schizophrenia. *Journal of Clinical Psychiatry* **68**, 368–379.

Marder SR, Vanputten T, Mintz J *et al.* (1984). Costs and benefits of 2 doses of fluphenazine. *Archives of General Psychiatry* **41**, 1025–1029.

McEvoy JP, Hogarty GE, Steingard S (1991). Optimal dose of neuroleptic in acute schizophrenia. *Archives of General Psychiatry* **48**, 740–745.

McEvoy JP, Lieberman JA, Stroup TS *et al.* (2006). Effectiveness of clozapine *vs.* olanzapine, quetiapine, and risperidone in patients with chronic schizophrenia who did not respond to prior atypical antipsychotic treatment. *American Journal of Psychiatry* **163**, 600–610.

McGorry PD (2005). Royal Australian and New Zealand College of Psychiatrists clinical practice guidelines for the treatment of schizophrenia and related disorders. *Australian and New Zealand Journal of Psychiatry* **39**, 1–30.

Moller HJ, Kissling W, Lang C *et al.* (1982). Efficacy and side effects of haloperidol in psychotic patients: oral *vs.* intravenous administration. *American Journal of Psychiatry* **139**, 1571–1575.

Muller N, Riedel M, Scheppach C *et al.* (2002). Beneficial antipsychotic effects of celecoxib add-on therapy compared to risperidone alone in schizophrenia. *American Journal of Psychiatry* **159**, 1029–1034.

Naber D, Hippius H (1990). The European experience with use of clozapine. *Hospital and Community Psychiatry* **41**, 886–890.

NICE (2003). *Schizophrenia: Full National Guideline on Core Interventions in Primary and Secondary Care.* London: National Institute for Clinical Excellence/Royal College of Psychiatrists.

Newcomer JW (2005). Second-generation (atypical) antipsychotics and metabolic effects – a comprehensive literature review. *CNS Drugs* **19**, 1–93.

Nolte S, Wong D, Latchford G (2004). Amphetamines for schizophrenia. *Cochrane Database of Systematic Reviews* **4**, CD004964.

Odejide OA, Aderounmu AF (1982). Double-blind placebo substitution: withdrawal of fluphenazine decanoate in schizophrenic patients. *Journal of Clinical Psychiatry* **43**, 195–196.

Omori IM, Wang J (2009). Sulpiride *vs.* placebo for schizophrenia. *Cochrane Database of Systematic Reviews* **2**, CD007811.

Patel MX, Taylor M, David AS (2009). Antipsychotic long-acting injections: mind the gap. *British Journal of Psychiatry* (Suppl.) **52**, S1–S4.

Paton C, Whittington C, Barnes TR (2007). Augmentation with a second antipsychotic in patients with schizophrenia who partially respond to clozapine – a meta-analysis. *Journal of Clinical Psychopharmacology* **27**, 198–204.

Pietzcker A, Gaebel W, Koepcke W *et al.* (1993). Intermittent *vs.* maintenance neuroleptic long-term treatment in schizophrenia – 2 years' results of a German multicenter study. *Journal of Psychiatric Research* **27**, 321–339.

Premkumar TS, Pick J (2006). Lamotrigine for schizophrenia. *Cochrane Database of Systematic Reviews* **4**, CD005962.

Raveendran NS, Tharyan P, Alexander J, Adams CE (2007). Rapid tranquillisation in psychiatric emergency settings in India: pragmatic randomised controlled trial of intramuscular olanzapine *vs.* intramuscular haloperidol plus promethazine. *British Medical Journal* **335**, 865.

Robinson D, Woerner MG, Alvir JM *et al.* (1999). Predictors of relapse following response from a first episode of schizophrenia or schizoaffective disorder. *Archives of General Psychiatry* **56**, 241–247.

Rosenheck R, Cramer J, Xu WC *et al.* (1997). A comparison of clozapine and haloperidol in hospitalized patients with refractory schizophrenia. *New England Journal of Medicine* **337**, 809–815.

Rosenheck R, Perlick D, Bingham S *et al.* (2003). Effectiveness and cost of olanzapine and haloperidol in the treatment of schizophrenia – a randomized controlled trial. *Journal of the American Medical Association* **290**, 2693–2702.

Rummel C, Kissling W, Leucht S (2006). Antidepressants for the negative symptoms of schizophrenia. *Cochrane Database of Systematic Reviews* 3, CD005581.

Rummel-Kluge C, Komossa K, Schwarz S et al. (2010). Second generation antipsychotic drugs and extrapyramidal side effects: a systematic review and meta-analysis of head-to-head comparisons. *Schizophrenia Bulletin*. Published online: 31 May 2010. doi:10.1093/schbul/sbq042.

Sampath G, Shah A, Krska J, Soni SD (1992). Neuroleptic discontinuation in the very stable schizophrenic patient – relapse rates and serum neuroleptic levels. *Human Psychopharmacology: Clinical and Experimental* 7, 255–264.

Schooler NR, Keith SJ, Severe JB et al. (1997). Relapse and rehospitalization during maintenance treatment of schizophrenia. *Archives of General Psychiatry* 54, 453–463.

See RE, Fido AA, Maurice M et al. (1999). Risperidone-induced increase of plasma norepinephrine is not correlated with symptom improvement in chronic schizophrenia. *Biological Psychiatry* 45, 1653–1656.

Sepehry AA, Potvin S, Elie R, Stip E (2007). Selective serotonin reuptake inhibitor (SSRI) add-on therapy for the negative symptoms of schizophrenia: a meta-analysis. *Journal of Clinical Psychiatry* 68, 604–610.

Shalev A, Hermesh H, Rothberg J, Munitz H (1993). Poor neuroleptic response in acutely exacerbated schizophrenic patients. *Acta Psychiatrica Scandinavica* 87, 86–91.

Shepherd M, Watt D, Falloon I, Smeeton N (1989). The natural history of schizophrenia: a five-year follow-up study of outcome and prediction in a representative sample of schizophrenics. *Psychological Medicine* (Suppl.) 15, 1–46.

Simpson GM, Mahmoud RA, Lasser RA et al. (2006). A 1-year double-blind study of 2 doses of long-acting risperidone in stable patients with schizophrenia or schizoaffective disorder. *Journal of Clinical Psychiatry* 67, 1194–1203.

Singh SP, Singh V, Kar N, Chan K (2010). Efficacy of antidepressants in treating the negative symptoms of chronic schizophrenia: meta-analysis. *British Journal of Psychiatry* 197, 174–179.

Siris SG (1991). Diagnosis of secondary depression in schizophrenia: implications for DSM–IV. *Schizophrenia Bulletin* 17, 75–98.

Smith RC, Infante M, Singh A, Khandat A (2001). The effects of olanzapine on neurocognitive functioning in medication-refractory schizophrenia. *International Journal of Neuropsychopharmacology* 4, 239–250.

Stip E, Sepehry AA, Chouinard S (2007). Add-on therapy with acetylcholinesterase inhibitors for memory dysfunction in schizophrenia: a systematic quantitative review, part 2. *Clinical Neuropharmacology* 30, 218–229.

Stone JM, Raffin M, Morrison P, McGuire PK (2010). The biological basis of antipsychotic response in schizophrenia. *Journal of Psychopharmacology* 24, 953–964.

Stroup TS, Lieberman JA, McEvoy JP et al. (2007). Effectiveness of olanzapine, quetiapine, and risperidone in patients with chronic schizophrenia after discontinuing perphenazine: a CATIE study. *American Journal of Psychiatry* 164, 415–427.

Suzuki T, Uchida H, Watanabe K et al. (2007). How effective is it to sequentially switch among olanzapine, quetiapine and risperidone? – A randomized, open-label study of algorithm-based antipsychotic treatment to patients with symptomatic schizophrenia in the real-world clinical setting. *Psychopharmacology* (Berlin) 195, 285–295.

Taylor DM, Smith L (2009). Augmentation of clozapine with a second antipsychotic – a meta-analysis of randomized, placebo-controlled studies. *Acta Psychiatrica Scandinavica* 119, 419–425.

Tharyan P, Adams CE (2005). Electroconvulsive therapy for schizophrenia. *Cochrane Database of Systematic Reviews* 2, CD000076.

Tiihonen J, Wahlbeck K, Kiviniemi V (2009). The efficacy of lamotrigine in clozapine-resistant schizophrenia: a systematic review and meta-analysis. *Schizophrenia Research* 109, 10–14.

Tollefson GD, Beasley CM, Tran PV et al. (1997). Olanzapine vs. haloperidol in the treatment of schizophrenia and schizoaffective and schizophreniform disorders: results of an international collaborative trial. *American Journal of Psychiatry* **154**, 457–465.

Tranulis C, Sepehry AA, Galinowski A, Stip E (2008). Should we treat auditory hallucinations with repetitive transcranial magnetic stimulation? A meta-analysis. *Canadian Journal of Psychiatry* **53**, 577–586.

Trikalinos TA, Churchill R, Ferri M *et al.* (2004). Effect sizes in cumulative meta-analyses of mental health randomized trials evolved over time. *Journal of Clinical Epidemiology* **57**, 1124–1130.

Tuominen HJ, Tiihonen J, Wahlbeck K (2006). Glutamatergic drugs for schizophrenia. *Cochrane Database of Systematic Reviews* **2**, CD003730.

Uchida H, Suzuki T, Takeuchi H *et al.* (2009). Low dose *vs.* standard dose of antipsychotics for relapse prevention in schizophrenia: meta-analysis. *Schizophrenia Bulletin.* Published online: 27 November 2009. doi :10.1093/schbul/sbpl49.

Volavka J, Czobor P, Sheitman B *et al.* (2002). Clozapine, olanzapine, risperidone, and haloperidol in the treatment of patients with chronic schizophrenia and schizoaffective disorder. *American Journal of Psychiatry* **159**, 255–262.

Volz A, Khorsand V, Gillies D, Leucht S (2007). *Benzodiazepines for Schizophrenia*. Cochrane Library. Chichester: John Wiley & Sons.

Wahlbeck K, Cheine M, Essali A, Adams C (1999). Evidence of clozapine's effectiveness in schizophrenia: a systematic review and meta-analysis of randomized trials. *American Journal of Psychiatry* **156**, 990–999.

Wang CY, Xiang YT, Cai ZJ *et al.* (2010). Risperidone maintenance treatment in schizophrenia. A randomised, controlled trial. *American Journal of Psychiatry* **167**, 676–685.

Waraich P, Adams C, Hammill K *et al.* (2002). Haloperidol dose for the acutely ill phase of schizophrenia. *Cochrane Database of Systematic Reviews* **2**, CD001951.

Whitehead C, Moss S, Cardno A, Lewis G (2003). Antidepressants for the treatment of depression in people with schizophrenia: a systematic review. *Psychological Medicine* **33**, 589–599.

Wirshing DA, Marshall BD, Green MF *et al.* (1999). Risperidone in treatment-refractory schizophrenia. *American Journal of Psychiatry* **156**, 1374–1379.

Wunderink L, Nienhuis FJ, Sytema S *et al.* (2007). Guided discontinuation *vs.* maintenance treatment in remitted first-episode psychosis: relapse rates and functional outcome. *Journal of Clinical Psychiatry* **68**, 654–661.

Zimbroff DL, Kane JM, Tamminga CA *et al.* (1997). Controlled, dose response study of sertindole and haloperidol in the treatment of schizophrenia. *American Journal of Psychiatry* **154**, 782–791.

Evidence-based pharmacotherapy of bipolar disorder

3

Matthew J. Taylor and John R. Geddes

Introduction

Recent years have seen a substantial expansion of the evidence base guiding the pharmacotherapy of bipolar disorder. Bipolar disorder has traditionally been relatively neglected in the research literature (Clement *et al.*, 2003), despite comprising a major source of disability worldwide (Lopez *et al.*, 2006), and being associated with higher rates of relapse than unipolar illness (Angst, 1995; Winokur *et al.*, 1993). Two threads contribute to an improved evidence base to guide pharmacological management. On the one hand, the increasing availability of systematic reviews and meta-analyses allows the existing literature to be better understood. Furthermore, independent, high-quality, randomized controlled trials have begun to provide answers to some of the important clinical questions in the management of both acute episodes of illness (Sachs *et al.*, 2003; van der Loos *et al.*, 2009), and in prevention of relapse (Geddes *et al.*, 2010).

While this review restricts itself to the pharmacotherapy of bipolar disorder, it is, of course, important to recognize that pharmacological agents need to be delivered as part of a coherent package of care that may also involve specific psychological therapies (Beynon *et al.*, 2008) and other psychological and social support. Bipolar disorder is also commonly accompanied by substantial comorbidity, including high rates of anxiety disorders and also of substance and alcohol-use disorders (Simon *et al.*, 2004). While the management of these other disorders is beyond the scope of this review, these are important to assess and treat where appropriate.

For the most part trials in bipolar disorder have predominantly included participants with bipolar I disorder. While there is increasing recognition of the importance of bipolar II, and many studies are in progress, it is still the case that to some extent management of this condition has to be guided by extrapolation from results obtained from trials including only patients with bipolar I. Where data are available specifically addressing the management of bipolar II disorder, this is highlighted. Here we consider evidence-based pharmacotherapy for the three main clinical scenarios – episodes of bipolar depression, manic or mixed episodes, and the prevention of relapse. Although drug combinations are often used in clinical practice, trials have tended to investigate monotherapy. A new generation of trials is now beginning to investigate the effectiveness of combination therapies and these are providing robust evidence to underpin clinical practice (e.g. BALANCE; Geddes *et al.*, 2010).

Essential Evidence-Based Psychopharmacology, Second Edition, ed. Dan J. Stein, Bernard Lerer, and Stephen M. Stahl. Published by Cambridge University Press. © Cambridge University Press.

Pharmacotherapy of bipolar depression

Episodes of depression are more frequent than mania in bipolar disorder (Judd *et al.*, 2002). The clinical features may be identical to those encountered in unipolar depression, although there is some evidence that so-called 'atypical' features are more common in bipolar I depression, i.e. hypersomnia, hyperphagia, and leaden paralysis, along with psychomotor retardation, psychotic features, and pathological guilt (Mitchell *et al.*, 2008). However, while bipolar and unipolar depression may present similarly, it is increasingly clear that their pharmacological management should be different. In new episodes of bipolar depression, the three approaches with the strongest evidence base at present are the use of quetiapine, lamotrigine, and the optimization of existing long-term treatments (Fig. 3.1). The evidence for the use of conventional antidepressants, such as selective serotonin reuptake inhibitors (SSRIs), in bipolar depression has weakened in recent years.

Quetiapine

Initial evidence for the efficacy of quetiapine in the treatment of bipolar depression came from the BOLDER I and BOLDER II studies. These multicenter randomized, placebo-controlled studies together included more than 1000 participants. Pooled analyses of data from these studies have been reported for participants with bipolar I ($n = 694$) (Weisler *et al.*, 2008) and bipolar II ($n = 351$) (Suppes *et al.*, 2008). In participants with bipolar I disorder, significant benefits were seen for fixed doses of 300 mg/day or 600 mg/day compared with placebo on the primary outcome of change from baseline in Montgomery–Åsberg Depression Rating Scale (MADRS) score (at week 8: quetiapine 300 mg/day $= -19.4$; 600 mg/day $= -19.6$; placebo $= -12.6$; $p < 0.001$ for each dose). Response rates at week 8 were also greater with quetiapine 300 mg/day (60.9%) or quetiapine 600 mg/day (61.4%) compared with placebo (38.7%) ($p < 0.001$ for each dose vs. placebo). Similar benefits were observed in bipolar II depression, with a mean change from baseline at week 8 for quetiapine 300 and 600 mg/day versus placebo -17.1 and -17.9 versus -13.3.

Results in a separate placebo-controlled trial (Suppes *et al.*, 2010) of quetiapine XR 300 mg/day in a mixed cohort of bipolar I and II participants ($n = 270$) were similar with response and remission rates at week 8 significantly higher with quetiapine XR (65.4% response, 54.1% remission) than with placebo (43.1% response, 39.4% remission). The recently published results of the EMBOLDEN I and II trials also appear supportive of the efficacy of quetiapine in bipolar depression. EMBOLDEN I (Young *et al.*, 2010) randomized participants with bipolar I or II depression to quetiapine, lithium, or placebo. Quetiapine was superior to both lithium and placebo over 8 weeks of treatment (Fig. 3.1). Similarly EMBOLDEN II (McElroy *et al.*, 2010), which randomized 740 participants with bipolar I or II depression between quetiapine, paroxetine, or placebo, found quetiapine to be the most effective of the treatments over 8 weeks. Taken together, the data from these five placebo-controlled trials (Fig. 3.1) indicate a rather consistent effect of quetiapine on response rates at both 300 mg (Relative risk (RR) 1.36, 95% confidence interval (CI) 1.24–1.49) and 600 mg (RR 1.34, 95% CI 1.21–1.48).

It is important to note that the efficacy of quetiapine does not appear to be a class effect generalizable to other atypical antipsychotic medications. For example, in analysis of two placebo-controlled randomized trials of aripiprazole for depression in bipolar I disorder

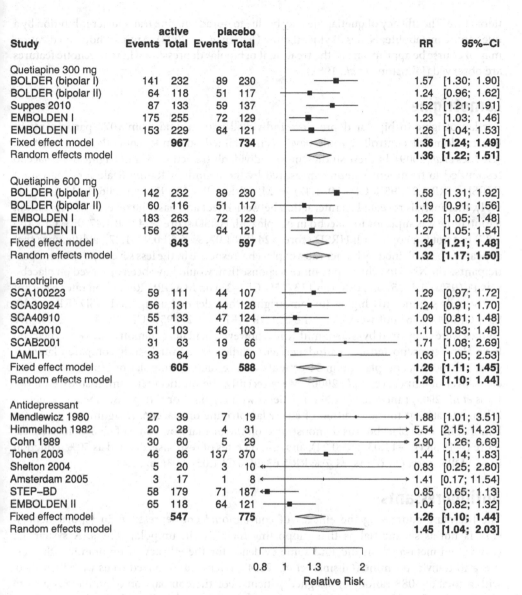

Study	active Events	Total	placebo Events	Total		RR	95%-CI
Quetiapine 300 mg							
BOLDER (bipolar I)	141	232	89	230		1.57	[1.30; 1.90]
BOLDER (bipolar II)	64	118	51	117		1.24	[0.96; 1.62]
Suppes 2010	87	133	59	137		1.52	[1.21; 1.91]
EMBOLDEN I	175	255	72	129		1.23	[1.03; 1.46]
EMBOLDEN II	153	229	64	121		1.26	[1.04; 1.53]
Fixed effect model		967		734		**1.36**	**[1.24; 1.49]**
Random effects model						**1.36**	**[1.22; 1.51]**
Quetiapine 600 mg							
BOLDER (bipolar I)	142	232	89	230		1.58	[1.31; 1.92]
BOLDER (bipolar II)	60	116	51	117		1.19	[0.91; 1.56]
EMBOLDEN I	183	263	72	129		1.25	[1.05; 1.48]
EMBOLDEN II	156	232	64	121		1.27	[1.05; 1.54]
Fixed effect model		843		597		**1.34**	**[1.21; 1.48]**
Random effects model						**1.32**	**[1.17; 1.50]**
Lamotrigine							
SCA100223	59	111	44	107		1.29	[0.97; 1.72]
SCA30924	56	131	44	128		1.24	[0.91; 1.70]
SCA40910	55	133	47	124		1.09	[0.81; 1.48]
SCAA2010	51	103	46	103		1.11	[0.83; 1.48]
SCAB2001	31	63	19	66		1.71	[1.08; 2.69]
LAMLIT	33	64	19	60		1.63	[1.05; 2.53]
Fixed effect model		605		588		**1.26**	**[1.11; 1.45]**
Random effects model						**1.26**	**[1.10; 1.44]**
Antidepressant							
Mendlewicz 1980	27	39	7	19		1.88	[1.01; 3.51]
Himmelhoch 1982	20	28	4	31		5.54	[2.15; 14.23]
Cohn 1989	30	60	5	29		2.90	[1.26; 6.69]
Tohen 2003	46	86	137	370		1.44	[1.14; 1.83]
Shelton 2004	5	20	3	10		0.83	[0.25; 2.80]
Amsterdam 2005	3	17	1	8		1.41	[0.17; 11.54]
STEP-BD	58	179	71	187		0.85	[0.65; 1.13]
EMBOLDEN II	65	118	64	121		1.04	[0.82; 1.32]
Fixed effect model		547		775		**1.26**	**[1.10; 1.44]**
Random effects model						**1.45**	**[1.04; 2.03]**

0.8 1 1.3 2
Relative Risk

Fig. 3.1. Forest plot of response rates in participants with bipolar depression in randomized placebo-controlled trials for quetiapine (300 mg and 600 mg), lamotrigine, and antidepressants. Study details as described in the text. Lamotrigine study identifiers as employed in Geddes *et al.* (2009). Additional antidepressant studies as described in Gijsman *et al.* (2004).

(Thase *et al.*, 2008) with a combined total of 749 participants, no significant difference was seen on the primary outcome of change in MADRS score at trial end-point, nor on secondary outcomes of response or remission rates. In a large trial ($n = 833$) comparing olanzapine, placebo, and olanzapine–fluoxetine combination treatment (Tohen *et al.*, 2003), while olanzapine was more effective than placebo, it was less effective than combination treatment with fluoxetine. The efficacy of quetiapine may be due to noradrenaline transporter inhibition by a quetiapine metabolite, N-desalkylquetiapine (Jensen *et al.*, 2008). Antipsychotic medication may of course be appropriate in the treatment of bipolar depression where psychotic features are observed (Johnstone *et al.*, 1988).

Lamotrigine

For lamotrigine in bipolar depression, individual patient data from 1072 participants in five randomized controlled trials have been obtained and independently meta-analyzed (Geddes *et al.*, 2009). In these studies, more individuals treated with lamotrigine than placebo responded to treatment whether measured by the Hamilton Rating Scale for Depression (HRSD) (RR 1.27, 95% CI 1.09–1.47) or MADRS (RR 1.22, 95% CI 1.06–1.41). Interestingly, this analysis revealed an interaction between effect and baseline severity of depression; lamotrigine was superior to placebo in people with HRSD score >24 (RR 1.47, 95% CI 1.16–1.87) but not in people with HRSD score <24 (RR 1.07, 95% CI 0.90–1.27), a difference that appears to be explained by higher rates of placebo-response in the less severely depressed participants. The NNT to achieve one more response than would have been observed on placebo was 11 (95% CI 7–25) on HRSD and 13 (95% CI 7–33) on MADRS. Remission rates were not statistically significantly higher for lamotrigine when defined using the HRSD (RR = 1.10, 95% CI 0.90–1.36) but were using the MADRS (RR = 1.21, 95% CI 1.03–1.42). These five studies were sponsored by GlaxoSmithKline, however, benefits of lamotrigine versus placebo have also been reported in two independent studies. One initial study compared lamotrigine, gabapentin, and placebo in 31 patients with refractory unipolar or bipolar illness in a cross-over design (Frye *et al.*, 2000). More recently, the multicenter LamLit study (van der Loos *et al.*, 2009) randomized 124 outpatients with bipolar I or II depression while receiving lithium treatment to the addition of either lamotrigine or placebo. A significant benefit of lamotrigine over placebo was demonstrated on the primary outcome of change in MADRS score (−15.38 *vs.* −11.03, *p* = 0.24), and also on rates of response, defined as 50% reduction in MADRS score, (51.6% *vs.* 31.7%; RR 1.63, 95% CI 1.05–2.53; Fig. 3.1).

Antidepressants

The literature addressing the efficacy of conventional antidepressants in bipolar depression is not as substantial as that supporting their use in unipolar illness. A systematic review and meta-analysis did find some evidence for the efficacy of imipramine, fluoxetine, and tranylcypromine (Gijsman *et al.*, 2004). Twelve randomized trials were identified, with a total of 1088 randomly assigned patients. For the comparison of antidepressants to placebo, data from four randomized trials (662 participants) indicated that those receiving antidepressants were more likely to respond than those receiving placebo (RR 1.86, 95% CI 1.49–2.30).

Antidepressants did not induce more switching to mania (the event rate for antidepressants was 3.8% and for placebo was 4.7%). While there was a trend for an increased risk of switching with tricyclic antidepressants (10%) than with other antidepressants (3.2%), manic switch is a rare event, so the statistical power to prove any effect was limited. It may also be important that 75% of patients in these studies were receiving a concurrent mood stabilizer or an atypical antipsychotic, which may have reduced the risk of emergent mania.

While these data were supportive of the role of antidepressants in bipolar depression, more recently, the large STEP-BD trial found no benefit (Sachs *et al.*, 2007). The STEP-BD acute depression comparison compared optimization of mood stabilizer plus the addition of either paroxetine or bupropion to mood stabilizer optimization alone. Forty-two of the 179 subjects (23.5%) receiving a mood stabilizer plus adjunctive antidepressant therapy had a durable recovery, as did 51 of the 187 subjects (27.3%) receiving a mood stabilizer plus a matching placebo, so no statistically significant difference was seen ($p = 0.40$). In keeping with previous data, there was no significant difference in the rates of treatment-emergent mania, hypomania, or mixed episodes between the patients receiving a mood stabilizer plus an antidepressant (10.1%) and those receiving a mood stabilizer plus placebo (10.7%).

In the EMBOLDEN II study (McElroy et al., 2010) of 740 patients which compared quetiapine, paroxetine, and placebo in bipolar depression, paroxetine was not superior to placebo on the primary outcome of change in MADRS score at week 8 ($p = 0.313$), nor were response or remission rates significantly different from placebo. Incorporating the data from these two large studies alongside two recent smaller studies and the four previously identified unsurprisingly suggests that the effect of conventional antidepressants on response rates in bipolar depression is more modest than it had appeared (RR 1.25; 95% CI 1.10–1.44), and the trial data are less consistent across studies than is the case for quetiapine or lamotrigine (Fig. 3.1).

Overall, if antidepressants are to be used on bipolar depression, to avoid manic switch they should be combined with an effective anti-manic agent, SSRIs should be used for preference, and tapered discontinuation should be carried out after remission in most cases.

Valproate

There is some emerging evidence of the efficacy of valproate in the treatment of acute episodes of bipolar depression. Studies in bipolar disorder have for the most part employed valproate in the form of divalproex (valproate semisodium). Here we use valproate to refer to all formulations of the molecule since valproic acid is assumed to be the active component.

A recent meta-analysis identified four small randomized placebo-controlled trials of valproate in bipolar I or bipolar II depression (Bond et al., 2009). Despite a small overall sample (total $n = 140$), participants receiving valproate were statistically more likely to respond to treatment than those receiving placebo (RR 2.10, 95% CI 1.10–4.03), and to achieve remission (RR 1.61, 95% CI 1.02–2.53). Both approaches seemed similarly well tolerated with no clear difference in numbers completing trials in either group (RR 1.13, 95% CI 0.85–1.51). Valproate therefore appears a promising prospect for the treatment of bipolar depression, although more randomized data will be needed to clarify the magnitude of its effect.

Other agents

The data investigating the efficacy of lithium in acute episodes of bipolar depression is rather limited (Bhagwagar & Goodwin, 2002), and in the EMBOLDEN I study (Young et al., 2010), lithium did not significantly differ from placebo. STEP-BD compared augmentation with inositol, risperidone, or lamotrigine as treatment options in cases where bipolar depression was refractory to treatment (Nierenberg et al., 2009). No significant differences between the three augmentation strategies were observed on the primary outcome (recovery sustained for 8 weeks) were observed, although a secondary analysis of symptom scores favored lamotrigine.

Non-pharmacological options, including specific psychotherapies, such as cognitive behavioral therapy, interpersonal therapy, family-focussed therapy, and electroconvulsive therapy, while potentially effective in bipolar depression, are beyond the scope of this review.

Pharmacotherapy of mania and mixed episodes

For the treatment of acute episodes of mania or mixed states, there are an increasing number of randomized trials to inform practice. A recent meta-analysis identified 38 such studies including over 10 000 patients (Yildiz *et al.*, 2011). First-line options are the use of antipsychotic medication or valproate alongside the optimization of any existing long-term treatment. The combination of lithium or valproate with an antipsychotic can be considered in severe cases. Short-term use of benzodiazepines for restoration of sleep–wake cycle or sedation may be required. Anti-manic agents may be discontinued once remission is achieved, or continuation as maintenance therapy may be considered.

Antipsychotics

Antipsychotic medications have long been used in the management of mania, although placebo-controlled trial data are generally lacking for the older, typical antipsychotics. The efficacy of many of the newer atypical agents has been demonstrated for this indication, and the use of haloperidol as an active comparator has also confirmed its efficacy. Risperidone, olanzapine, aripiprazole, quetiapine, and ziprasidone are all superior to placebo as monotherapy in mania (Perlis *et al.*, 2006), and similar effect sizes are seen with asenapine, cariprazine, and paliperidone (Yildiz *et al.*, 2011). There are some data to suggest that the combination of an antipsychotic with lithium or valproate may be best where partial response is observed or symptoms have broken through monotherapy (Sachs *et al.*, 2002; Smith *et al.*, 2007).

While overall tolerability of atypical and typical antipsychotics is generally similar (Geddes *et al.*, 2000), there may be a benefit from the lower risk of extrapyramidal side-effects with the newer agents, since some data suggest people with bipolar disorder may be more vulnerable to motor side-effects than those with schizophrenia (Gao *et al.*, 2008).

Valproate

When the use of valproate in mania was systematically reviewed and meta-analyzed (Macritchie *et al.*, 2003), data from three randomized trials (316 participants) indicated that valproate was more efficacious than placebo in the treatment of mania. A separate post-hoc analysis of the same trial data found that response to valproate appears to depend on serum level, with the greatest effect at serum levels of 94 ug/ml or above (Allen *et al.*, 2006). Three further placebo-controlled randomized trials have since been reported (Bowden *et al.*, 2006; Hirschfeld *et al.*, 2010; Tohen *et al.*, 2008) in which more than 850 patients participated. Although only one of these trials (Bowden *et al.*, 2006) showed a statistically significant difference, taken together the six studies in total indicate an increased response rate with valproate *vs.* placebo (RR 1.46. CI 1.26–1.70). No clear difference in efficacy between valproate and active comparators such as olanzapine, lithium, or carbamazepine has been demonstrated.

Other agents

Lithium has efficacy in the acute treatment of mania. Meta-analysis of two randomized trials (Smith *et al.*, 2007) found that participants receiving lithium were more likely to respond than were those receiving placebo (RR 1.89, 95% CI 1.40–2.57). One possible complication of initiating treatment with lithium during an episode of mania may be the high risks of relapse observed on rapid discontinuation (Goodwin, 1994). Furthermore, a comparison of the antipsychotic, chlorpromazine, with lithium favored the antipsychotic in the most severe cases (Prien *et al.*, 1972).

Carbamazepine is rarely advocated for the treatment of mania, although it does have some anti-manic effect (Okuma *et al.*, 1990; Weisler *et al.*, 2006). Enzyme interactions complicate its use in combination with other medications. While the related molecule, oxcarbazepine, has fewer such interactions, one recent study found it was of no benefit (Wagner *et al.*, 2006).

Tamoxifen, the estrogen receptor modulator and protein kinase C inhibitor, is showing early promise for the treatment of mania as both monotherapy (Yildiz *et al.*, 2008; Zarate *et al.*, 2007) and an adjunct to lithium (Amrollahi *et al.*, 2011) although total numbers of patients treated remain small.

Pharmacotherapy of relapse prevention

The prevention of episodes of illness forms a major component of the treatment of bipolar disorder. Traditionally, particularly in European guidelines, prophylactic medication has often been reserved for cases where multiple episodes of illness occur in rapid succession (Grunze *et al.*, 2004), however a case can be made for considering preventative medication after a single severe manic episode (Goodwin, 2009). Observational studies have found that with each episode of illness subsequent symptom-free periods decrease, which suggests that avoiding early relapse may help secure a more benign course of illness (Kessing *et al.*, 1998). Risk of relapse remains high in bipolar disorder even after several years without episodes of mood disorder, so very extended prescribing may be required.

Agents for preventing relapse in bipolar disorder have often been known as 'mood stabilizers,' and there has been an implication that they will be equally effective against both manic and depressive poles of illness. Increasing evidence suggests that agents differ in their relative efficacy against mood elevation and depression, as will be seen below.

The gold standard long-term treatment for bipolar disorder remains lithium, either as monotherapy or in combination with other agents. Where avoidance of mania is particularly important, alternatives include the atypical antipsychotics, aripiprazole, quetiapine, and olanzapine, and valproate. To avoid depression both quetiapine and lamotrigine may be of benefit.

Lithium

Lithium prevents relapses into mania and depression. A meta-analysis of five randomized trials (Geddes *et al.*, 2004) with 770 participants found that participants randomized to lithium rather than placebo had a reduced risk of relapse into mania (RR 0.62, 95% CI 0.40–0.95) and a trend towards avoidance of depression (RR 0.72, 95% CI 0.49–1.07). There are also data from meta-analysis of randomized trials (Cipriani *et al.*, 2005) to indicate that lithium reduces suicide rates in bipolar disorder (odds ratio (OR) 0.26, 95% CI 0.09–0.77), and also reduces overall mortality (OR 0.42, 95% CI 0.21–0.87).

Recently, the BALANCE trial (Geddes *et al.*, 2010) compared outcomes in 330 participants randomized to either lithium, valproate, or lithium/valproate combination and found that both lithium and lithium/valproate combination were superior to valproate alone in preventing relapse. A 41% relative benefit of the combination over valproate monotherapy was seen irrespective of baseline severity of illness, was maintained for up to 2 years, and was most apparent in prevention of manic relapse. Further information to inform the role of lithium treatment in bipolar disorder may become available from ongoing studies such as LitMUS (Nierenberg et al., 2009).

Use of lithium can be complicated by the risk of (particularly manic) relapse and hospital admission on rapid discontinuation (Johnson & McFarland, 1996). Unless lithium use is maintained for at least 2 years, the benefits of treatment may be outweighed by this complication (Goodwin, 1994).

Valproate

Valproate does appear to reduce relapse rates in bipolar disorder. In one three-arm randomized trial ($n = 372$) (Bowden et al., 2000), comparing valproate with lithium and with placebo in maintenance treatment, valproate was superior to placebo in preventing relapse (OR 0.51, 95% CI 0.30–0.87). Considering depression and mania separately, there was a significant effect on depressive relapse (OR 0.32, 95% CI 0.15–0.69), but the effect on mania did not reach statistical significance (OR 0.74, 95% CI 0.30–1.38).

Valproate has been compared with lithium in randomized trials. A meta-analysis of two studies (Beynon et al., 2009; Bowden et al., 2000; Calabrese et al., 2005) found no significant difference in relapse rates (OR 1.37, 95% CI 0.84–2.24). As noted above, the evidence from the recent BALANCE trial indicates that valproate may be less effective than lithium or in particular lithium/valproate combination (Fig. 3.2).

Olanzapine

A meta-analysis of five randomized trials of olanzapine in the maintenance treatment of bipolar disorder (Cipriani et al., 2010), identified two that provided data comparing the efficacy of olanzapine to that of placebo. Olanzapine monotherapy was superior to placebo in avoiding relapse (RR 0.58, 95% CI 0.49–0.69, $n = 361$), but superiority could not be demonstrated when administered alongside lithium or valproate (RR 0.94, 95% CI 0.52–1.71, $n = 99$).

In the study of olanzapine monotherapy (Tohen et al., 2005), participants who had responded to olanzapine in acute phase open-label treatment were randomized to either continue or switch to placebo. Thus potentially, apparent treatment effects could be inflated by any rebound deterioration on discontinuation of active treatment.

Quetiapine

Two large randomized trials of similar design have investigated quetiapine in maintenance treatment alongside lithium or valproate semisodium (Suppes et al., 2009; Vieta et al., 2008). In these studies, after clinical response to quetiapine in an open-label acute phase, participants were randomized to continue quetiapine or to switch to placebo. The primary outcome was time to any relapse (depression, mania, or mixed episode). In one study, with 708 participants randomized (Vieta et al., 2008), quetiapine extended the time to relapse (Hazard Ratio (HR) 0.28, 95% CI 0.21–0.37), and fewer relapses were observed compared with placebo (18.5% vs. 49.0%). Effects were seen on both time to relapse into mania (HR 0.30, 95% CI 0.20–0.44), and depressive relapse (HR 0.26, 0.17–0.41).

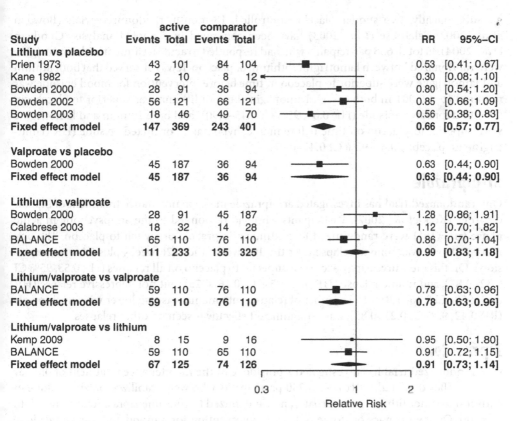

Study	active		comparator		RR	95%–CI
	Events	Total	Events	Total		
Lithium vs placebo						
Prien 1973	43	101	84	104	0.53	[0.41; 0.67]
Kane 1982	2	10	8	12	0.30	[0.08; 1.10]
Bowden 2000	28	91	36	94	0.80	[0.54; 1.20]
Bowden 2002	56	121	66	121	0.85	[0.66; 1.09]
Bowden 2003	18	46	49	70	0.56	[0.38; 0.83]
Fixed effect model	**147**	**369**	**243**	**401**	**0.66**	**[0.57; 0.77]**
Valproate vs placebo						
Bowden 2000	45	187	36	94	0.63	[0.44; 0.90]
Fixed effect model	**45**	**187**	**36**	**94**	**0.63**	**[0.44; 0.90]**
Lithium vs valproate						
Bowden 2000	28	91	45	187	1.28	[0.86; 1.91]
Calabrese 2003	18	32	14	28	1.12	[0.70; 1.82]
BALANCE	65	110	76	110	0.86	[0.70; 1.04]
Fixed effect model	**111**	**233**	**135**	**325**	**0.99**	**[0.83; 1.18]**
Lithium/valproate vs valproate						
BALANCE	59	110	76	110	0.78	[0.63; 0.96]
Fixed effect model	**59**	**110**	**76**	**110**	**0.78**	**[0.63; 0.96]**
Lithium/valproate vs lithium						
Kemp 2009	8	15	9	16	0.95	[0.50; 1.80]
BALANCE	59	110	65	110	0.91	[0.72; 1.15]
Fixed effect model	**67**	**125**	**74**	**126**	**0.91**	**[0.73; 1.14]**

0.3   1   2
Relative Risk

Fig. 3.2. Forest plot of relapse rates in bipolar disorder in randomized trials comparing lithium and valproate (divalproex, valproate semisodium) to placebo and each other. Study details as described in the text or as described in Geddes *et al.* (2004).

In the second study, with 628 participants randomized (Suppes *et al.*, 2009), results were similar. In those receiving quetiapine, time to relapse was delayed (HR 0.32, 95% CI 0.24–0.42), relapses were less frequent (20.3% *vs.* 52.1%), with the protective effect seen for both manic and depressive relapses.

These data support the potential of quetiapine to protect against relapse into both poles of the illness, although as for olanzapine, interpretation is complicated by issues of potential withdrawal and rebound effects.

Lamotrigine

Three published randomized trials have investigated lamotrigine maintenance therapy in participants who have responded to lamotrigine in open-label acute phase treatment. One study of 182 participants with rapid-cycling bipolar disorder compared lamotrigine to placebo (Calabrese *et al.*, 2000). No significant difference was observed between groups on the primary outcome of time before additional pharmacotherapy was required for emerging symptoms of a mood episode, however, numbers of participants completing the entire 6-month trial without relapse favored lamotrigine (41% *vs.* 26%, $p = 0.03$).

Subsequently, two similar placebo-controlled, 18-month, randomized trials (Bowden *et al.*, 2003; Calabrese *et al.*, 2003) have been combined in a pooled analysis (Goodwin *et al.*, 2004). In total, 638 participants who had responded to acute treatment with lamotrigine were randomized between lamotrigine, lithium, or placebo. It was observed that both lithium and lamotrigine were superior to placebo in time before intervention for mood episode was required ($p < 0.001$ in both cases). Lamotrigine but not lithium was superior to placebo in time to depressive episode (HR 0.64, 95% CI 0.45–0.90), and both lithium and lamotrigine were superior to placebo on time before manic, hypomanic, or mixed episode (HR (lamotrigine *vs.* placebo) 0.64, 95% CI 0.42–0.97).

Aripiprazole

One randomized trial has investigated aripiprazole in the maintenance treatment of bipolar disorder (Keck *et al.*, 2007). Participants who had responded to the antipsychotic in acute phase (n = 161) were randomized to continue aripiprazole or switch to placebo. The primary outcome was time to relapse over the 100-week study (26 weeks plus 74-week extension). On this measure, aripiprazole was superior to placebo on all relapses (HR 0.53, 95% CI 0.32–0.87), and manic relapse (HR 0.35, 95% CI 0.16–0.75), but not depressive relapse (HR 0.81, 95% CI 0.36–1.81). The number of relapses into mania was also lower with aripiprazole (RR 0.42, 95% CI 0.21–0.85), but no significant effect was seen on other relapses.

Ziprasidone

One randomized trial has investigated ziprasidone in the maintenance treatment of bipolar disorder (Bowden *et al.*, 2010), with 240 participants who were stabilized on ziprasidone in addition to either lithium or valproate, and randomized to continue ziprasidone or switch to placebo. On the primary outcome of time to intervention for a mood episode, ziprasidone was superior to placebo. Further analyses indicated that this effect was driven by prevention of mania rather than of depression.

Other agents

Carbamazepine appears less effective in preventing relapse in bipolar disorder than lithium (Greil *et al.*, 1997; Hartong *et al.*, 2003). The use of carbamazepine is complicated by its effects on the metabolism of other agents. Oxcarbazepine appears less prone to such interactions, and may be considered as an alternative to carbamazepine by extrapolation, although direct evidence is currently lacking (Vasudev *et al.*, 2008).

Clozapine may have a role in treatment-resistant bipolar disorder (Suppes *et al.*, 1999).

There are some patients for whom long-term antidepressant treatment appears well tolerated. There is some evidence that imipramine reduces rates of depressive relapse (Beynon *et al.*, 2009), although in practice its use is likely to be limited by the concerns of manic switch noted above.

Combination treatments

The combination of multiple agents for relapse prevention in bipolar disorder is widespread in practice, although traditionally the evidence base has been rather limited. As noted above, the results of the BALANCE trial (Geddes *et al.*, 2010) support the benefits of a combination of lithium and valproate over valproate alone as maintenance therapy. It is interesting to also note that quetiapine, for example, appears to confer additional benefits when prescribed alongside lithium or valproate. It is hoped that future studies will clarify further which combinations of agents are optimal in terms of efficacy and tolerability.

Conclusions

The evidence base to guide pharmacotherapy of bipolar disorder is increasing. Strong evidence guides first-line choices for episodes of bipolar depression, manic or mixed episodes, and for relapse prevention. Future studies may clarify the comparative effectiveness of alternative therapies, and also clarify whether particular combinations of agents will prove more effective than monotherapy.

Statement of Interest

John Geddes has received research funding from MRC, ESRC, NIHR, Stanley Medical Research Institute and has received donations of drugs supplies for trials from Sanofi-Aventis and GSK. He has acted as an expert witness for Dr. Reddys. Dr. Taylor's spouse is an employee of GSK.

References

Allen MH, Hirschfeld RM, Wozniak PJ et al. (2006). Linear relationship of valproate serum concentration to response and optimal serum levels for acute mania. *American Journal of Psychiatry* 163 (2), 272–275.

Amrollahi Z, Rezaei F, Salehi B et al. (2011). Double-blind, randomized, placebo-controlled 6-week study on the efficacy and safety of the tamoxifen adjunctive to lithium in acute bipolar mania. *Journal of Affective Disorders* 129 (1–3), 327–331.

Angst J (1995). [Epidemiology of the bipolar spectrum]. *Encephale* 21(Spec No. 6), 37–42.

Beynon S, Soares-Weiser K, Woolacott N et al. (2008). Psychosocial interventions for the prevention of relapse in bipolar disorder: systematic review of controlled trials. *British Journal of Psychiatry* 192, 5–11.

Beynon S, Soares-Weiser K, Woolacott N et al. (2009). Pharmacological interventions for the prevention of relapse in bipolar disorder: a systematic review of controlled trials. *Journal of Psychopharmacology* 23, 574–591.

Bhagwagar Z, Goodwin GM (2002). Role of mood stabilizers in bipolar disorder. *Expert Reviews in Neurotherapeutics* 2, 239–248.

Bond DJ, Lam RW, Yatham LN (2009). Divalproex sodium versus placebo in the treatment of acute bipolar depression: A systematic review and meta-analysis. *Journal of Affective Disorders* 124, 228–234.

Bowden CL, Calabrese JR, McElroy SL et al. (2000). A randomized, placebo-controlled 12-month trial of divalproex and lithium in treatment of outpatients with bipolar I disorder. Divalproex Maintenance Study Group. *Archives of General Psychiatry* 57, 481–489.

Bowden CL, Calabrese JR, Sachs G et al. (2003) A placebo-controlled 18-month trial of lamotrigine and lithium maintenance treatment in recently manic or hypomanic patients with bipolar I disorder. *Archives of General Psychiatry* 60, 392–400.

Bowden CL, Mosolov S, Hranov L et al. (2010) Efficacy of valproate versus lithium in mania or mixed mania: a randomized, open 12-week trial. *International Clinical Psychopharmacology* 25(2), 60–67.

Bowden CL, Swann AC, Calabrese JR et al. (2006). A randomized, placebo-controlled, multicenter study of divalproex sodium extended release in the treatment of acute mania. *Journal of Clinical Psychiatry* 67,1501–1510.

Calabrese JR, Bowden CL, Sachs G et al. (2003). A placebo-controlled 18-month trial of lamotrigine and lithium maintenance treatment in recently depressed patients with bipolar I disorder. *Journal of Clinical Psychiatry* 64, 1013–1024.

Calabrese JR, Shelton MD, Rapport DJ et al. (2005). A 20-month, double-blind, maintenance trial of lithium versus divalproex in rapid-cycling bipolar disorder. *American Journal of Psychiatry* **162**, 2152–2161.

Calabrese JR, Suppes T, Bowden CL *et al.* (2000). A double-blind, placebo-controlled, prophylaxis study of lamotrigine in rapid-cycling bipolar disorder. Lamictal 614 Study Group. *Journal of Clinical Psychiatry* **61**, 841–850.

Cipriani A, Pretty H, Hawton K, Geddes JR (2005). Lithium in the prevention of suicidal behavior and all-cause mortality in patients with mood disorders: a systematic review of randomized trials. *American Journal of Psychiatry* **162**, 1805–1819.

Cipriani A, Rendell J, Geddes JR (2010). Olanzapine in the long-term treatment of bipolar disorder: a systematic review and meta-analysis. *Journal of Psychopharmacology* **24**,1729–1738.

Clement S, Singh SP, Burns T (2003). Status of bipolar disorder research. Bibliometric study. *British Journal of Psychiatry* **182**, 148–152.

Frye MA, Ketter TA, Kimbrell TA *et al.* (2000). A placebo-controlled study of lamotrigine and gabapentin monotherapy in refractory mood disorders. *Journal of Clinical Psychopharmacology* **20**, 607–614.

Gao K, Kemp DE, Ganocy SJ *et al.* (2008). Antipsychotic-induced extrapyramidal side effects in bipolar disorder and schizophrenia: a systematic review. *Journal of Clinical Psychopharmacology* **28**, 203–209.

Geddes J, Freemantle N, Harrison P, Bebbington P (2000). Atypical antipsychotics in the treatment of schizophrenia: systematic overview and meta-regression analysis. *British Medical Journal* **321**(7273), 1371–1376.

Geddes JR, Burgess S, Hawton K *et al.* (2004). Long-term lithium therapy for bipolar disorder: systematic review and meta-analysis of randomized controlled trials. *American Journal of Psychiatry* **161**, 217–222.

Geddes JR, Calabrese JR, Goodwin GM (2009). Lamotrigine for treatment of bipolar depression: independent meta-analysis and meta-regression of individual patient data from five randomised trials. *British Journal of Psychiatry* **194**, 4–9.

Geddes JR, Goodwin GM, Rendell J *et al.* (2010). Lithium plus valproate combination therapy versus monotherapy for relapse prevention in bipolar I disorder (BALANCE): a randomised open-label trial. *Lancet* **375**(9712), 385–395.

Gijsman HJ, Geddes JR, Rendell JM *et al.* (2004). Antidepressants for bipolar depression: a systematic review of randomized, controlled trials. *American Journal of Psychiatry* **161**, 1537–1547.

Goodwin, GM (1994). Recurrence of mania after lithium withdrawal. Implications for the use of lithium in the treatment of bipolar affective disorder. *British Journal of Psychiatry* **164**, 149–152.

Goodwin GM (2009). Evidence-based guidelines for treating bipolar disorder: revised second edition – recommendations from the British Association for Psychopharmacology. *Journal of Psychopharmacology* **23**, 346–388.

Goodwin GM, Bowden CL, Calabrese JR *et al.* (2004). A pooled analysis of 2 placebo-controlled 18-month trials of lamotrigine and lithium maintenance in bipolar I disorder. *Journal of Clinical Psychiatry* **65**, 432–441.

Greil W, Ludwig-Mayerhofer W, Erazo N *et al.* (1997). Lithium versus carbamazepine in the maintenance treatment of bipolar disorders – a randomised study. *Journal of Affective Disorders* **43**, 151–161.

Grunze H, Kasper S, Goodwin G *et al.* (2004). The World Federation of Societies of Biological Psychiatry (WFSBP) guidelines for the biological treatment of bipolar disorders, part III: maintenance treatment. *World Journal of Biological Psychiatry* **5**(3), 120–135.

Hartong EG, Moleman P, Hoogduin CA *et al.* (2003). Prophylactic efficacy of lithium versus carbamazepine in treatment-naive bipolar patients. *Journal of Clinical Psychiatry* **64**, 144–151.

Hirschfeld RM, Bowden CL, Wozniak P, Collins M (2010). A randomized, placebo-controlled, multicenter study of divalproex sodium extended-release in the acute treatment of mania. *Journal of Clinical Psychiatry* **71**, 426–432.

Jensen NH, Rodriguiz RM, Caron MG *et al.* (2008). N-desalkylquetiapine, a potent norepinephrine reuptake inhibitor and partial 5-HT1A agonist, as a putative mediator of quetiapine's antidepressant activity. *Neuropsychopharmacology* 33, 2303–2312.

Johnson RE, McFarland BH (1996). Lithium use and discontinuation in a health maintenance organization. *American Journal of Psychiatry* 153, 993–1000.

Johnstone EC, Crow TJ, Frith CD, Owens DG (1988). The Northwick Park "functional" psychosis study: diagnosis and treatment response. *Lancet* 2(8603), 119–125.

Judd LL, Akiskal HS, Schettler PJ et al. (2002). The long-term natural history of the weekly symptomatic status of bipolar I disorder. *Archives of General Psychiatry* 59, 530–537.

Keck PE Jr, Calabrese JR, McIntyre RS et al. (2007). Aripiprazole monotherapy for maintenance therapy in bipolar I disorder: a 100-week, double-blind study versus placebo. *Journal of Clinical Psychiatry* 68, 1480–1491.

Kessing LV, Andersen PK, Mortensen PB, Bolwig TG (1998). Recurrence in affective disorder. I. Case register study. *British Journal of Psychiatry* 172, 23–28.

Lopez AD, Mathers CD, Ezzati M et al. (2006). *Global Burden of Disease and Risk Factors.* Washington, DC: World Bank.

Macritchie K, Geddes JR, Scott J et al. (2003). Valproate for acute mood episodes in bipolar disorder. *Cochrane Database of Systematic Reviews* 1, CD004052.

McElroy SL, Weisler RH, Chang W et al. (2010). A double-blind, placebo-controlled study of quetiapine and paroxetine as monotherapy in adults with bipolar depression (EMBOLDEN II). *Journal of Clinical Psychiatry* 71, 163–174.

Mitchell PB, Goodwin GM, Johnson GF, Hirschfeld RM (2008). Diagnostic guidelines for bipolar depression: a probabilistic approach. *Bipolar Disorders* 10(1 Pt 2), 144–152.

Nierenberg AA, Sylvia LG, Leon AC et al. (2009). Lithium treatment – moderate dose use study (LiTMUS) for bipolar disorder: rationale and design. *Clinical Trials* 6, 637–648.

Okuma T, Yamashita I, Takahashi R et al. (1990). Comparison of the antimanic efficacy of carbamazepine and lithium carbonate by double-blind controlled study. *Pharmacopsychiatry* 23(3), 143–150.

Perlis RH, Welge JA, Vornik LA et al. (2006). Atypical antipsychotics in the treatment of mania: a meta-analysis of randomized, placebo-controlled trials. *Journal of Clinical Psychiatry* 67, 509–516.

Prien RF, Caffey EM Jr, Klett CJ (1972). Comparison of lithium carbonate and chlorpromazine in the treatment of mania. Report of the Veterans Administration and National Institute of Mental Health Collaborative Study Group. *Archives of General Psychiatry* 26, 146–153.

Sachs GS, Grossman F, Ghaemi SN et al. (2002). Combination of a mood stabilizer with risperidone or haloperidol for treatment of acute mania: a double-blind, placebo-controlled comparison of efficacy and safety. *American Journal of Psychiatry* 159, 1146–1154.

Sachs GS, Nierenberg AA, Calabrese JR et al. (2007). Effectiveness of adjunctive antidepressant treatment for bipolar depression. *New England Journal of Medicine* 356(17), 1711–1722.

Sachs GS, Thase ME, Otto MW et al. (2003). Rationale, design, and methods of the systematic treatment enhancement program for bipolar disorder (STEP-BD) *Biological Psychiatry* 53(11), 1028–1042.

Simon NM, Otto MW, Wisniewski SR et al. (2004). Anxiety disorder comorbidity in bipolar disorder patients: data from the first 500 participants in the Systematic Treatment Enhancement Program for Bipolar Disorder (STEP-BD) *American Journal of Psychiatry* 161, 2222–2229.

Smith LA, Cornelius V, Warnock A et al. (2007). Pharmacological interventions for acute bipolar mania: a systematic review of randomized placebo-controlled trials. *Bipolar Disorders* 9, 551–560.

Suppes T, Datto C, Minkwitz M et al. (2010). Effectiveness of the extended release formulation of quetiapine as monotherapy for the treatment of acute bipolar depression. *Journal of Affective Disorders* 121, 106–115.

Suppes T, Hirschfeld RM, Vieta E et al. (2008). Quetiapine for the treatment of bipolar II depression: analysis of data from two randomized, double-blind, placebo-controlled studies. *World Journal of Biological Psychiatry* 9, 198–211.

Suppes T, Vieta E, Liu S et al. (2009). Maintenance treatment for patients with bipolar I disorder: results from a North American study of quetiapine in combination with lithium or divalproex (trial 127). American Journal of Psychiatry 166, 476–488.

Suppes T, Webb A, Paul B et al. (1999). Clinical outcome in a randomized 1-year trial of clozapine versus treatment as usual for patients with treatment-resistant illness and a history of mania. American Journal of Psychiatry 156, 1164–1169.

Thase ME, Jonas A, Khan A et al. (2008). Aripiprazole monotherapy in nonpsychotic bipolar I depression: results of 2 randomized, placebo-controlled studies. Journal of Clinical Psychopharmacology 28, 13–20.

Tohen M, Greil W, Calabrese JR et al. (2005). Olanzapine versus lithium in the maintenance treatment of bipolar disorder: a 12-month, randomized, double-blind, controlled clinical trial. American Journal of Psychiatry 162, 1281–1290.

Tohen M, Vieta E, Calabrese J et al. (2003). Efficacy of olanzapine and olanzapine-fluoxetine combination in the treatment of bipolar I depression. Archives of General Psychiatry 60, 1079–1088.

Tohen M, Vieta E, Goodwin GM et al. (2008). Olanzapine versus divalproex versus placebo in the treatment of mild to moderate mania: a randomized, 12-week, double-blind study. Journal of Clinical Psychiatry 69, 1776–1789.

van der Loos ML, Mulder PG, Hartong EG et al. (2009). Efficacy and safety of lamotrigine as add-on treatment to lithium in bipolar depression: a multicenter, double-blind, placebo-controlled trial. Journal of Clinical Psychiatry 70, 223–231.

Vasudev A, Macritchie K, Watson S et al. (2008). Oxcarbazepine in the maintenance treatment of bipolar disorder. Cochrane Database of Systematic Reviews 1, CD005171.

Vieta E, Suppes T, Eggens I et al. (2008). Efficacy and safety of quetiapine in combination with lithium or divalproex for maintenance of patients with bipolar I disorder (international trial 126). Journal of Affective Disorders 109, 251–263.

Wagner KD, Kowatch RA, Emslie GJ et al. (2006). A double-blind, randomized, placebo-controlled trial of oxcarbazepine in the treatment of bipolar disorder in children and adolescents. American Journal of Psychiatry 163, 1179–1186.

Weisler RH, Calabrese JR, Thase ME et al. (2008). Efficacy of quetiapine monotherapy for the treatment of depressive episodes in bipolar I disorder: a post hoc analysis of combined results from 2 double-blind, randomized, placebo-controlled studies. Journal of Clinical Psychiatry 69, 769–782.

Weisler RH, Hirschfeld R, Cutler AJ et al. (2006). Extended-release carbamazepine capsules as monotherapy in bipolar disorder: pooled results from two randomised, double-blind, placebo-controlled trials. CNS Drugs 20, 219–231.

Winokur G, Coryell W, Keller M et al. (1993). A prospective follow-up of patients with bipolar and primary unipolar affective disorder. Archives of General Psychiatry 50, 457–465.

Yildiz A, Guleryuz S, Ankerst DP, Ongür D, Renshaw PF. (2008). Protein kinase C inhibition in the treatment of mania: a double-blind, placebo-controlled trial of tamoxifen. Archives of General Psychiatry 65, 255–263.

Yildiz A, Vieta E, Leucht S, Baldessarini RJ (2011). Efficacy of antimanic treatments: meta-analysis of randomized, controlled trials. Neuropsychopharmacology 36, 375–389.

Young AH, McElroy SL, Bauer M et al. (2010). A double-blind, placebo-controlled study of quetiapine and lithium monotherapy in adults in the acute phase of bipolar depression (EMBOLDEN I). Journal of Clinical Psychiatry 71, 150–162.

Zarate CA Jr, Singh JB, Carlson PJ et al. (2007). Efficacy of a protein kinase C inhibitor (tamoxifen) in the treatment of acute mania: a pilot study. Bipolar Disorder 9, 561–570.

Evidence-based pharmacotherapy of major depressive disorder

Jamie M. Dupuy, Michael J. Ostacher, Jeffrey Huffman, Roy H. Perlis, and Andrew A. Nierenberg

Introduction

Major depressive disorder (MDD) is estimated by the World Health Organization to be a leading cause for loss of disability-adjusted life years. In the USA, the 2001 National Comorbidity Survey showed overall lifetime prevalence estimates for MDD of 16.2% (Kessler et al., 2003). Over 50% of respondents with MDD received some type of treatment in the 12 months before their interview. However, only about one-fifth of patients received "adequate" treatment during that time, indicating that more efforts are required at improving access to and utilization of care. Even for patients who are treated, pharmacotherapy is not uniformly effective. Many episodes do not completely respond to initial antidepressant, response may be delayed for weeks or months, and residual symptoms may cause significant morbidity. In this paper, we review the evidence for first-line treatment of MDD, and strategies for patients with treatment-resistant depression.

Methods

For the purposes of this review, we searched MEDLINE and PsycINFO for controlled trials published in English between January 1981 and October 2010, in which adults with MDD were randomly assigned to receive medication, placebo, or active comparator drugs, and for all meta-analyses of pharmacotherapy for MDD. The number of published randomized placebo-controlled trials (RCTs) of antidepressants for the acute treatment of MDD is too vast to allow discussion of each study. In order to recommend first-line treatment for MDD, we examined meta-analyses of RCTs of antidepressant drugs for MDD as a statistical means of weighing the relative efficacy of antidepressants that have not been compared directly. Because placebo response rates in antidepressant trials tend to be high, many positive trials have small effect sizes, and meta-analysis of multiple trials may be used to determine whether drug–placebo differences are meaningful.

First-line treatment for MDD

Although an array of options exists for first-line treatment of MDD, no single agent has distinguished itself as clearly superior. Selective serotonin reuptake inhibitors (SSRIs) are still the most widely prescribed antidepressants, due to safety, tolerability, and cost. However, newer agents have gained in market share, as patients and clinicians search for treatment options while struggling to contain costs. Many trials have investigated the efficacy of SSRIs compared with other antidepressants.

SSRIs vs. tricyclic antidepressants (TCAs)

A Cochrane Collaboration meta-analysis identified 98 trials comparing SSRIs with other antidepressants, and failed to detect any clinically significant difference in efficacy between SSRIs and TCAs (Geddes et al., 2002). Another Cochrane Collaboration meta-analysis investigated the tolerability and efficacy of the TCA amitriptyline in comparison with other antidepressants and SSRIs, and found no difference in overall efficacy between amitriptyline and other TCAs or the SSRI comparators, but tolerability and acceptability measures favored SSRIs (Guaiana et al., 2007). SSRIs also demonstrate efficacy for depression, without clear evidence of superiority over older drugs, when studied in particular patient subgroups. A smaller meta-analysis including 365 SSRI-treated geriatric depressed patients found SSRIs and TCAs to be equally efficacious (Wilson et al., 2003).

SSRIs demonstrate benefit over older medications in tolerability and acceptability. A Cochrane Collaboration review identified 136 randomized trials in which SSRIs and TCAs were compared among depressed patients, and found a modest but significant difference favoring SSRIs in terms of discontinuation of treatment (Barbui et al., 2003). SSRIs have the advantage of safety and tolerability over TCAs and monoamine oxidase inhibitors (MAOIs), and remain the treatment choice for MDD.

SSRIs vs. newer-generation antidepressants

Antidepressants with dual-action and triple-action mechanisms have proved effective for depression in both outpatient and inpatient settings, and in placebo-controlled and comparator trials. Data suggest that these newer-generation antidepressants improve response over SSRIs. For example, a meta-analysis of 93 trials of treatment for MDD with antidepressants that have serotonergic plus noradrenergic action showed that these drugs were slightly more efficacious in achieving clinical response than were SSRIs (response rate of 63% vs. 59%) (Papakostas et al., 2007a). However, the number needed to treat (NNT) statistic was 24. In addition, some studies have shown that mirtazapine offers an earlier onset of response than SSRIs (Versiani et al., 2005), but use of this medication may be limited by its side-effect profile (Papakostas et al., 2008).

Overall, efforts at distinguishing efficacy and acceptability between SSRIs and newer antidepressants have been limited by the lack of RCTs examining direct, head-to-head comparisons between medications. In 2009, Cipriani and colleagues conducted a systematic review of 117 RCTs comparing 12 new-generation antidepressants, in terms of efficacy and acceptability, as monotherapy for the acute-phase treatment of MDD, with outcome measures at 8 weeks (Cipriani et al., 2009). Data from 25 928 individual subjects were included in the study, of which approximately two-thirds were women. In analyzing the data, the authors used number of patients who responded as a measure of "efficacy," and number of patients who dropped out as a measure of "acceptability." Direct pair-wise comparisons of efficacy and acceptability were performed, as well as a multiple-treatments meta-analysis. The authors found that, in terms of response, mirtazapine, escitalopram, venlafaxine, and sertraline were more efficacious than duloxetine, fluoxetine, fluvoxamine, paroxetine, and reboxetine [odds ratio (OR) 1.22–2.03]. In terms of acceptability, the better-tolerated drugs were escitalopram, sertraline, citalopram, and bupropion. In a complex statistical analysis combining and comparing both response rates and discontinuation rates, the authors conclude that sertraline and escitalopram, followed by mirtazapine and venlafaxine, have better risk–benefit profiles than other antidepressants. Considering the additional element of cost, the authors suggest that sertraline might be the best first choice for treating moderate to severe depression.

This study was limited by the lack of data from direct comparisons between the medications. In the absence of head-to-head comparisons, the authors analyzed comparative efficacy by using fluoxetine as a reference drug. This statistical method has the advantage of using available data to draw inferences about drugs that have never been directly compared. However, the results must be interpreted with caution, and must not be viewed as having the same validity that analysis of results from RCTs would provide. In addition, these authors interpreted data from studies of different patient populations, and compared outcomes measured by different rating scales. They used response rate as a dichotomous variable, rather than change in score on symptom rating scales, which could have inflated differences between treatments. The use of discontinuation rate as a proxy for tolerability and safety is problematic as well, since different medications can cause widely varying side-effects or adverse events.

To illustrate the difficulty in interpreting the data, we next consider another large-scale meta-analysis comparing second-generation antidepressants, by Gartlehner *et al.* (2008), who used similar methods but came to a somewhat different conclusion. Their analysis of 203 studies produced a conclusion that there are no substantial differences in comparative efficacy and effectiveness of second-generation antidepressants for the treatment of MDD. However, there were differences identified among individual drugs. For example, bupropion had fewer sexual side-effects, and mirtazapine had a faster onset of action, compared with some of the SSRIs. In subgroup analyses, no patient factors were identified that could allow prediction of response or non-response to an individual drug.

Subpopulations and predictors of response

Symptom severity at baseline

In studies of antidepressants, baseline symptom severity may affect treatment outcome, such that more severely depressed patients have a more robust response (Khan *et al.*, 2002; Kirsch *et al.*, 2008). However, the generalizability of these data has been limited by exclusion of patients with "minor" depression, or less severe major depressive symptomatology. In a 2010 meta-analysis, Fournier and colleagues combined data from six RCTs that included patients with the lower range of baseline symptom severity (Hamilton Rating Scale for Depression (HRSD or HAMD) scores from the low teens) (Fournier *et al.*, 2010). The authors analyzed individual patient data, allowing for a "mega-analysis." The authors employed a severity × treatment interaction statistic, and concluded that the efficacy of antidepressant medication for depression varies considerably as a function of symptom severity. The advantage over placebo was non-existent or negligible among patients with mild, moderate, and even severe baseline symptoms, while the advantage over placebo was large for patients with very severe symptoms. This result is consistent with the findings of Khan *et al.* and Kirsch *et al.* summarized above. A limitation was that Fournier's analysis interpreted data from small subpopulations of patients with minor depression or mild–moderate depression, and the results may not be generalizable to this population in clinical practice. Additionally, it should be noted that of the thousands of clinical trials of antidepressants, very few have included patients with mild or moderate depression. This lack of evidence for antidepressant effect should not be misinterpreted as negative evidence. As nearly half of outpatients meeting diagnostic criteria for MDD have symptoms in the mild–moderate range (Zimmerman *et al.*, 2002), it is clear that this question has significant clinical implications, and requires further investigation.

For those patients who do have severe and melancholic forms of depression, limited data are available to determine whether one antidepressant or class is preferable to another. In a study of depressed inpatients, one large meta-analysis found TCAs to have a small amount of benefit over SSRIs (Geddes *et al.*, 2002). The authors caution that this difference was attributed to a one-point difference on the HAMD, and may be due to chance. Meta-analysis showed that while depressed inpatients responded better to TCAs *vs.* SSRIs, the SSRIs were moderately more tolerable (Anderson, 1998, 2000). In the STAR*D study, nearly a quarter of subjects had melancholic features at baseline, and these patients had higher severity scores, higher current suicidal risk, higher rates of previous suicide attempts, and more psychiatric comorbidity at enrolment (McGrath *et al.*, 2008). After initial treatment with citalopram, patients with melancholic features showed a 24% decrease in remission rate relative to patients without melancholic features. Together, the findings above suggest that the presence of melancholic features may be a negative prognostic factor for SSRI treatment, particularly among inpatients, but, in light of the STAR*D findings, perhaps in outpatients as well. However, it is not clear whether the STAR*D Level 1 (citalopram treatment) finding can be generalized to include response to other SSRIs. For example, as patients with melancholic features participated in subsequent levels of treatment in STAR*D, it did not appear that they responded differentially to sertraline *vs.* bupropion-SR or venlafaxine-SR (Rush *et al.*, 2008). The limitations of the STAR*D study included lack of placebo control, and lack of structured diagnostic algorithms to ascertain and track melancholic features.

Patients at risk of suicide

Patients with MDD are at higher risk of suicide, and guidelines indicate that patients should be assessed for suicide at the start of treatment and regularly over the course of treatment (Fochtman & Gelenberg, 2005). In 2005, Fergusson and colleagues conducted a large meta-analysis of RCTs comparing SSRIs with placebo or an active comparator, to investigate this association (Fergusson *et al.*, 2005). The authors examined 702 clinical trials, comprised of 87 650 patients, and included trials of SSRIs for MDD, but nearly 60% of included trials had investigated SSRIs for other clinical conditions. In meta-analysis, the authors found a significant increase in the odds of suicide attempts [OR 2.28, 95% confidence interval (CI) 1.14–4.55, NNT to harm 684] for patients receiving SSRIs compared with placebo. In the pooled analysis of SSRIs *vs.* TCAs, there was no difference in the odds ratio of suicide attempts (OR 0.88, 95% CI 0.54–1.42). Notably, the authors reported, "Estimates for patients with major depression favored a decrease in suicides with SSRIs, whereas patients with depression and other clinical indications may have as much as an eightfold increase in the rates of suicide." This meta-analysis had several limitations, including that only about half of the trials included directly reported rates of suicide attempts, and most trials included small numbers of patients followed for short durations (average of 10 weeks), making it difficult to analyze longer-term outcomes. And, as Mulder and colleagues point out, much of the evidence used to assess risk of suicidality is generated by industry-sponsored antidepressant trials, which typically exclude patients with high-risk factors including current suicidal ideation, substance abuse, or comorbid personality disorders (Mulder *et al.*, 2008). This practice essentially produces studies of depressed patients without suicidal ideation or recent attempts, and biases trials to detect emerging suicidal ideation and behavior, as well as making the data difficult to generalize to outpatients seen in clinical practice.

In a prospective trial, Mulder and colleagues followed a group of unselected outpatients who were started on antidepressants, for a 6-month study period (Mulder *et al.*, 2008). The study population included patients with comorbid Axis I and II disorders, and suicidal ideation at study entry. Patients were randomly assigned to fluoxetine or nortriptyline, and clinicians were allowed to titrate doses or make augmentation or switching decisions based on clinical response. One hundred and seventy-six patients completed follow-up at 6 months. The proportion of patients with significant suicidal ideation (Montgomery–Åsberg Depression Rating Scale (MADRS) suicide item score $\geq$ 3) fell from 47% to 14% during the first 3 weeks of the trial. Around 10% of patients did have "emergent" suicidality, but of these, it was found that nearly three-quarters did have suicidal ideation during the 6 months prior to study entry. Excluding those with prior suicidal ideation, only 3% of patients had emergent suicidal ideation for the first time after starting antidepressants. The authors firmly conclude that antidepressant use is associated with a reduction in suicidal ideation and attempts.

The Mulder study supports the findings of other investigators, who, in epidemiological studies, found decreased rates of suicide associated with prescriptions of antidepressants (Gibbons *et al.*, 2005, 2006; Nakagawa *et al.*, 2007). An interesting study by Gibbons and colleagues examined epidemiological data for suicide rates among adolescents in 2003–2005, after US and European regulators issued warnings about a possible association between antidepressants and suicide risk (Gibbons *et al.*, 2007). Subsequent to the warning, antidepressant prescriptions decreased by about 20% in the USA and the Netherlands. During that period, youth suicide rates increased strikingly in both countries. Again, the epidemiological data appear to support the utility of SSRIs and newer-generation antidepressants in reducing risk for suicide across age groups. However, much debate continues about the risk for suicide among child and adolescent patients who are prescribed antidepressants, and the US Food and Drug Administration (FDA) "black box" warning was extended in 2006 to include young adults (Leon, 2007). While the data may be conflicting, it is without question that any patient at risk of suicide requires careful monitoring and ongoing assessment of risk. (See below for a discussion of the antisuicidal properties of lithium.)

Timing of clinical improvement

The delayed onset of antidepressant therapeutic effect is an obstacle in the treatment of depression. The full therapeutic effect of antidepressants may take many weeks to develop, leaving patients to endure long periods of depressive symptomatology before making subsequent treatment decisions. Recently, data have emerged that re-examine the necessity of waiting 8–12 weeks for a full antidepressant trial, and challenge the notion that early responders are experiencing a placebo effect. For example, in a meta-analysis of eight studies ($n = 7121$ patients), Papakostas and colleagues compared early sustained response rates between antidepressant- and placebo-treated adults with MDD (Papakostas *et al.*, 2006). Sustained early response, defined as clinical improvement not followed by worsening of symptoms, was more likely among antidepressant-treated patients than among patients receiving placebo at weeks 1 or 2 (OR 1.50 and 2.06, respectively). The authors conclude that a "true" antidepressant response can occur within the first 1 or 2 weeks of treatment. An earlier study of response to fluoxetine showed that more than half of eventual responders will show response by week 2, and over 75% respond by week 4; conversely, if patients had not experienced onset of response by weeks 4–6, they were unlikely to respond by the end of the 8-week study period (Nierenberg et al., 2000). In addition, a study of 182 outpatients showed that earlier clinical improvement with fluoxetine predicted greater symptom resolution at 8 weeks (Papakostas et al., 2007b). This study was limited by lack of a placebo comparator group, and lack of follow-up for a longer duration.

Wade et al. (2009) performed a pooled analysis of four RCTs of escitalopram vs. a comparator antidepressant in MDD. Onset of improvement at week 2 was correlated with response at week 8: 80% of patients with onset at week 2 responded by week 8, but among those without onset of improvement at week 2, only 43% responded by week 8. Of those who did not show improvement at week 4, only 13% had responded at week 8. In this meta-analysis the authors also showed that response at week 8 predicted a greater probability of achieving remission, and completing 6 months of treatment.

Thus the emerging data suggest that early response is predictive of longer-term treatment outcomes. The application of these data to clinical practice is not as clear, as the clinical trials have been limited by lack of placebo control, and lack of longer-term follow-up. More studies in this line of inquiry could prove very valuable to patients, should there come a time when the data support evolving the treatment strategy at the earliest possible opportunity.

Continuation and maintenance treatment

After resolution of an acute episode, the period of time to continue antidepressant treatment has not been definitively determined. Longitudinal, naturalistic follow-up data of patients who recover from an index episode of MDD found that 85% of subjects had a recurrence over the 15-year study (Mueller et al., 1999). After remission of an acute episode, the most robust predictor of relapse is having had a prior episode (Coryell et al., 1991; Keller et al., 1983; Maj et al., 1992; Mueller et al., 1999; Roy-Byrne et al., 1985; Simpson et al., 1997). A 10-year follow-up study of 318 subjects after an index episode of depression found that the risk of recurrence increases with each subsequent episode (Solomon et al., 2000). Another strong predictor of recurrence is severity of illness in the acute episode. Angst et al.'s (2003) 40-year follow-up of patients initially hospitalized for unipolar or bipolar depression found steady recurrence rates over the study for this more severely ill population, and suggests that maintenance treatment is warranted for more severely ill patients.

Residual symptoms after remission of an acute episode also predict recurrence (Judd et al., 1998; Nierenberg et al., 2010). Kennedy & Paykel (2004) followed up with 60 severely and recurrently depressed patients, at 8–10 years after remission from an index episode of depression. The presence of significant residual symptoms predicted more time with depressive symptoms, as well as impaired social functioning and reduced quality of life. In the STAR*D trial, at 1-year follow-up, over 90% of patients who had remitted with citalopram had at least one residual symptom, and, concordant with other findings, patients with more residual symptom domains had a higher probability of relapse (Nierenberg et al., 2010). In contrast, those patients with complete resolution of their symptoms have a longer time to next episode than those patients who do have residual depressive symptoms (Pintor et al., 2003).

Most antidepressants have been studied in continuation after resolution of an acute depressive episode, and appear superior to placebo for preventing relapse (Weihs et al., 2002).

A thoughtful and rigorous pooled analysis of 31 trials of antidepressant continuation up to 36 months found that the benefit of antidepressants over placebo was sustained no matter what the length of continuation (Geddes et al., 2003). Most of the studies examined were of 12 months duration, so the authors suggest that the data for longer continuation be confirmed. Patients with shorter (1–2 months) and longer (4–6 months) treatment before randomization to continued antidepressant, and from 6 months to 36 months of follow-up after randomized treatment, all appeared to have similar reductions in proportional risk. The results for different classes of antidepressants were similar, suggesting that all antidepressants that are effective in treating depression will be effective for maintenance treatment. To examine the efficacy and effectiveness of second-generation antidepressants in preventing relapse and recurrence during continuation and maintenance phases of treatment, Hansen et al. (2008) assembled a large meta-analysis of 23 placebo-controlled, and four active comparator trials. Pooled data for the class of second-generation antidepressants compared with placebo suggested a large effect size, and the NNT to prevent both relapse and recurrence was five patients, suggesting the overall benefit of these medications for continuation and maintenance.

Treatment-resistant depression

A significant proportion of patients do not respond to initial antidepressant treatment. Before switching or augmenting antidepressants, initial treatment must be optimized; under-utilization and under-dosing of antidepressants for MDD have been documented repeatedly. "Pseudoresistance," as this phenomenon has been termed, is the result of inadequate dosing or inadequate treatment duration, and must be differentiated from true treatment resistance (Nierenberg & Amsterdam, 1990). Under-prescribing is as ineffective over the long term as no pharmacological treatment at all (Leon et al., 2003).

Antidepressant switching

A review of the evidence for switching pharmacotherapy after a first trial with a SSRI examined eight RCTs and 23 open studies (Ruhe et al., 2006). A limitation of this review, and indeed of most studies of this patient population, is that definitions of response, remission rate, and treatment-resistant depression differed. Response rates and remission rates varied widely between the included studies, from 12–86% and 5–39%, respectively. The authors concluded that no unequivocal evidence is available to prove differences in outcome between switches within classes or between classes of antidepressants.

In STAR*D, 727 patients were randomly assigned to the switch strategy option in Level 2, after failing to remit with Level 1 treatment (citalopram) (Rush et al., 2008). The overall remission rate in Level 2 was about 31% (Rush et al., 2006a). About one-quarter of patients who switched to another SSRI (sertraline), a serotonin norepinephrine reuptake inhibitor (SNRI) (venlafaxine-XR), or a norepinephrine dopamine reuptake inhibitor (NDRI) (bupropion-SR) achieved remission with the second antidepressant, and the overall side-effect burden and rate of serious adverse events did not differ (Rush et al., 2006b). Clinical symptom patterns or demographic measures were not useful for predicting which patients would respond to any particular medication (Rush et al., 2008). In Level 3, about 14% of participants achieved remission (Rush et al., 2006a). Patients entering this level could be considered treatment-resistant, having failed to achieve remission with two different antidepressant regimens. As a strategy, switching to a third antidepressant monotherapy resulted in lower remission rates than in the first two levels (< 20%) (Fava *et al.*, 2006). There were no statistically significant differences in remission between a second monotherapy switch to mirtazapine (12%) or nortriptyline (20%), and both were equally tolerable (Fava *et al.*, 2006). Patients entering Level 4 had failed three consecutive antidepressant trials, and were considered to have highly treatment-resistant illness. About 13% of subjects achieved remission in this level (Rush *et al.*, 2006b), and there was no significant difference in remission between those who switched to the MAOI tranylcypromine (7%), or those who switched to venlafaxine-XR plus mirtazapine (14%) (McGrath *et al.*, 2006). However, interpretation of the efficacy of tranylcypromine is limited by its poor tolerability; nearly half of patients receiving the MAOI discontinued the medication before 6 weeks. There are many valid criticisms of STAR*D. These include use of lower-than-recommended medication dosages in later levels, broadly inclusive enrolment criteria that may have dampened effect sizes, and underpowered trials in the later levels of the study.

Antidepressant augmentation

Additional antidepressants

A double-blind, placebo-controlled trial of mirtazapine augmentation of patients who remained depressed on antidepressant monotherapy was performed (Carpenter *et al.*, 2002). Twenty-six patients were randomized to receive mirtazapine or placebo for 4 weeks. Response to mirtazapine was marked, with a response rate of 64% (7/11) for those on drug compared with 20% for placebo (3/15) ($p = 0.043$). The remission rate was 45.4% for drug and 13.3% for placebo. Aside from its small size, a limitation of this study is the wide range of doses of a broad array of antidepressants that were augmented with mirtazapine. It is difficult to state whether one antidepressant or class of antidepressant is more likely to benefit from mirtazapine augmentation.

STAR*D allowed an RCT of adding a second antidepressant to an ineffective first antidepressant. The Level 2 switching strategy randomly assigned patients to augmentation of citalopram (a SSRI) with bupropion-SR (a NDRI) or buspirone (a partial agonist at the 5-HT_{1A} receptor) (Trivedi *et al.*, 2006). Both augmentation strategies led to similar rates of remission, 30% each, as measured by reduction in HAMD scores. However, bupropion-SR was associated with a greater reduction in the Quick Inventory of Depressive Symptomatology – Self Report (QIDS-SR), a patient self-report of depression symptoms, and also was somewhat better tolerated by patients over buspirone.

Atypical antipsychotics

The 1990s saw the introduction of second-generation antipsychotic drugs, with an advantage over typical antipsychotics in the lower likelihood for extrapyramidal side-effects (Correll *et al.*, 2004). These medications block central dopamine receptors, but have significant heterogeneity in their mechanisms of action, a number of which suggest antidepressant properties; e.g. serotonin 5-HT_2 receptor antagonist and 5-HT_{1A} and dopamine receptor partial agonist activity (DeBattista & Hawkins, 2009).

A meta-analysis by Nelson & Papakostas (2009) reviewed RCTs of acute-phase treatment with atypical antipsychotic augmentation in patients with MDD, in addition to other unpublished data. In meta-analysis of the data, the authors found that augmentation with atypical antipsychotics was significantly more effective than placebo, for outcome measures of response (OR 1.69) and remission (OR 2.00). No significant differences in efficacy were found between the four atypical agents studied (olanzapine, risperidone, quetiapine, aripiprazole). The atypical antipsychotics as a class did show significantly higher rates of discontinuation for adverse effects, and this result was seen in studies of short duration (4–12 weeks). Longer-term effects of atypical antipsychotics can include weight gain and metabolic syndrome, and extrapyramidal side-effects including tardive dyskinesia, or rare events including neuroleptic malignant syndrome. Thus safety and tolerability, as well as the significant economic cost should be considered when evaluating augmenting strategies for MDD. Finally, the efficacy of these agents for continuation and maintenance therapy is yet to be studied.

Lithium

Until the advent of atypical antipsychotics, lithium had been the most-studied medication for antidepressant augmentation (Nelson & Papakostas, 2009). Early studies of lithium augmentation demonstrated benefit compared with placebo when added to TCAs for partial response, but there had until recently been no studies of lithium augmentation in patients with a history of non-response to multiple antidepressants. In a 2003 study, Nierenberg and colleagues treated 35 treatment-resistant subjects prospectively with nortriptyline for 6 weeks (Nierenberg et al., 2003). Those who tolerated the medication but did not respond were then randomized to receive lithium or placebo augmentation for another 6 weeks. At that time, 12.5% of lithium-augmented patients showed a response, vs. 20% of placebo-augmented patients, a non-significant difference between lithium and placebo. The authors concluded that the utility of lithium augmentation may be restricted to patients with depression refractory to a single medication. A meta-analysis of lithium augmentation for unipolar and bipolar patients with major depression was conducted by Crossley & Bauer (2007). In the meta-analysis of 10 augmentation studies, the data suggest that lithium is an effective augmenting strategy, with an OR of 3.11. A limitation of this meta-analysis was that included studies were not limited to patients with treatment-resistant depression, and combined patients with unipolar and bipolar depression.

Lithium has long been postulated to have antisuicidal properties. A meta-analysis of the antisuicidal effect of lithium in patients with recurrent MDD concludes that the overall risk for suicide or attempt was 88.5% lower in patients taking lithium vs. those without lithium (Guzzetta et al., 2007). The effect was observed even in two studies that selected patients with high risk for suicide. Limitations of the study were relatively small number of trials included, with a small number of patients contributing data ($n = 78$), and that in some studies, suicide was observed incidentally, rather than as an outcome measure. However, the data are consistent with earlier findings that lithium reduces suicide rates in patients with bipolar disorder or other psychiatric illness. An RCT investigating the effect of adjunctive lithium treatment in the prevention of suicidal behavior was published in 2008 (Lauterbach et al., 2008). In this study, 167 patients with a suicide attempt in the past 3 months, in the context of a depressed episode, were treated with either lithium or placebo, and followed for 12 months. Seventy-six percent of patients had MDD, and the others had adjustment disorders or dysthymia; nearly three-quarters of patients had comorbid psychiatric or substance-use disorders as well. Lithium and placebo were studied as add-on treatments, and patients received usual clinical care in community settings. The composite primary outcome measure was the occurrence of a suicide attempt or completed suicide during the follow-up period. Over the study period, there were 17 suicide attempts or completions, seven in the lithium group and 10 in the placebo group. Survival analysis showed no significant difference of suicidal acts between the lithium- and placebo-treated groups. However, in post-hoc analysis, it was revealed that all completed suicides occurred in the placebo group, accounting for a significant difference in the incidence rates. The authors conclude that lithium may be effective in reducing the risk of completed suicide in adults with depressive disorders. This was the first prospective RCT examining suicide as an outcome measure in a sample of depressed patients at high risk for suicide. Although the findings were limited by small sample size, this study adds to the body of evidence suggesting an antisuicidal effect of lithium, and should encourage further investigation.

Lamotrigine

A few small studies have shown some efficacy for lamotrigine as an augmenting agent for antidepressants in patients with treatment-resistant depression. In one study, 23 patients with treatment failure for MDD were selected to receive treatment with fluoxetine, and randomized to concomitant treatment with lamotrigine or placebo (Barbosa et al., 2003). Lamotrigine at 100 mg was statistically superior to placebo on the outcome measure of Clinical Global Impression (CGI) scale scores, but failed to separate from placebo on the primary outcome measure, HAMD scores. The study was limited by small sample size and inclusion of bipolar II and MDD patients.

In an open-label trial of lithium vs. lamotrigine for treatment-resistant depression, 34 patients were randomized to receive one or the other as antidepressant augmentation (Schindler & Anghelescu, 2007). In both groups, clinically significant reductions in HAMD scores were achieved, and there was no statistically significant difference between the groups. Twenty-three percent of the lamotrigine group and 18% of the lithium group achieved remission. This study was limited by small sample size and non-blinded observations, but the results suggest that further investigation of lamotrigine augmentation is warranted.

Triiodothyronine (T3)

Triiodothyronine (T3) has been well-studied in antidepressant non-responders. A meta-analysis by Altshuler and colleagues found that the pooled, weighted effect size of the addition of T3 to TCAs in non-refractory patients was 0.58 (Altshuler et al., 2001). Five of the six randomized trials of T3 found benefit in augmentation. All of the trials, however, took place between 1969 and 1974, in patients prescribed relatively low doses of TCAs. Whether the effect would have been apparent in subjects with higher TCA dosing is unclear. While most of the published data support the use of T3 as augmentation for TCAs, some more recent studies have shown moderate efficacy of T3 augmentation for SSRIs (Abraham et al., 2006; Iosifescu et al., 2005).

A recent prospective, placebo-controlled pilot study was performed to evaluate the utility of T3 in accelerating antidepressant response under naturalistic conditions (Posternak et al., 2008). Fifty consecutive outpatients who were diagnosed with MDD and started on antidepressants were concurrently randomized to receive T3 or placebo, and followed for 6 weeks. Response rates, defined as a > 50% reduction in MADRS scores, were higher for the adjunctive cohort after weeks 1 and 2, and the authors conclude that T3 may be used to accelerate the antidepressant response; further investigation is needed.

S-adenosyl methionine (SAMe)

S-adenosyl methionine (SAMe) has been studied previously for its antidepressant properties, and has been prescribed in Europe since the 1970s. SAMe was initially studied in its parenteral forms; these early studies demonstrated efficacy vs. placebo, and also suggested that SAMe was similar in efficacy to TCAs (see Papakostas, 2009, for a review). When a stable oral form of SAMe became available for study, three RCTs demonstrated its comparable efficacy to TCAs, and two studies demonstrated efficacy superior to placebo (Papakostas, 2009). In a 2002 meta-analysis by the Agency for Healthcare Research and Quality, results of studies in which SAMe was administered orally, intramuscularly, and intravenously were combined, and supported the conclusion that SAMe was similarly effective to TCAs (effect size 0.08, 95% CI −0.17 to 0.32), and superior to placebo (effect size 0.65) for the treatment of depression (Hardy et al., 2002).

More recent data support the use of SAMe as an antidepressant augmentation strategy. Papakostas and colleagues presented a RCT focusing on the use of oral SAMe for antidepressant augmentation in patients with MDD who were SRI non-responders (Papakostas et al., 2010). Seventy-three patients were randomized to adjunctive placebo or 800–1600 mg/day SAMe. The response rate (the primary outcome measure) for SAMe-treated patients was 36.1%, which differed significantly from the response rate for placebo-treated patients, 17.6%. Discontinuation rates for side-effects were similar in both groups. Replication and further studies are needed, but this first randomized and placebo-controlled study demonstrates a promising finding for the use of SAMe as an antidepressant augmentation strategy.

In summary, after an initial trial of antidepressant monotherapy, both switching and augmenting are reasonable next steps for patients who fail to achieve remission. One advantage to switching medication is to avoid polypharmacy and its inherent risk for side-effects or adverse events. An advantage to augmenting is to continue any partial response that might have occurred as a therapeutic effect of the initial antidepressant agent. Evidence-supported augmenting strategies include addition of atypical antipsychotics, an antidepressant with a different mechanism of action, lithium, T3, or SAMe.

Emerging evidence

Agomelatine

The development of agomelatine, a melatonin receptor agonist and a $5\text{-}HT_{2C}$ receptor antagonist, has added a new approach to treating depression. The drug increases monoaminergic transmission, and through its effect on melatonin receptors, contributes to improvements in sleep onset and quality. Two recent RCTs found significant improvements in HAMD scores over the 8-week study periods (Stahl et al., 2010; Zajecka et al., 2010). The studies conflicted in determining the effective dose of agomelatine, with Stahl et al. reporting 25 mg was more efficacious, and Zajecka et al. reporting efficacy with only a 50-mg dose. Both studies observed transient aminotransferase elevations in the 50-mg groups. In a longer, 24-week study of agomelatine responders, subjects were randomized to continue treatment with agomelatine or to placebo; over the study period, the relapse rate for agomelatine-treated patients was 21.7%, compared with 46.6% for placebo-treated patients (Goodwin et al., 2009). Previous studies with agomelatine reported a superior sexual side-effect profile with agomelatine compared with other antidepressants, specifically venlafaxine XR (Kennedy et al., 2008), and paroxetine (Montejo et al., 2010).

Glutamatergic agents

Converging lines of evidence suggest that the glutamatergic system plays a role in the pathophysiology of MDD, and treatments targeting this system are already being studied for their effect on depressive symptomatology (Hashimoto, 2009; Sanacora, 2009). Several known mood-modulating medications act on the glutamatergic system: lamotrigine affects glutamate release, ketamine and memantine antagonize the NMDA receptor, and the antioxidant N-acetyl-L-cysteine (NAC) activates the cystine-glutamate antiporter. Early studies of ketamine by Zarate *et al.* (2006a) demonstrated a robust and very rapid antidepressant response to an intravenous infusion of ketamine in patients with treatment-resistant depression. Patients were randomized to an infusion of ketamine or placebo on 2 days, 1 week apart. Fifty percent of patients met response criteria within 2 h, and 71% within 24 h; the effect was significantly different from outcome measures of the placebo group, and was sustained at 7 days post-treatment. A study of memantine, a NMDA receptor antagonist, failed to separate from placebo on MADRS scores at 8 weeks (Zarate *et al.*, 2006b). Finally, riluzole, a drug used for the treatment of amyotrophic lateral sclerosis, affects both glutamate release and reuptake, and has shown some effect on depressive symptoms in treatment-resistant depression, both when used as augmentation and as monotherapy (Sanacora, 2009). Agents that affect glutamatergic neurotransmission will continue to be an active topic for study in the treatment of MDD.

Pramipexole

Pramipexole is a pre-synaptic dopamine agonist, with a preference for the D_3 receptor subtype. In addition to potentiating dopamine receptors, pramipexole has a suppressive effect on REM sleep, and has demonstrated neurotrophic effects as well. A meta-analysis by Aiken in 2007 reviewed the literature supporting its use in psychiatric conditions (Aiken, 2007). Aiken identified three placebo-controlled trials, but pooled data for all treated subjects in both prospective and retrospective studies, and found large effect sizes in unipolar and bipolar depression. In the only controlled trial of patients with unipolar MDD, Corrigan *et al.* (2000) compared pramipexole as monotherapy to 20 mg fluoxetine, and placebo, in 174 patients. In this industry-sponsored study, pramipexole improved scores on HAMD, MADRS, and CGI, in a statistically significant finding at 8 weeks. The most improvement was seen in patients taking the 5-mg dose, although more patients at this dose range dropped out. Other studies of mood symptoms in bipolar depression and in Parkinson's disease show improvement in pramipexole-treated patients (Aiken, 2007). More study is needed to show efficacy, and the authors raise concern over previously reported adverse effects including sleep attacks, compulsive behavior, mania, and psychosis in other patient populations.

Modafinil

Modafinil is an analeptic (wake-promoting) agent that has FDA approval for narcolepsy and shift-work sleep disorder, and as adjunctive treatment for obstructive sleep apnea/hypopnea syndrome. Its novel mechanism of action includes increased release of monoamines, as well as increased localized histamine release in the hypothalamus; investigators have hoped to see a benefit of modafinil on residual depressive symptoms, in particular in measures of fatigue. Small studies of open-label treatment, and a small RCT, have had positive results for augmentation of antidepressants (DeBattista *et al.*, 2003, 2004; Rasmussen *et al.*, 2005). In 2005, Fava and colleagues reported an RCT of 311 outpatients who had partial response to SSRI monotherapy, and had persistent fatigue and sleepiness (Fava *et al.*, 2005). The dual treatment group reported improved scores on the Brief Fatigue Inventory that separated from placebo by the end of the 8-week trial. In addition, patients in the dual-treatment group had greater improvements on CGI scores, and a (non-significant) trend towards greater improvement on HAMD scores. Finally, in a meta-analysis of 33 double-blind, placebo-controlled trials of modafinil for *any* clinical indication, the authors concluded that there is some evidence for modafinil's off-label use as an adjunct to antidepressants in depressive disorders, for treatment of depressed mood and depression-related fatigue and sleepiness (Ballon & Feifel, 2006).

Galantamine

Galantamine is an acetylcholinesterase inhibitor that modulates activity at nicotine receptor sites. It is approved for treatment of Alzheimer disease, but as findings emerged showing improvement in mood symptoms among galantamine-treated patients with mild cognitive impairment, interest developed in studying the medication as an adjunct therapy for depression (Elgamal & MacQueen, 2008). Two small RCTs have been published to date. In 2008, Elgamal and colleagues reported on a trial of 20 patients with MDD, not in an acute episode, who were randomized to placebo or galantamine (up to 16 mg) as augmentation to their current antidepressants (Elgamal & MacQueen, 2008). Although the antidepressant effect did not separate from placebo overall, certain patients with higher symptom severity at study entry did show some response. The galantamine-treated group did show improvement in cognitive scales, but the results were not statistically significant. This study was limited by the small sample size, and the study of patients without acute mood symptoms at study entry. Another small study investigated galantamine augmentation of antidepressant treatment in older adults with MDD (Holtzheimer *et al.*, 2008). Thirty-eight non-demented older adults were randomized to galantamine or placebo augmentation of standard antidepressant therapy (citalopram or venlafaxine XR). The study period was 24 weeks, and failed to demonstrate a benefit of galantamine that separated from placebo. Galantamine-treated patients were more likely to withdraw early from the study. However, there was some evidence that galantamine-treated patients had lower depression scores at week 2 of treatment. These small pilot studies suggest that further investigation is warranted.

Pharmacogenetics

Much attention has been focused on testing individual patients for genetic markers that may predict antidepressant response, and the hope has been to more closely match patients with suitable and effective treatments. Several recent studies have suggested that response to antidepressants may have a genetic basis (see McMahon *et al.*, 2006; Perlis *et al.*, 2008; Serretti *et al.*, 2007; and recently published results of the Genome-based Therapeutic Drugs for Depression study; Uher *et al.*, 2009). However, replication of the findings has been difficult to achieve. Genetic studies require large, well-characterized populations, as the effects of a single gene are very small and difficult to detect. Thus it has been difficult to generalize results to various minority racial-ethnic groups, as most association studies have used White samples. In addition, any single gene is likely to exert only a small effect, and useful pharmacogenetic testing would require incorporating and interpreting results from multiple loci. Finally, considerations of cost and access will become relevant as testing improves and becomes commercially available (Perlis *et al.*, 2009). However, pharmacogenetic testing has already become a reality in other fields of medicine, and it seems inevitable that we will soon use genetic markers to predict risk and outcomes in psychiatric conditions as well.

Conclusions

SSRIs and newer agents have proven to be safe and effective alternatives to the older antidepressants; these agents are all suitable for first-line use in patients with MDD. Each medication's unique side-effect profile should guide drug selection for individual patients. In this economic age, cost should be considered as well, both from an individual patient perspective, and from an aggregate perspective. For depressive episodes not responding to initial therapy, no single strategy – whether switching to a different drug of the same class, switching to a different class of drug, or augmenting with an additional agent – has been clearly established as superior. As augmenting agents, atypical antipsychotics, lithium, and T3 have been studied the most extensively, and shown to have benefit. However, their risks and side-effect profiles may make them less attractive to patients, and patient preference and safety should determine treatment decisions for refractory or chronic MDD.

To have advantages over existing drugs, novel antidepressants must have a more rapid onset of action, higher rates of response and remission, or marked improvements in tolerability and ease of use. Some of the novel agents, targeting other neurotransmitter systems such as glutamate, show promise in producing early response. The use of biomarkers, including pharmacogenetic testing, may one day provide more accurate predictors of response or adverse outcomes, allowing targeted treatments and the promise of personalized medicine.

Acknowledgements

Supported in part by the National Institute on Alcoholism and Alcohol Abuse (Grant K23AA016340–01A1), and the Scholars in Clinical Science Program of Harvard Catalyst/The Harvard Clinical and Translational Science Center (Award #UL1 RR 025758 and financial contributions from Harvard University and its affiliated academic health care centres) (Dr Ostacher). The content is solely the responsibility of the authors and does not necessarily represent the official views of Harvard Catalyst, Harvard University and its affiliated academic health care centres, the National Center for Research Resources or the National Institutes of Health.

Statement of interest

Dr. Ostacher has received research support from Pfizer, and has served on the advisory/consulting boards of Pfizer, Schering-Plough, and Concordant Rater Systems. He has received speaker's fees from AstraZeneca, Bristol–Myers Squibb, Eli Lilly & Company, GlaxoSmithKline, Janssen Pharmaceutica, Pfizer, and Massachusetts General Psychiatry Academy.

Dr. Perlis has received honoraria, consulting, or speaker's fees from AstraZeneca, Bristol-Myers Squibb, Eli Lilly & Co., GlaxoSmithKline, Pfizer, Proteus Biomedical, and Concordant Rater Systems. He holds patents and receives royalties with Concordant Rater Systems.

Dr. Nierenberg is a full-time employee of the Massachusetts General Hospital (MGH). He has served as a consultant to the American Psychiatric Association (only travel expenses paid), Appliance Computing Inc. (Mindsite), Brandeis University. Through the

MGH Clinical Trials Network and Institute, he has consulted for Brain Cells, Inc., Dianippon Sumitomo/Sepracor Novartis, PGx Health, Shire, Schering-Plough, Targacept, and Takeda/Lundbeck Pharmaceuticals. He received grant/research support through MGH from NIMH, PamLabs, Pfizer Pharmaceuticals, and Shire. He received honoraria from Belvior Publishing, University of Texas Southwestern Dallas, Hillside Hospital, American Drug Utilization Review, American Society for Clinical Psychopharmacology, Baystate Medical Center, Columbia University, IMEDEX, MJ Consulting, New York State, MBL Publishing, Physicians Postgraduate Press, SUNY Buffalo, University of Wisconsin, and the University of Pisa. Dr. Nierenberg is a presenter for the Massachusetts General Hospital Psychiatry Academy (MGHPA). The education programs conducted by the MGHPA were supported through Independent Medical Education (IME) grants from the following pharmaceutical companies in 2008: AstraZeneca, Eli Lilly, and Janssen Pharmaceuticals; in 2009 AstraZeneca, Eli Lilly, and Bristol–Myers Squibb. No speakers' bureaus or boards since 2003. He is on the advisory boards of Appliance Computing, Inc., Brain Cells, Inc., Eli Lilly and Company, and Takeda/Lundbeck and Targacept. Dr. Nierenberg owns stock options in Appliance Computing, Inc. and Brain Cells, Inc. Through MGH, he is named for copyrights to the Clinical Positive Affect Scale and the MGH Structured Clinical Interview for the Montgomery–Åsberg Depression Scale exclusively licensed to the MGH Clinical Trials Network and Institute (CTNI). Also, through MGH, Dr. Nierenberg has a patent extension application for the combination of buspirone, bupropion, and melatonin for the treatment of depression.

References

Abraham G, Milev R, Stuart Lawson J (2006). T3 augmentation of SSRI resistant depression. *Journal of Affective Disorders* **91**, 211–215.

Aiken CB (2007). Pramipexole in psychiatry: a systematic review of the literature. *Journal of Clinical Psychiatry* **68**, 1230–1236.

Altshuler LL, Bauer M, Frye MA *et al.* (2001). Does thyroid supplementation accelerate tricyclic antidepressant response? A review and meta-analysis of the literature. *American Journal of Psychiatry* **158**, 1617–1622.

Anderson IM (1998). SSRIs *vs.* tricyclic antidepressants in depressed inpatients: a meta-analysis of efficacy and tolerability. *Depression and Anxiety* **7** (Suppl. 1), 11–17.

Anderson IM (2000). Selective serotonin reuptake inhibitors *vs.* tricyclic antidepressants: a meta-analysis of efficacy and tolerability. *Journal of Affective Disorders* **58**, 19–36.

Angst J, Gamma A, Sellaro R et al. (2003). Recurrence of bipolar disorders and major depression. A life-long perspective. *European Archives of Psychiatry and Clinical Neuroscience* **253**, 236–240.

Ballon JS, Feifel D (2006). A systematic review of modafinil: potential clinical uses and mechanisms of action. *Journal of Clinical Psychiatry* **67**, 554–566.

Barbosa L, Berk M, Vorster M (2003). A double-blind, randomized, placebo-controlled trial of augmentation with lamotrigine or placebo in patients concomitantly treated with fluoxetine for resistant major depressive episodes. *Journal of Clinical Psychiatry* **64**, 403–407.

Barbui C, Hotopf M, Freemantle N et al. (2003). Treatment discontinuation with selective serotonin reuptake inhibitors (SSRIs) *vs.* tricyclic antidepressants (TCAs). *Cochrane Database of Systematic Reviews* **3**, CD002791.

Carpenter LL, Yasmin S, Price LH (2002). A double-blind, placebo-controlled study of antidepressant augmentation with mirtazapine. *Biological Psychiatry* **51**, 183–188.

Cipriani A, Furukawa TA, Salanti G et al. (2009). Comparative efficacy and acceptability of 12 new-generation antidepressants: a multiple-treatments meta-analysis. *Lancet* **373**, 746–758.

Correll CU, Leucht S, Kane JM (2004). Lower risk for tardive dyskinesia associated with second-generation antipsychotics: a systematic review of one-year studies. *American Journal of Psychiatry* **161**, 414–415.

Corrigan MH, Denahan AQ, Wright CE *et al.* (2000). Comparison of pramipexole, fluoxetine, and placebo in patients with major depression. *Depression and Anxiety* **11**, 58–65.

Coryell W, Endicott J, Keller MB (1991). Predictors of relapse into major depressive disorder in a nonclinical population. *American Journal of Psychiatry* **148**, 1353–1358.

Crossley NA, Bauer M (2007). Acceleration and augmentation of antidepressants with lithium for depressive disorders: two meta-analyses of randomized, placebo-controlled trials. *Journal of Clinical Psychiatry* **68**, 935–940.

DeBattista C, Doghramji K, Menza MA *et al.* (2003). Adjunct modafinil for the short-term treatment of fatigue and sleepiness in patients with major depressive disorder: a preliminary double-blind, placebo-controlled study. *Journal of Clinical Psychiatry* **64**, 1057–1064.

DeBattista C, Hawkins J (2009). Utility of atypical antipsychotics in the treatment of resistant unipolar depression. *CNS Drugs* **23**, 369–377.

DeBattista C, Lembke A, Solvason HB *et al.* (2004). A prospective trial of modafinil as an adjunctive treatment of major depression. *Journal of Clinical Psychopharmacology* **24**, 87–90.

Elgamal S, MacQueen G (2008). Galantamine as an adjunctive treatment in major depression. *Journal of Clinical Psychopharmacology* **28**, 357–359.

Fava M, Rush AJ, Wisniewski SR *et al.* (2006). A comparison of mirtazapine and nortriptyline following two consecutive failed medication treatments for depressed outpatients: a STAR*D report. *American Journal of Psychiatry* **163**, 1161–1172.

Fava M, Thase ME, DeBattista C (2005). A multicenter, placebo-controlled study of modafinil augmentation in partial responders to selective serotonin reuptake inhibitors with persistent fatigue and sleepiness. *Journal of Clinical Psychiatry* **66**, 85–93.

Fergusson D, Doucette S, Cranley Glass K, Shapiro S *et al.* (2005). Association between suicide attempts and selective serotonin reuptake inhibitors: systematic review of randomized controlled trials. *British Medical Journal* **330**, 396.

Fochtman LJ, Gelenberg AJ (2005). *Guideline Watch: Practice Guideline for the Treatment of Patients with Major Depressive Disorder*, 2nd edn. American Psychiatric Association (http://www.psychiatryonline.com/pracGuide/loadGuidelinePdf.aspx?file=MDD.watch).

Fournier JC, DeRubeis RJ, Hollon SD *et al.* (2010). Antidepressant drug effects and depression severity: a patient-level meta-analysis. *Journal of the American Medical Association* **303**, 47–53.

Gartlehner G, Gaynes BN, Hansen RA *et al.* (2008). Comparative benefits and harms of second-generation antidepressants: background paper for the American College of Physicians. *Annals of Internal Medicine* **149**, 734–750.

Geddes JR, Carney SM, Davies C *et al.* (2003). Relapse prevention with antidepressant drug treatment in depressive disorders: a systematic review. *Lancet* **361**, 653–661.

Geddes JR, Freemantle N, Mason J *et al.* (2002). Selective serotonin reuptake inhibitors (SSRIs) for depression. *Cochrane Database of Systematic Reviews* **2**, CD00185.

Gibbons RD, Brown CH, Hur K *et al.* (2007). Early evidence on the effects of regulators' suicidality warnings on SSRI prescriptions and suicide in children and adolescents. *American Journal of Psychiatry* **164**, 1356–1363.

Gibbons RD, Hur K, Bhaumik DK, Mann JJ (2005). The relationship between antidepressant medication use and rate of suicide. *Archives of General Psychiatry* **62**, 165–172.

Gibbons RD, Hur K, Bhaumik DK, Mann JJ (2006). The relationship between antidepressant prescription rates and rate of early adolescent suicide. *American Journal of Psychiatry* **163**, 1898–1904.

Goodwin GM, Emsley R, Rembry S *et al.* (2009). Agomelatine prevents relapse in patients with major depressive disorder without evidence of a discontinuation syndrome: a

24-week randomized, double-blind, placebo-controlled trial. *Journal of Clinical Psychiatry* **70**, 1128–1137.

Guaiana G, Barbui C, Hotopf M (2007). Amitriptyline for depression. *Cochrane Database of Systematic Reviews* **3**, CD004186.

Guzzetta F, Tondo L, Centorrino F, Baldessarini RJ (2007). Lithium treatment reduces suicide risk in recurrent major depressive disorder. *Journal of Clinical Psychiatry* **68**, 380–383.

Hansen R, Gaynes B, Thieda P et al. (2008). Meta-analysis of major depressive disorder relapse and recurrence with second-generation antidepressants. *Psychiatric Services* **59**, 1121–1130.

Hardy M, Coulter I, Morton SC et al. (2002). S-adenosyl-methionine for treatment of depression, osteoarthritis, and liver disease (publication number, 02-E04). Rockville, MD: Agency for Healthcare Research and Quality, US Department of Health and Human Services.

Hashimoto K (2009). Emerging role of glutamate in the pathophysiology of major depressive disorder. *Brain Research Reviews* **61**, 105–123.

Holtzheimer 3rd PE, Meeks TW, Kelley ME et al. (2008). A double blind, placebo-controlled pilot study of galantamine augmentation of antidepressant treatment in older adults with major depression. *International Journal of Geriatric Psychiatry* **23**, 625–631.

Iosifescu DV, Nierenberg AA, Mischoulon D et al. (2005). An open study of triiodothyronine augmentation of selective serotonin reuptake inhibitors in treatment-resistant major depressive disorder. *Journal of Clinical Psychiatry* **66**, 1038–1042.

Judd L, Akiskal HS, Maser JD et al. (1998). A prospective 12-year study of subsyndromal and syndromal depressive symptoms in unipolar major depressive disorders. *Journal of Affective Disorders* **50**, 97–108.

Keller MB, Lavori PW, Lewis CE, Klerman GL (1983). Predictors of relapse in major depressive disorder. *Journal of the American Medical Association* **250**, 3299–3304.

Kennedy N, Paykel ES (2004). Residual symptoms at remission from depression: impact on long-term outcome. *Journal of Affective Disorders* **80**, 135–144.

Kennedy SH, Rizvi S, Fulton K, Rasmussen J (2008). A double-blind comparison of sexual functioning, antidepressant efficacy, and tolerability between agomelatine and venlafaxine XR. *Journal of Clinical Psychopharmacology* **28**, 329–333.

Kessler RC, Berglund P, Demler O et al. (2003). The epidemiology of major depressive disorder: results from the National Comorbidity Survey Replication (NCS-R). *Journal of the American Medical Association* **289**, 3095–3105.

Khan A, Leventhal RM, Khan SR, Brown WA (2002). Severity of depression and response to antidepressants and placebo: an analysis of the Food and Drug Administration database. *Journal of Clinical Psychopharmacology* **22**, 40–45.

Kirsch I, Deacon BJ, Huedo-Medina TB et al. (2008). Initial severity and antidepressant benefits: a meta-analysis of data submitted to the Food and Drug Administration. *PLoS Medicine/Public Library of Science* **5**, e45.

Lauterbach E, Felber W, Muller-Oerlinghausen B et al. (2008). Adjunctive lithium treatment in the prevention of suicidal behaviour in depressive disorders: a randomised, placebo-controlled, 1-year trial. *Acta Psychiatrica Scandinavica* **118**, 469–479.

Leon AC (2007). The revised warning for antidepressants and suicidality: unveiling the black box of statistical analyses. *American Journal of Psychiatry* **164**, 1786–1789.

Leon AC, Solomon DA, Mueller TI et al. (2003). A 20-year longitudinal observational study of somatic antidepressant treatment effectiveness. *American Journal of Psychiatry* **160**, 727–733.

Maj M, Veltro F, Pirozzi R et al. (1992). Pattern of recurrence of illness after recovery from an episode of major depression: a prospective study. *American Journal of Psychiatry* **149**, 795–800.

McGrath PJ, Khan AY, Trivedi MH et al. (2008). Response to a selective serotonin reuptake inhibitor (citalopram) in major depressive disorder with melancholic features: a STAR*D report. *Journal of Clinical Psychiatry* **69**, 1847–1855.

McGrath PJ, Stewart JW, Fava M et al. (2006). Tranylcypromine *vs.* venlafaxine plus mirtazapine following three failed antidepressant medication trials for depression: a STAR*D report. *American Journal of Psychiatry* **163**, 1531–1541.

McMahon FJ, Buervenich S, Charney D *et al.* (2006). Variation in the gene encoding the serotonin 2A receptor is associated with outcome of antidepressant treatment. *American Journal of Human Genetics* **78**, 804–814.

Montejo AL, Prieto N, Terleira A *et al.* (2010). Better sexual acceptability of agomelatine (25 and 50 mg) compared with paroxetine (20 mg) in healthy male volunteers. An 8-week, placebo-controlled study using the PRSEXDQ-SALSEX scale. *Journal of Psychopharmacology* **24**, 111–120.

Mueller TI, Leon AC, Keller MB *et al.* (1999). Recurrence after recovery from major depressive disorder during 15 years of observational follow-up. *American Journal of Psychiatry* **156**, 1000–1006.

Mulder RT, Joyce PR, Frampton CM *et al.* (2008). Antidepressant treatment is associated with a reduction in suicidal ideation and suicide attempts. *Acta Psychiatrica Scandinavica* **118**, 116–122.

Nakagawa A, Grunebaum MF, Ellis SP *et al.* (2007). Association of suicide and antidepressant prescription rates in Japan, 1999–2003. *Journal of Clinical Psychiatry* **68**, 908–916.

Nelson JC, Papakostas GI (2009). Atypical antipsychotic augmentation in major depressive disorder: a meta-analysis of placebo-controlled randomized trials. *American Journal of Psychiatry* **166**, 980–991.

Nierenberg AA, Amsterdam JD (1990). Treatment-resistant depression: definition and treatment approaches. *Journal of Clinical Psychiatry* **51** (Suppl.), 39–47.

Nierenberg AA, Farabaugh AH, Alpert JE *et al.* (2000). Timing of onset of antidepressant response with fluoxetine treatment. *American Journal of Psychiatry* **157**, 1423–1428.

Nierenberg AA, Husain MM, Trivedi MH *et al.* (2010). Residual symptoms after remission of major depressive disorder with citalopram and risk of relapse: a STAR*D report. *Psychological Medicine* **40**, 41–50.

Nierenberg AA, Papakostas GI, Petersen T *et al.* (2003). Lithium augmentation of nortriptyline for subjects resistant to multiple antidepressants. *Journal of Clinical Psychopharmacology* **23**, 92–95.

Papakostas GI (2009). The role of S-adenosyl methionine in the treatment of depression. *Journal of Clinical Psychiatry* **70** (Suppl. 5), 18–22.

Papakostas GI, Homberger CH, Fava M (2008). A meta-analysis of clinical trials comparing mirtazapine with selective serotonin reuptake inhibitors for the treatment of major depressive disorder. *Journal of Psychopharmacology* **22**, 843–848.

Papakostas GI, Mischoulon D, Shyu I *et al.* (2010). S-adenosyl methionine (SAMe) augmentation of serotonin reuptake inhibitors for antidepressant nonresponders with major depressive disorder: a double-blind, randomized clinical trial. *American Journal of Psychiatry* **167**, 942–948.

Papakostas GI, Perlis RH, Scalia MJ *et al.* (2006). A meta-analysis of early sustained response rates between antidepressants and placebo for the treatment of major depressive disorder. *Journal of Clinical Psychopharmacology* **26**, 56–60.

Papakostas GI, Peterson T, Sklarsky KG *et al.* (2007*b*). Timing of clinical improvement and symptom resolution in the treatment of major depressive disorder. *Psychiatry Research* **149**, 195–200.

Papakostas GI, Thase ME, Fava M *et al.* (2007*a*). Are antidepressant drugs that combine serotonergic and noradrenergic mechanisms of action more effective than the selective serotonin reuptake inhibitors in treating major depressive disorder? A meta-analysis of studies of newer agents. *Biological Psychiatry* **62**, 1217–1227.

Perlis RH, Moorjani P, Fagerness J *et al.* (2008). Pharmacogenetic analysis of genes implicated in rodent models of antidepressant response: association of TREK 1 and treatment resistance in the STAR(*)D study. *Neuropsychopharmacology* **33**, 2810–2819.

Perlis RH, Patrick A, Smoller JW, Wang PS (2009). When is pharmacogenetic testing for antidepressant response ready for the clinic? A cost-effectiveness analysis based on data from the STAR*D study. *Neuropsychopharmacology* **34**, 2227–2236.

Pintor L, Gasto C, Navarro V et al. (2003). Relapse of major depression after complete and partial remission during a 2-year follow-up. Journal of Affective Disorders 73, 237–244.

Posternak M, Novak S, Stern R et al. (2008). A pilot effectiveness study: placebo-controlled trial of adjunctive L-triiodothyronine (T3) used to accelerate and potentiate the antidepressant response. International Journal of Neuropsychopharmacology 11, 15–25.

Rasmussen NA, Schroder P, Olsen LR et al. (2005). Modafinil augmentation in depressed patients with partial response to antidepressants: a pilot study on self-reported symptoms covered by the Major Depression Inventory (MDI) and the Symptoms Checklist (SCL-92). Nordic Journal of Psychiatry 59, 173–178.

Roy-Byrne P, Post RM, Uhde TW et al. (1985). The longitudinal course of recurrent affective illness: life chart data from research patients at the NIMH. Acta Psychiatrica Scandinavica (Suppl.) 7, 3–34.

Ruhe HG, Huyser J, Swinkels JA, Schene AH (2006). Switching antidepressants after a first selective serotonin reuptake inhibitor in major depressive disorder: a systematic review. Journal of Clinical Psychiatry 67, 1836–1855.

Rush AJ, Trivedi MH, Wisniewski SR et al. (2006a). Acute and longer-term outcomes in depressed outpatients requiring one or several treatment steps: a STAR*D report. American Journal of Psychiatry 163, 1905–1917.

Rush AJ, Trivedi MH, Wisniewski SR et al. (2006b). Bupropion-SR, sertraline, or venlafaxine-XR after failure of SSRIs for depression. New England Journal of Medicine 354, 1231–1242.

Rush AJ, Wisniewski SR, Warden D et al. (2008). Selecting among second-step antidepressant medication monotherapies: predictive value of clinical, demographic, or first-step treatment features. Archives of General Psychiatry 65, 870–880.

Sanacora G (2009). Do glutamatergic agents represent a new class of antidepressant drugs? Part 1. Journal of Clinical Psychiatry 70, 1473–1474.

Schindler F, Anghelescu IG (2007). Lithium vs. lamotrigine augmentation in treatment resistant unipolar depression: a randomized, open-label study. International Clinical Psychopharmacology 22, 179–182.

Serretti A, Kato M, De Ronchi D, Kinoshita T (2007). Meta-analysis of serotonin transporter gene promoter polymorphism (5-HTTLPR) association with selective serotonin reuptake inhibitor efficacy in depressed patients. Molecular Psychiatry 12, 247–257.

Simpson HB, Nee JC, Endicott J (1997). First-episode major depression: few sex differences in course. Archives of General Psychiatry 54, 633–639.

Solomon DA, Keller MB, Leon AC et al. (2000). Multiple recurrences of major depressive disorder. American Journal of Psychiatry 157, 229–233.

Stahl SM, Fava M, Trivedi MH et al. (2010). Agomelatine in the treatment of major depressive disorder: an 8-week, multicenter, randomized, placebo-controlled trial. Journal of Clinical Psychiatry 71, 616–626.

Trivedi MH, Fava M, Wisniewski SR, Thase ME (2006). Medication augmentation after the failure of SSRIs for depression. New England Journal of Medicine 354, 1243–1252.

Uher R, Huczo-Diaz P, Perroud N et al. (2009). Genetic predictors of response to antidepressants in the GENDEP project. Pharmacogenomics Journal 4, 225–233.

Versiani M, Moreno R, Ramakers-van Moorsel CJ, Schutte AJ (2005). Comparative Efficacy Antidepressants Study Group. Comparison of the effects of mirtazapine and fluoxetine in severely depressed patients. CNS Drugs 19, 137–146.

Wade AG, Schlaepfer TE, Andersen HF, Kilts CD (2009). Clinical milestones predict symptom remission over 6-month and choice of treatment of patients with major depressive disorder (MDD). Journal of Psychiatric Research 43, 568–575.

Weihs KL, Houser T, Batey SR et al. (2002). Continuation phase treatment with bupropion SR effectively decreases the risk for relapse of depression. Biological Psychiatry 51, 753–761.

Wilson K, Mottram P, Sivanranthan A, Nightingale A (2003). Antidepressants *vs.* placebo for the depressed elderly. *Cochrane Database of Systematic Reviews* 2, CD000561.

Zajecka J, Schatzberg A, Stahl S *et al.* (2010). Efficacy and safety of agomelatine in the treatment of major depressive disorder: a multicenter, randomized, double-blind, placebo-controlled trial. *Journal of Clinical Psychopharmacology* 30, 135–144.

Zarate CA Jr, Singh JB, Carlson PJ *et al.* (2006a). A randomized trial of an N-methyl-D-aspartate antagonist in treatment-resistant major depression. *Archives of General Psychiatry* 63, 856–864.

Zarate CA, Singh JB, Quiroz JA *et al.* (2006b). A double-blind, placebo-controlled study of memantine in the treatment of major depression. *American Journal of Psychiatry* 163, 153–155.

Zimmerman M, Posternak MA, Chelminski I (2002). Symptom severity and exclusion from antidepressant efficacy trials. *Journal of Clinical Psychopharmacology* 22, 610–614.

Evidence-based pharmacotherapy of panic disorder

Neeltje M. Batelaan, Anton J. L. M. Van Balkom, and
Dan J. Stein

Introduction

Panic disorder is a common mental disorder that is associated with significant morbidity.
Fortunately, effective treatments for panic disorder are available, and include both medication and cognitive–behavioral therapy (CBT). Ongoing research on the pharmacotherapy of
panic disorder makes it timely to update an evidence-based approach to the pharmacotherapy of panic disorder (Bakker *et al.*, 2005). Here we briefly emphasize the importance of
adequate care before reviewing the available pharmacological evidence on treating panic disorder, focusing in particular on (1) the optimal first-line pharmacotherapy of panic disorder,
(2) the optimal duration of maintenance therapy, and (3) the optimal approach to pharmacotherapy in the treatment-refractory patient. To reveal relevant research conducted since the
publication of Bakker *et al.* (2005), a MEDLINE search (2003–2010) using the terms 'panic'
and 'treatment' was undertaken.

Importance of adequate care

Panic disorder is a common mental disorder, with a 12-month prevalence rate of 1.8% (Goodwin *et al.*, 2005). Only a minority of those affected receive adequate care. The main reason is
that not all patients seek help. It may take years before individuals with panic disorder seek
help; only about one third of those affected seek help within the year of onset (Wang *et al.*,
2005*a*). The gap between those affected and those seeking help for panic disorder is about
50% (Kohn *et al.*, 2004; Wang *et al.*, 2005*b*).

When seeking help, individuals with panic disorder frequently turn to medical special-
ists or to emergency units (Hirschfeld, 1996; Katerndahl & Realini, 1995; Leon *et al.*, 1995;
Rees *et al.*, 1998; Salvador-Carulla *et al.*, 1995), likely due to the predominance of physical
symptoms. Misdiagnosis by the general practitioner (Rees *et al.*, 1998) or by the cardiologist
at the emergency unit is common (Harvison *et al.*, 2004; Kuijpers *et al.*, 2000). Thus, even
those who seek help often go unrecognized.

Once the correct diagnosis has been made, delivery of care is often not in concordance
with the advice provided in practice guidelines (Bruce *et al.*, 2003). It is regrettable that only
a minority of individuals with panic disorder receive evidence-based treatment, given the
unfavorable long-term course of panic disorder and the impact of panic on daily life. We
briefly discuss these aspects below.

Essential Evidence-Based Psychopharmacology, Second Edition, ed. Dan J. Stein, Bernard Lerer,
and Stephen M. Stahl. Published by Cambridge University Press. © Cambridge University Press.

Course

The course of panic disorder in the general population may be chronic or recurrent (Batelaan *et al.*, 2010*a*, 2010*b*; Eaton *et al.*, 1998; Kessler *et al.*, 2006; Wittchen *et al.*, 2008). In addition, comorbid disorders tend to develop during the course of panic disorder (de Graaf *et al.*, 2003; Johnson *et al.*, 1990; Kessler *et al.*, 1998; Wittchen *et al.*, 2003). Finally, it should be noted that even when panic symptoms remit, other psychiatric pathology may be present (Wittchen *et al.*, 2008).

Impact

Panic disorder has a negative impact on well-being and on health perception (Katerndahl & Realini, 1997; Klerman *et al.*, 1991), and is associated with impaired functioning (Kessler *et al.*, 2006; Wittchen *et al.*, 1998) and absence from work (Alonso *et al.*, 2004; Kouzis & Eaton, 1994, 1997). In addition, panic disorder may be associated with suicidal ideation and/or attempts (Cougle *et al.*, 2009; Goodwin & Roy-Byrne, 2006; Lepine *et al.*, 1993; Weissman *et al.*, 1989), though the impact of comorbid disorders on this association is a matter of debate (Hornig & McNally, 1995) and though the evidence that panic disorder causes suicidality remains unclear (Sareen *et al.*, 2005*a*). Panic disorder is also associated with medical morbidity, including cardiovascular disease (Chen *et al.*, 2009; Gomez-Caminero *et al.*, 2005; Sareen *et al.*, 2005*b*; Smoller *et al.*, 2007). Some studies report increased mortality rates in individuals with panic disorder as a result of suicide (Coryell *et al.*, 1982) or cardiovascular disease (Coryell *et al.*, 1982; Grasbeck *et al.*, 1996; Smoller *et al.*, 2007). Finally, panic disorder causes considerable economic costs to society, both compared with healthy persons and to other psychiatric disorders (Andlin-Sobocki & Wittchen, 2005; Batelaan *et al.*, 2007; Salvador-Carulla *et al.*, 1995).

Available pharmacological evidence

Pharmacological agents with sufficient evidence to support their use in the treatment of panic disorder include antidepressants (the SSRIs, the SNRI venlafaxine, several TCAs and the irreversible MAO-inhibitor phenelzine), and benzodiazepines. First, we will review antidepressants and benzodiazepines with regard to efficacy in acute and long-term treatment, the side-effects and risks involved, drop-out rates, onset of action and efficacy in comorbid conditions. This comparison will be used to determine which agents should be considered first-line treatments. Subsequently we will review data on optimal duration of maintenance therapy and optimal approach to pharmacotherapy of the treatment-refractory patient.

Antidepressants

Efficacy in acute phase treatment

Antidepressants acting on the serotonergic system are effective in treating panic disorder. These include the SSRIs (citalopram, fluvoxamine, fluoxetine, paroxetine, and sertraline) (Bakker *et al.*, 2002; Hoehn-Saric *et al.*, 1993; Lecrubier *et al.*, 1997; Michelson *et al.*, 1998; Pollack *et al.*, 1998; Stahl *et al.*, 2003; Wade *et al.*, 1997), the TCAs imipramine and clomipramine (Cross National Collaborative Panic Study, 1992; Papp *et al.*, 1997) the SNRI venlafaxine (Bradwejn *et al.*, 2005; Liebowitz *et al.*, 2009; Pollack *et al.*, 2007*a*, 2007*b*), and the irreversible MAO-inhibitor phenelzine (Sheehan *et al.*, 1980; Tyrer *et al.*, 1973).

Table 5.1. Dosage of drugs effective in panic disorder (in mg/day).

Drug name		Start	Mean	Maximum
Antidepressants				
SSRI				
	citalopram	10	20–30	60
	escitalopram	5	10	20
	fluoxetine	20	20	60
	fluvoxamine	50	100–150	300
	paroxetine	10	20–40	60
	sertraline	50	100	200
SNRI				
	venlafaxine	37.5	75–150	225
TCA				
	clomipramine	25	100–150	250
	imipramine	25	100–150	300
Benzodiazepines				
	alprazolam	1.5	4–6	*
	clonazepam	1	2–3	*
	diazepam	5–10	40–50	*
	lorazepam	1	2–4	*
MAO-inhibitor				
	phenelzine	10	40–60	*

* Only use mean dosage.

During the past few years the SSRIs paroxetine controlled-release formulation (paroxetine CR) and escitalopram, and the SNRI venlafaxine extended-release (venlafaxine XR) have been thoroughly investigated in panic disorder. Three double-blind placebo-controlled trials investigating paroxetine CR were pooled, allowing analysis of a total study population of 889 panic disorder patients. Paroxetine CR (25–75 mg/day) was superior to placebo on the primary outcome measure, percentage of patients who were free of panic attacks in the 2 weeks prior to end-point (Sheehan *et al.*, 2005). In a 10-week randomized controlled double-blind trial (total $n = 366$; $n = 128$ with escitalopram), escitalopram (5–10 mg/day) was more effective than placebo (Stahl *et al.*, 2003). Finally, the SNRI venlafaxine XR (75–225 mg/day) has been found significantly more effective than placebo in several randomized controlled double-blind trials (Bradwejn *et al.*, 2005; Liebowitz *et al.*, 2009; Pollack *et al.*, 2007a, 2007b; see for an overview Kjernisted & McIntosh, 2007). The daily dosages of these antidepressants when used for panic disorder are similar to those used for major depressive disorder (see Table 5.1).

Efficacy in long-term treatment

The SSRIs (i.e. citalopram, fluvoxamine, and paroxetine) (Holland *et al.*, 1994; Lecrubier & Judge, 1997; Lepola *et al.*, 1998) and the TCAs (Curtis *et al.*, 1993; Lecrubier & Judge, 1997; Mavissakalian & Perel, 1992) all remain effective in the treatment of panic disorder over the long term (follow-up periods up until 2 years). Recently, a 6-month placebo-controlled discontinuation study found that time to relapse was significantly longer in the venlafaxine XR group than the placebo-group (Ferguson *et al.*, 2007). No studies investigating the long-term efficacy of phenelzine have been conducted.

Side-effects and risks involved

Side-effects of antidepressants partly differ across various classes of antidepressants (American Psychiatric Association, 2009). The most common side-effects of the SSRIs include headaches, irritability, gastrointestinal complaints, insomnia, sexual dysfunction, weight gain, increased anxiety, drowsiness, and tremor. The most common side-effects of venlafaxine as reported in panic-disorder patients are nausea, dry mouth, constipation, anorexia, insomnia, sweating, somnolence, tremor, and sexual dysfunction. Monitoring of blood pressure is advised given the increase in blood pressure that is sometimes observed. In TCAs the most commonly reported side-effects in panic-disorder patients are anticholinergic effects, increased sweating, sleep disturbance, orthostatic hypotension and dizziness, fatigue and weakness, cognitive disturbance, weight gain, and sexual dysfunction. Specific concern is needed when treating elderly patients with TCAs as orthostatic hypotension may result in falls. In addition, arrhythmias may occur in patients with preexisting cardiac conduction abnormalities, and in case of an overdose. The irreversible MAO-inhibitor phenelzine has an unfavorable side-effect profile, including hypotension, weight gain, sexual dysfunction, paresthesia, myoclonic jerks, dry mouth, edema, and sleeping problems. Probably more important, to avoid life-threatening hypertensive crisis, adherence to a strict tyramine low diet is required (Rosenberg, 1999). To prevent side-effects, it is advised to start treatment with antidepressants at a lower dosage. Of special importance is the finding that panic symptoms often increase in the first weeks of treatment with SSRIs, venlafaxine, or TCAs. This may be partly due to misinterpreting physical side-effects as symptoms of a panic attack. Psycho-education should aim to prevent such misinterpretations, and slow dose titration is recommended. To lower anxiety symptoms and to achieve a more rapid stabilization of panic symptoms, temporary addition of benzodiazepines during the initial phase of antidepressant treatment can also be considered (Goddard et al., 2001; Pollack et al., 2003).

Drop-out rates

During SSRI treatment of panic disorder 18% of patients drop out prematurely (Bakker et al., 2002). The recently investigated agents paroxetine CR, escitalopram, and venlafaxine are all well tolerated in panic-disorder patients, and hence, reported drop-out rates were relatively low: 11% of patients treated with paroxetine CR (Sheehan et al., 2005), 6.3% of patients treated with escitalopram (Stahl et al., 2003) and ranging from 1–12% of patients treated with venlafaxine (Kjernisted & McIntosh, 2007). With TCAs, about 30% of patients drop out of treatment (Bakker et al., 2002). Due to the unfavorable side-effect profile of MAO-inhibitors, drop-out rates are high.

Onset of action

For all antidepressants, onset of action in panic disorder is relatively slow. As a result, an assessment of outcome should be made only after several weeks of treatment.

Efficacy in comorbid conditions

Antidepressants are effective for a range of anxiety disorders and depressive disorder, which are commonly comorbid with panic disorder (Bandelow et al., 2008).

Benzodiazepines

Efficacy in acute phase treatment

The benzodiazepines alprazolam, clonazepam, diazepam, and lorazepam are superior to placebo in the acute phase treatment of panic disorder (Cross National Collaborative Panic Study, 1992; van Balkom et al., 1997, 1995). The mean dosages of the benzodiazepines used in acute treatment are provided in Table 5.1.

Efficacy in long-term treatment

Controlled studies up until 32 weeks with alprazolam (Ballenger, 1991; Burrows et al., 1993), and an open study with clonazepam lasting over one year (Pollack et al., 1986) showed that these benzodiazepines are efficacious in maintenance treatment. Sometimes the daily dosage could be reduced whilst remaining efficacious.

Side-effects and risks involved

Side-effects of benzodiazepines include sedation, fatigue, ataxia, slurred speech, memory impairment, and weakness (American Psychiatric Association, 2009). Usually, treatment is started at a low dose to diminish side-effects. Caution is advised in prescribing benzodiazepines in elderly patients because of a higher risk of falls, and in patients driving vehicles because of a higher risk of motor vehicle accidents. When prescribed for long-term use, dependence may occur. Hypothetically, this may have two adverse consequences: dose escalation and problems withdrawing the medication. While dose escalation does not appear a common consequence of long-term benzodiazepine use, problems when discontinuing benzodiazepines are frequently reported, especially during the last half of the taper period (American Psychiatric Association, 2009).

Drop-out rates

In panic disorder trials, drop-out rates due to side-effects are about 15% for benzodiazepines (Landelijke Stuurgroep Multidisciplinaire Richtlijnontwikkeling in de GGZ, 2009).

Onset of action

Benzodiazepines have a fast onset of action, i.e. they show effects as soon as an effective dose is administered (Burrows & Norman, 1999).

Efficacy in comorbid conditions

Benzodiazepines are generally thought ineffective for comorbid depressive disorders (Bandelow et al., 2008).

Optimal first-line pharmacotherapy

With regard to efficacy in acute treatment, comparable efficacy has been revealed when directly comparing antidepressants (imipramine) and benzodiazepines (alprazolam, clonazepam) (van Balkom et al., 1995), SSRIs and TCAs (Bakker et al., 1999, 2002; Lecrubier et al.,

1997; Otto *et al.*, 2001; Wade *et al.*, 1997), and when comparing various SSRIs (Dannon *et al.*, 2007). In one study, a high dosage of venlafaxine (225 mg) proved to be superior to paroxetine 40 mg on the primary outcome measure (percentage of patients free from full-symptom panic attacks) and on one of the secondary outcome measures (improvement on the Panic Disorder Severity Scale) (Pollack *et al.*, 2007*a*). In panic disorder, only one trial administered either escitalopram, citalopram, or placebo. However, in this trial no direct comparisons between escitalopram and citalopram were made (Stahl *et al.*, 2003). As described above, both antidepressants (SSRIs, SNRI venlafaxine, and TCAs) and benzodiazepines remain effective over the long term.

Given the comparable efficacy of the pharmacological classes described above in acute phase treatment and the efficacy in long-term treatment, other considerations determine which agent should be considered the first-line pharmacotherapy of panic disorder. These include side-effects and risks involved, drop-out rates, the time of onset of action, and efficacy in comorbid symptomatology.

Considering these aspects, both SSRIs and venlafaxine should be considered first-line agents. Given the slow onset of action and the potential for increased anxiety during the initial phase of treatment with antidepressants, temporary co-administration of a benzodiazepine should be considered. SSRIs and venlafaxine are effective in acute and long-term treatment, have an acceptable side-effect profile, acceptable drop-out rate, and are effective in comorbid depression. Direct comparisons between SSRIs and venlafaxine with regard to onset of action, side-effect profile, or drop-out rates have not been made in panic disorder. Likewise, direct comparisons of the tolerability profile and onset of action of recently investigated agents (paroxetine CR and escitalopram) and other SSRIs are lacking.

TCAs may have a slower onset than SSRIs (Lecrubier *et al.*, 1997). In addition, TCAs have a less tolerable side-effect profile than SSRIs given that they have more anticholinergic effects, and are generally less safe than SSRIs. Finally, reported drop-out rates are higher in TCAs compared with SSRIs (Bakker *et al.*, 2002).

Benzodiazepines have a faster onset of action and have lower drop-out rates compared with TCAs (van Balkom *et al.*, 1995). The tolerability of benzodiazepines is usually good, but patients may suffer from drowsiness and cognitive side-effects. Another disadvantage is that these drugs may lead to benzodiazepine dependence. Moreover, benzodiazepines are generally thought ineffective with regard to comorbid psychopathology such as depressive disorders, whereas antidepressants are effective (Bandelow *et al.*, 2008). This is of importance, because depressive disorders often complicate panic disorder (Ravelli *et al.*, 1998). In summary, benzodiazepines as a monotherapy should not be regarded as a first-line treatment in view of their side-effect profile (which includes dependence) and in view of their lack of efficacy in treating comorbid conditions.

The irreversible MAO-inhibitor phenelzine should be prescribed only in case of severe and treatment-refractory panic disorder given the side-effect profile and risks involved, and the high drop-out rates.

Optimal duration of pharmacotherapy

Considering the long-lasting, often relapsing course of panic disorder, optimizing the long-term outcome and thus reducing the vulnerability to relapse should be a main goal of treatment (Andrews, 2003; Batelaan *et al.*, 2010*a*; Fava & Mangelli, 1999). Discontinuation of pharmacotherapy frequently results in relapse (Ferguson *et al.*, 2007; Lecrubier & Judge,

1997; Lotufo-Neto et al., 2001; Marks et al., 1993; Mavissakalian & Perel, 1999; Noyes Jr. et al., 1989, 1991; Rapaport et al., 2001; Spiegel et al., 1994). For example, 37% of patients experienced a relapse within 10 weeks after discontinuing clomipramine, and another 43% of patients within about 1.5 years (Lotufo-Neto et al., 2001), over one-third relapsed within the first year of imipramine discontinuation (Mavissakalian & Perel, 1999), and half of those who discontinued venlafaxine relapsed within half a year (Ferguson et al., 2007).

The consistent finding that maintenance pharmacotherapy may prevent relapse when compared with medication discontinuation (Donovan et al., 2010) can be considered an argument to continue pharmacotherapy for a longer period. Another argument for continuing pharmacotherapy is that during maintenance treatment, further improvements can be seen (Ballenger, 2000; Lecrubier & Judge, 1997). However, many remitted patients discontinue antidepressant treatment. Studies investigating treatment adherence of anxiety-disorder patients and, more specifically of panic-disorder patients, reported that more than half of the patients are non-compliant or interrupt treatment within several months to years (Stein et al., 2006; Toni et al., 2004).

A crucial question is what the optimal duration of pharmacotherapy is, such that patients can discontinue pharmacotherapy relatively safely (i.e. without a substantial risk to relapse), and do not take medication longer than necessary. Research with regard to the optimum duration of pharmacotherapy is sparse; results so far, however, do not indicate the existence of a "safe" period to withdraw from medication. In a study conducted by Mavissakalian and Perel, the duration of treatment with imipramine following response was not associated with relapse: relapse occurred as frequently after 6 months of treatment as after 12 to 30 months of treatment (Mavissakalian & Perel, 2002). In addition, Choy and colleagues reported that even after 3 years of sustained remission while taking medication, relapse occurs more often and earlier in those who discontinue medication compared with those who continue pharmacological treatment (Choy et al., 2007). However, because this is a naturalistic study, a firm causal relation cannot be presumed.

Given the limited empirical data available, international guidelines differ slightly in their recommendations on maintenance treatment. Whereas the guideline from the American Psychiatric Association refrains from recommendations (American Psychiatric Association, 2009), most guidelines refer to expert consensus and suggest continuation for at least a year (Andrews, 2003; Bandelow et al., 2008; Landelijke Stuurgroep Multidisciplinaire Richtlijn-ontwikkeling in de GGZ, 2009), though a shorter period has also been suggested (Baldwin et al., 2005; Canadian Psychiatric Association, 2006).

When medication is being discontinued, consensus advice is to taper down the medication gradually over weeks to months (American Psychiatric Association, 2009; Andrews, 2003; Baldwin et al., 2005; Landelijke Stuurgroep Multidisciplinaire Richtlijnontwikkeling in de GGZ, 2009) to reduce the likelihood of discontinuation symptoms and to monitor for early signs of relapse.

To reduce the risk for relapse and optimize the long-term outcome in panic disorder, research on the optimal duration of pharmacotherapy should be conducted, as well as research on how to optimize treatment adherence. In addition, other lines of research may also be fruitful.

First, predictors for relapse should be identified, because those at the highest risk for relapse may benefit most from long-term maintenance treatment, and it can be hypothesized that patients at the highest risk for relapse are more motivated for long-term maintenance treatment. In addition, costs of long-term maintenance treatment for those at highest risk to relapse may well be acceptable given the costs associated with recurrence of panic disorder.

Second, the question of whether maintenance treatment with lower dosages will suffice to maintain acute phase improvements is worthy of further study, given previous results of a small study in which patients maintained their improvement when imipramine was continued at half the dosage (Mavissakalian & Perel, 1992), and studies indicating that the daily dosage of benzodiazepines can be reduced whilst remaining efficacious (Ballenger, 1991; Burrows *et al.*, 1993; Pollack *et al.*, 1986).

Third, providing psychotherapy to panic-disorder patients may also be beneficial in enhancing the long-term outcome for several reasons, the most important reason being that the effects of cognitive–behavioral therapy (CBT) may be maintained over time (Bakker *et al.*, 1998; Fava *et al.*, 2001; Oei *et al.*, 1999; Peter *et al.*, 2008). In addition, some evidence indicates that a CBT relapse prevention program provided after acute phase treatment prevents relapse in patients with panic disorder (Wright *et al.*, 2000) and that adding brief psychodynamic psychotherapy to clomipramine treatment may reduce relapse rates in panic disorder (Wiborg & Dahl, 1996). Finally, a few studies have shown that CBT may also prevent relapse or worsening of panic in patients who discontinue pharmacological treatment (Bruce *et al.*, 1999; Choy *et al.*, 2007; Furukawa *et al.*, 2007; Schmidt *et al.*, 2002; Spiegel *et al.*, 1994; Whittal *et al.*, 2001).

Optimal approach to pharmacotherapy in the treatment-refractory patient

Despite the availability of treatments with reported efficacy, a substantial number of panic-disorder patients do not respond, or respond partially to treatment. For example, Pollack *et al.* (2007*b*) reported response rates between 70–80% and remission rates around 45% during the acute treatment of panic disorder with venlafaxine, thereby underscoring the need for additional treatment strategies to achieve full remission. There are however few data to guide clinicians in next-step treatment strategies (Ipser *et al.*, 2006). The approach to treatment-refractory patients may consist of optimizing the current treatment, switching to another agent or treatment modality, or augmentation.

Optimizing treatment

With regard to optimizing the current pharmacotherapy, it may be useful to investigate whether the patient is adhering to the treatment regimen, given the high rates of non-compliance with pharmacological treatment. In addition, it should be noted that during maintenance treatment, further improvements may occur (Ballenger, 2000; Lecrubier & Judge, 1997). With regard to the dosage, assessing the blood level of imipramine may be helpful (Mavissakalian & Perel, 1995). By contrast, a small study reported that an increased dosage of an SSRI was no more effective than continuing the previous dosage (Simon *et al.*, 2009*b*), a finding that is in line with recent research on the absence of additional effects when increasing the SSRI dose in depressed patients (Ruhe *et al.*, 2009).

Switching

Switching within or between classes of pharmacological agents seems a reasonable option. Based on safety and tolerability issues described above, we propose the following steps: SSRI or venlafaxine, another SSRI or venlafaxine, clomipramine or imipramine, benzodiazepine, MAO-inhibitor. Switching to another treatment modality with proven efficacy in treating panic disorder, such as CBT, is also a reasonable option. CBT is effective in panic disorder (Furukawa et al., 2007), and positive effects have been reported of CBT in studies with panic-disorder patients who failed to respond adequately to pharmacological treatment (Rodrigues et al., 2011).

In addition, a wide range of other pharmacological agents has been suggested for the treatment of panic disorder. These include SNRIs other than venlafaxine (Blaya et al., 2007; Simon et al., 2009a), the selective noradrenergic reuptake inhibitor reboxetine (Bertani et al., 2004; Dannon et al., 2002; Seedat et al., 2003; Versiani et al., 2002), GABA-ergic treatment including vigabatrin and tiagabine (Pande et al., 2000; Zwanzger & Rupprecht, 2005; Zwanzger et al., 2009a), the reversible MAO-inhibitor moclobemide (Kruger & Dahl, 1999; Loerch et al., 1999; Ross et al., 2010; Tiller et al., 1999; Uhlenhuth et al., 2002), other antidepressants including mirtazepine, buproprion, trazodone (American Psychiatric Association, 2009), anticonvulsants (Mula et al., 2007; Papp, 2006), the antipsychotic olanzapine (Hollifield et al., 2005), and antihypertensives (American Psychiatric Association, 2009). None of these agents can be considered as first-line options for the pharmacological treatment of panic disorder because they are insufficiently investigated or because results were inconsistent. To determine their role in treating panic disorder, randomized controlled trials of sufficient sample sizes are needed to verify results and to compare both efficacy and tolerability with more established treatments. A clinician could potentially consider prescribing these agents in treatment-refractory patients, prioritizing those agents for which there is the most data on efficacy and tolerability.

The agents for which there are most data on efficacy and tolerability are the SNRIs milnacipran and duloxetine and the selective noradrenergic reuptake inhibitor reboxetine. This is not very surprising given the efficacy of the SNRI venlafaxine in the treatment of panic disorder and the noradrenergic role in the pathophysiology of panic disorder. Small open-label studies showed positive results for the SNRIs milnacipran (Blaya et al., 2007) and duloxetine (Simon et al., 2009a). Reboxetine has been investigated in several small studies. In a single-blind, cross-over study, reboxetine was as effective as citalopram with regard to panic, though less effective than citalopram with regard to co-occurring depressive symptoms (Seedat et al., 2003). In a single blind, randomized trial ($n = 68$), paroxetine showed larger effects on panic attacks than reboxetine, but no differences were found on anticipatory anxiety and avoidance (Bertani et al., 2004). In a double-blind randomized controlled trial reboxetine was more effective as compared to a placebo-group (Versiani et al., 2002). Finally, in a small open-label study, reboxetine showed positive effects for patients who had not responded to an SSRI (Dannon et al., 2002). Given these preliminary results, both these SNRIs and reboxetine might be an option when prescribing off-label agents in treatment-refractory patients.

Other treatment modalities with insufficient evidence to date can also be considered in treatment-refractory patients. It should be stressed that, given the design and size of the studies, these results also should be viewed as preliminary. Risk–benefit ratios should be taken into account. Options include repetitive transcranial magnetic stimulation and aerobic exercise. Repetitive transcranial magnetic stimulation has shown some beneficial effects for panic disorder in several small and open studies (Pigot et al., 2008; Zwanzger et al., 2009b). With regard to aerobic exercise, it was found that subsequent to exercise, panic-disorder patients had less frequent panic when challenged with carbon dioxide (Esquivel et al., 2008) or cholecystokinin tetrapeptide (CCK-4) as compared with controls who had no exercise or only very light exercise (Strohle *et al.*, 2009). In an early study aerobic exercise indeed reduced panic symptoms, but later and less effectively than medication (Broocks *et al.*, 1998). Results of a recent randomized controlled trial of aerobic exercise in panic-disorder patients were disappointing (Wedekind *et al.*, 2010).

Augmentation

Pharmacological treatment can be augmented by the use of additional medications, or by other treatment modalities. The incremental efficacy of combined psychotherapy (most often CBT) and antidepressant treatment was investigated in a Cochrane review including 21 trials in panic disorder (Furukawa *et al.*, 2007). The authors concluded that in the short term, combined therapy was superior to medication alone, as well as to psychotherapy alone. These findings were irrespective of the kind of antidepressant (TCA versus SSRI), irrespective of the presence of agoraphobia, and irrespective of the presence of comorbid depression. Six months after terminating treatment, combination therapy was more effective than medication alone, but was as effective as psychotherapy alone. This finding should be interpreted with some caution, given the naturalistic nature of the follow-up period, with a substantial proportion of patients receiving treatment of some kind (Furukawa *et al.*, 2007). Insufficient data are available to determine whether combining benzodiazepines and psychotherapy is beneficial or not (Watanabe *et al.*, 2007).

Augmenting benzodiazepines to antidepressant treatment is an option as this appeared equally effective compared with adding CBT to antidepressants in panic disorder. It should be noted though, that effects of both strategies were small in this study (Simon *et al.*, 2009*b*). In addition, augmentation of antidepressants with an antipsychotic has been suggested for refractory panic-disorder patients (Hoge *et al.*, 2008; Saito & Miyaoka, 2007; Sepede *et al.*, 2006; Simon *et al.*, 2006). Risk–benefit ratios should be carefully considered given the adverse effects of antipsychotics. D-cycloserine, a partial agonist of the N-methyl-D-aspartate glutamatergic receptor, has recently received attention because it may enhance fear extinction during exposure therapy (Hofmann, 2007). A small ($n = 31$) randomized, double-blind, placebo-controlled trial in which interoceptive exposure was augmented with either low doses of D-cycloserine or placebo showed that panic-disorder patients who received D-cycloserine had better outcomes, both at post-treatment, and at 1-month follow-up (Otto *et al.*, 2010).

Conclusion

Panic disorder is a prevalent and disabling disorder that can be treated effectively. However, only a minority of those suffering from panic disorder appear to be adequately treated. The first-line pharmacotherapy for panic disorder has been SSRIs for some time, and there is now sufficient evidence to indicate that the SNRI venlafaxine should also be considered as a first-line agent. Less is known about how improvements can be maintained and how relapses can be prevented in patients who have responded well to medication in the acute phase. In general, however, most treatment recommendations are conservative, advising at least a year of antidepressant treatment. Likewise, relatively little is known about how best to manage treatment-refractory panic disorder. Nevertheless, current options include a range of switching and augmentation strategies. Further research comparing these options is needed.

Statement of interest

Dr. Batelaan has received consultancy honoraria from Lundbeck. Dr. van Balkom has received research grants and/or consultancy honoraria from GlaxoSmithKline, Servier, Solvay, and Wyeth. Dr. Stein has received research grants and/or consultancy honoraria from AstraZeneca, Eli-Lilly, GlaxoSmithKline, Jazz Pharmaceuticals, Johnson & Johnson, Lundbeck, Orion, Pfizer, Pharmacia, Roche, Servier, Solvay, Sumitomo, Takeda, Tikvah, and Wyeth.

References

Alonso J, Angermeyer MC, Bernert S et al. (2004). Disability and quality of life impact of mental disorders in Europe: results from the European Study of the Epidemiology of Mental Disorders (ESEMeD) project. *Acta Psychiatrica Scandinavica* **420** (Suppl.), 38–46.

American Psychiatric Association (2009). *Practice Guidelines for the Treatment of Patients with Panic Disorder, 2nd edn.* Washington, DC: American Psychiatric Association.

Andlin-Sobocki P, Wittchen HU (2005). Cost of anxiety disorders in Europe. *European Journal of Neurology* **12** (Suppl. 1), 39–44.

Andrews G (2003). Australian and New Zealand clinical practice guidelines for the treatment of panic disorder and agoraphobia. *Australian and New Zealand Journal of Psychiatry* **37**, 641–656.

Bakker A, van Balkom AJ, Spinhoven P (2002). SSRIs *vs.* TCAs in the treatment of panic disorder: a meta-analysis. *Acta Psychiatrica Scandinavica* **106**, 163–167.

Bakker A, van Balkom AJ, Spinhoven P et al. (1998). Follow-up on the treatment of panic disorder with or without agoraphobia: a quantitative review. *Journal of Nervous and Mental Disease* **186**, 414–419.

Bakker A, van Balkom AJ, Stein DJ (2005). Evidence-based pharmacotherapy of panic disorder. *International Journal of Neuropsychopharmacology* **8**, 473–482.

Bakker A, van Dyck R, Spinhoven P, van Balkom AJ (1999). Paroxetine, clomipramine, and cognitive therapy in the treatment of panic disorder. *Journal of Clinical Psychiatry* **60**, 831–838.

Baldwin DS, Anderson IM, Nutt DJ et al. (2005). Evidence-based guidelines for the pharmacological treatment of anxiety disorders: recommendations from the British Association for Psychopharmacology. *Journal of Psychopharmacology* **19**, 567–596.

Ballenger JC (1991). Long-term pharmacologic treatment of panic disorder. *Journal of Clinical Psychiatry* **52** (Suppl.), 18–23.

Ballenger JC (2000). Panic disorder and agoraphobia. In Gelder MG, Lopez-lbor JJ, Andreasen NC (Eds.), *New Oxford Textbook of Psychiatry* (pp. 807–822). Oxford: Oxford University Press.

Bandelow B, Zohar J, Hollander E et al. (2008). World Federation of Societies of Biological Psychiatry (WFSBP) Guidelines for the pharmacological treatment of anxiety, obsessive-compulsive and post-traumatic stress disorders – first revision. *World Journal of Biological Psychiatry* **9**, 248–312.

Batelaan N, Smit F, de Graaf R et al. (2007). Economic costs of full-blown and subthreshold panic disorder. *Journal of Affective Disorders* **104**, 127–136.

Batelaan NM, de Graaf R, Penninx BW et al. (2010a). The 2-year prognosis of panic episodes in the general population. *Psychological Medicine* **40**, 147–157.

Batelaan NM, de Graaf R, Spijker J et al. (2010b). The course of panic attacks in individuals with panic disorder and subthreshold panic disorder: a population-based study. *Journal of Affective Disorders* **121**, 30–38.

Bertani A, Perna G, Migliarese G et al. (2004). Comparison of the treatment with paroxetine and reboxetine in panic disorder: a randomized, single-blind study. *Pharmacopsychiatry* **37**, 206–210.

Blaya C, Seganfredo AC, Dornelles M et al. (2007). The efficacy of milnacipran in panic disorder: an open trial. *International Clinical Psychopharmacology* **22**, 153–158.

Bradwejn J, Ahokas A, Stein DJ et al. (2005). Venlafaxine extended-release capsules in panic disorder: flexible-dose, double-blind, placebo-controlled study. *British Journal of Psychiatry* **187**, 352–359.

Broocks A, Bandelow B, Pekrun G et al. (1998). Comparison of aerobic exercise, clomipramine, and placebo in the treatment of panic disorder. *American Journal of Psychiatry* **155**, 603–609.

Bruce SE, Vasile RG, Goisman RM et al. (2003). Are benzodiazepines still the medication of choice for patients with panic disorder with or without agoraphobia? *American Journal of Psychiatry* **160**, 1432–1438.

Bruce TJ, Spiegel DA, Hegel MT (1999). Cognitive-behavioral therapy helps prevent relapse and recurrence of panic disorder following alprazolam discontinuation: a long-term follow-up of the Peoria and Dartmouth studies. *Journal of Consulting and Clinical Psychology* **67**, 151–156.

Burrows GD, Judd FK, Norman TR (1993). Long-term drug treatment of panic disorder. *Journal of Psychiatric Research* **27** (Suppl. 1), 111–125.

Burrows GD, Norman TR (1999). The treatment of panic disorder with benzodiazepines. In Nutt DJ, Ballenger JC, Lepine JP (Eds.), *Panic Disorder: Clinical Diagnosis, Management and Mechanisms* (pp. 145–158). London: Martin Dunitz.

Canadian Psychiatric Association (2006). Clinical practice guidelines. Management of anxiety disorders. *Canadian Journal of Psychiatry* **51** (Suppl.), 9–91.

Chen YH, Tsai SY, Lee HC, Lin HC (2009). Increased risk of acute myocardial infarction for patients with panic disorder: a nationwide population-based study. *Psychosomatic Medicine* **71**, 798–804.

Choy Y, Peselow ED, Case BG et al. (2007). Three-year medication prophylaxis in panic disorder: to continue or discontinue? A naturalistic study. *Comprehensive Psychiatry* **48**, 419–425.

Coryell W, Noyes R, Clancy J (1982). Excess mortality in panic disorder. A comparison with primary unipolar depression. *Archives of General Psychiatry* **39**, 701–703.

Cougle JR, Keough ME, Riccardi CJ, Sachs-Ericsson N (2009). Anxiety disorders and suicidality in the National Comorbidity Survey – Replication. *Journal of Psychiatric Research* **43**, 825–829.

Cross National Collaborative Panic Study (1992). Drug treatment of panic disorder. Comparative efficacy of alprazolam, imipramine, and placebo. Cross-National Collaborative Panic Study, Second Phase Investigators. *British Journal of Psychiatry* **160**, 191–202.

Curtis GC, Massana J, Udina C et al. (1993). Maintenance drug therapy of panic disorder. *Journal of Psychiatric Research* **27** (Suppl. 1), 127–142.

Dannon PN, Iancu I, Grunhaus L (2002). The efficacy of reboxetine in the treatment-refractory patients with panic disorder: an open label study. *Human Psychopharmacology* **17**, 329–333.

Dannon PN, Iancu I, Lowengrub K et al. (2007). A naturalistic long-term comparison study of selective serotonin reuptake inhibitors in the treatment of panic disorder. *Clinical Neuropharmacology* **30**, 326–334.

de Graaf R, Bijl RV, Spijker J et al. (2003). Temporal sequencing of lifetime mood disorders in relation to comorbid anxiety and substance use disorders – findings from the Netherlands Mental Health Survey and Incidence Study. *Social Psychiatry and Psychiatric Epidemiology* **38**, 1–11.

Donovan MR, Glue P, Kolluri S, Emir B (2010). Comparative efficacy of antidepressants in preventing relapse in anxiety disorders – a meta-analysis. *Journal of Affective Disorders* **123**, 9–16.

Eaton WW, Anthony JC, Romanoski A et al. (1998). Onset and recovery from panic disorder in the Baltimore Epidemiologic Catchment Area follow-up. *British Journal of Psychiatry* **173**, 501–507.

Esquivel, G, Az-Galvis J, Schruers K et al. (2008). Acute exercise reduces the effects of a 35% CO_2 challenge in patients with panic disorder. *Journal of Affective Disorders* **107**, 217–220.

Fava GA, Mangelli L (1999). Subclinical symptoms of panic disorder: new insights into pathophysiology and treatment. *Psychotherapy and Psychosomatics* **68**, 281–289.

Fava GA, Rafanelli C, Grandi S et al. (2001). Long-term outcome of panic disorder with agoraphobia treated by exposure. *Psychological Medicine* **31**, 891–898.

Ferguson JM, Khan A, Mangano R et al. (2007).
Relapse prevention of panic disorder in adult
outpatient responders to treatment with
venlafaxine extended release. Journal of
Clinical Psychiatry 68, 58–68.

Furukawa TA, Watanabe N, Churchill R (2007).
Combined psychotherapy plus
antidepressants for panic disorder with or
without agoraphobia. Cochrane Database of
Systematic Reviews 1, CD004364.

Goddard AW, Brouette T, Almai A et al. (2001).
Early coadministration of clonazepam with
sertraline for panic disorder. Archives of
General Psychiatry 58, 681–686.

Gomez-Caminero A, Blumentals WA, Russo LJ
et al. (2005). Does panic disorder increase
the risk of coronary heart disease? A cohort
study of a national managed care database.
Psychosomatic Medicine 67, 688–691.

Goodwin RD, Faravelli C, Rosi S et al. (2005).
The epidemiology of panic disorder and
agoraphobia in Europe. European
Neuropsychopharmacology 15, 435–443.

Goodwin RD, Roy-Byrne P (2006). Panic and
suicidal ideation and suicide attempts:
results from the National Comorbidity
Survey. Depression and Anxiety 23,
124–132.

Grasbeck A, Rorsman B, Hagne NO, Isberg PE
(1996). Mortality of anxiety syndromes in a
normal population. The Lundby Study.
Neuropsychobiology 33, 118–126.

Harvison KW, Woodruff-Borden J, Jeffery SE
(2004). Mismanagement of panic disorder in
emergency departments: contributors, costs,
and implications for integrated models of
care. Journal of Clinical Psychology and
Medicine 11, 217–232.

Hirschfeld RM (1996). Panic disorder:
diagnosis, epidemiology, and clinical course.
Journal of Clinical Psychiatry 57 (Suppl. 10),
3–8.

Hoehn-Saric R, McLeod DR, Hipsley PA (1993).
Effect of fluvoxamine on panic disorder.
Journal of Clinical Psychopharmacology 13,
321–326.

Hofmann SG (2007). Enhancing exposure-
based therapy from a translational research
perspective. Behaviour Research and Therapy
45, 1987–2001.

Hoge EA, Worthington JJ 3rd, Kaufman RE
et al. (2008). Aripiprazole as augmentation
treatment of refractory generalized anxiety

disorder and panic disorder. CNS Spectrums
13, 522–527.

Holland Rl, Fawcett J, Hoehn-Saric R (1994).
Long-term treatment of panic disorder with
fluvoxamine in out-patients who had
completed double-blind trials.
Neuropsychopharmacology 10 (Suppl. 3), 102.

Hollifield M, Thompson PM, Ruiz JE,
Uhlenhuth EH (2005). Potential effectiveness
and safety of olanzapine in refractory panic
disorder. Depression and Anxiety 21,
33–40.

Hornig CD, McNally RJ (1995). Panic disorder
and suicide attempt. A reanalysis of data
from the Epidemiologic Catchment Area
study. British Journal of Psychiatry 167,
76–79.

Ipser JC, Carey P, Dhansay Y et al. (2006).
Pharmacotherapy augmentation strategies in
treatment-resistant anxiety disorders.
Cochrane Database of Systematic Reviews 4,
CD005473.

Johnson J, Weissman MM, Klerman GL (1990).
Panic disorder, comorbidity, and suicide
attempts. Archives of General Psychiatry 47,
805–808.

Katerndahl DA, Realini JP (1995). Where do
panic attack sufferers seek care? Journal of
Family Practice 40, 237–243.

Katerndahl DA, Realini JP (1997). Quality of life
and panic-related work disability in subjects
with infrequent panic and panic disorder.
Journal of Clinical Psychiatry 58, 153–158.

Kessler RC, Chiu WT, Jin R et al. (2006). The
epidemiology of panic attacks, panic
disorder, and agoraphobia in the National
Comorbidity Survey Replication. Archives of
General Psychiatry 63, 415–424.

Kessler RC, Stang PE, Wittchen HU et al. (1998).
Lifetime panic-depression comorbidity in
the National Comorbidity Survey. Archives of
General Psychiatry 55, 801–808.

Kjernisted K, McIntosh D (2007). Venlafaxine
extended release (XR) in the treatment of
panic disorder. Therapeutics and Clinical Risk
Management 3, 59–69.

Klerman GL, Weissman MM, Ouellette R et al.
(1991). Panic attacks in the community.
Social morbidity and health care utilization.
Journal of the American Medical Association
265, 742–746.

Kohn R, Saxena S, Levav I, Saraceno B (2004).
The treatment gap in mental health care.

Bulletin of the World Health Organization 82, 858–866.

Kouzis AC, Eaton WW (1994). Emotional disability days: prevalence and predictors. *American Journal of Public Health* 84, 1304–1307.

Kouzis AC, Eaton WW (1997). Psychopathology and the development of disability. *Social Psychiatry and Psychiatric Epidemiology* 32, 379–386.

Kruger MB, Dahl AA (1999). The efficacy and safety of moclobemide compared to clomipramine in the treatment of panic disorder. *European Archives of Psychiatry and Clinical Neuroscience* 249, S19–S24.

Kuijpers PM, Honig A, Griez EJ et al. (2000). [Panic disorder in patients with chest pain and palpitations: an often unrecognized relationship]. *Nederlands Tijdschrift voor Geneeskunde* 144, 732–736.

Landelijke Stuurgroep Multidisciplinaire Richtlijnontwikkeling in de GGZ (2009). *Angststoornissen: Paniekstoornis en PTSS (eerste revisie)*. Utrecht: Trimbos-instituut.

Lecrubier Y, Bakker A, Dunbar G, Judge R (1997). A comparison of paroxetine, clomipramine and placebo in the treatment of panic disorder. Collaborative Paroxetine Panic Study Investigators. *Acta Psychiatrica Scandinavica* 95, 145–152.

Lecrubier Y, Judge R (1997). Long-term evaluation of paroxetine, clomipramine and placebo in panic disorder. Collaborative Paroxetine Panic Study Investigators. *Acta Psychiatrica Scandinavica* 95, 153–160.

Leon AC, Portera L, Weissman MM (1995). The social costs of anxiety disorders. *British Journal of Psychiatry* 27 (Suppl.), 19–22.

Lepine JP, Chignon JM, Teherani M (1993). Suicide attempts in patients with panic disorder. *Archives of General Psychiatry* 50, 144–149.

Lepola UM, Wade AG, Leinonen EV et al. (1998). A controlled, prospective, 1-year trial of citalopram in the treatment of panic disorder. *Journal of Clinical Psychiatry* 59, 528–534.

Liebowitz MR, Asnis G, Mangano R, Tzanis E (2009). A double-blind, placebo-controlled, parallel-group, flexible-dose study of venlafaxine extended release capsules in adult outpatients with panic disorder. *Journal of Clinical Psychiatry* 70, 550–561.

Loerch B, Graf-Morgenstern M, Hautzinger M et al. (1999). Randomised placebo-controlled trial of moclobemide, cognitive-behavioural therapy and their combination in panic disorder with agoraphobia. *British Journal of Psychiatry* 174, 205–212.

Lotufo-Neto F, Bernik M, Ramos RT et al. (2001). A dose-finding and discontinuation study of clomipramine in panic disorder. *Journal of Psychopharmacology* 15, 13–17.

Marks IM, Swinson RP, Basoglu M et al. (1993). Alprazolam and exposure alone and combined in panic disorder with agoraphobia. A controlled study in London and Toronto. *British Journal of Psychiatry* 162, 776–787.

Mavissakalian M, Perel JM (1992). Clinical experiments in maintenance and discontinuation of imipramine therapy in panic disorder with agoraphobia. *Archives of General Psychiatry* 49, 318–323.

Mavissakalian MR, Perel JM (1995). Imipramine treatment of panic disorder with agoraphobia: dose ranging and plasma level-response relationships. *American Journal of Psychiatry* 152, 673–682.

Mavissakalian MR, Perel JM (1999). Long-term maintenance and discontinuation of imipramine therapy in panic disorder with agoraphobia. *Archives of General Psychiatry* 56, 821–827.

Mavissakalian MR, Perel JM (2002). Duration of imipramine therapy and relapse in panic disorder with agoraphobia. *Journal of Clinical Psychopharmacology* 22, 294–299.

Michelson D, Lydiard RB, Pollack MH et al. (1998). Outcome assessment and clinical improvement in panic disorder: evidence from a randomized controlled trial of fluoxetine and placebo. The Fluoxetine Panic Disorder Study Group. *American Journal of Psychiatry* 155, 1570–1577.

Mula M, Pini S, Cassano GB (2007). The role of anticonvulsant drugs in anxiety disorders: a critical review of the evidence. *Journal of Clinical Psychopharmacology* 27, 263–272.

Noyes R Jr, Garvey MJ, Cook B, Suelzer M (1991). Controlled discontinuation of benzodiazepine treatment for patients with panic disorder. *American Journal of Psychiatry* 148, 517–523.

Noyes R Jr, Garvey MJ, Cook BL, Samuelson L (1989). Problems with tricyclic antidepressant use in patients with panic disorder or agoraphobia: results of a naturalistic follow-up study. *Journal of Clinical Psychiatry* 50, 163–169.

Oei TPS, Llamas M, Devilly GJ (1999). The efficacy and cognitive processes of cognitive behaviour therapy in the treatment of panic disorder with agoraphobia. *Behavioural and Cognitive Psychotherapy* 27, 63–88.

Otto MW, Tolin DF, Simon NM et al. (2010). Efficacy of d-cycloserine for enhancing response to cognitive-behavior therapy for panic disorder. *Biological Psychiatry* 67, 365–370.

Otto MW, Tuby KS, Gould RA et al. (2001). An effect-size analysis of the relative efficacy and tolerability of serotonin selective reuptake inhibitors for panic disorder. *American Journal of Psychiatry* 158, 1989–1992.

Pande AC, Pollack MH, Crockatt J et al. (2000). Placebo-controlled study of gabapentin treatment of panic disorder. *Journal of Clinical Psychopharmacology* 20, 467–471.

Papp LA (2006). Safety and efficacy of levetiracetam for patients with panic disorder: results of an open-label, fixed-flexible dose study. *Journal of Clinical Psychiatry* 67, 1573–1576.

Papp LA, Schneier FR, Fyer AJ et al. (1997). Clomipramine treatment of panic disorder: pros and cons. *Journal of Clinical Psychiatry* 58, 423–425.

Peter H, Bruckner E, Hand I et al. (2008). Treatment outcome of female agoraphobics 3–9 years after exposure in vivo: a comparison with healthy controls. *Journal of Behaviour Therapy and Experimental Psychiatry* 39, 3–10.

Pigot M, Loo C, Sachdev P (2008). Repetitive transcranial magnetic stimulation as treatment for anxiety disorders. *Expert Review of Neurotherapeutics* 8, 1449–1455.

Pollack M, Mangano R, Entsuah R et al. (2007*a*). A randomized controlled trial of venlafaxine ER and paroxetine in the treatment of outpatients with panic disorder. *Psychopharmacology* 194, 233–242.

Pollack MH, Lepola U, Koponen H et al. (2007*b*). A double-blind study of the efficacy of venlafaxine extended-release, paroxetine, and placebo in the treatment of panic disorder. *Depression and Anxiety* 24, 1–14.

Pollack MH, Otto MW, Worthington JJ et al. (1998). Sertraline in the treatment of panic disorder: a flexible-dose multicenter trial. *Archives of General Psychiatry* 55, 1010–1016.

Pollack MH, Simon NM, Worthington JJ et al. (2003). Combined paroxetine and clonazepam treatment strategies compared to paroxetine monotherapy for panic disorder. *Journal of Psychopharmacology* 17, 276–282.

Pollack MH, Tesar GE, Rosenbaum JF, Spier SA (1986). Clonazepam in the treatment of panic disorder and agoraphobia: a one-year follow-up. *Journal of Clinical Psychopharmacology* 6, 302–304.

Rapaport MH, Wolkow R, Rubin A et al. (2001). Sertraline treatment of panic disorder: results of a long-term study. *Acta Psychiatrica Scandinavica* 104, 289–298.

Ravelli A, Bijl RV, van Zessen G (1998). Comorbiditeit van psychiatrische stoornissen in de Nederlandse bevolking: Resultaten van de Netherlands Mental Health Survey and Incidence Study (NEMESIS). *Tijdschrift voor Psychiatrie* 40, 531–544.

Rees CS, Richards JC, Smith LM (1998). Medical utilisation and costs in panic disorder: a comparison with social phobia. *Journal of Anxiety Disorders* 12, 421–435.

Rodrigues H, Figueira I, Goncalves R et al. (2011). CBT for pharmacotherapy non-remitters – a systematic review of a next-step strategy. *Journal of Affective Disorders* 129, 219–228.

Rosenberg R (1999). Treatment of panic disorder with tricyclics and MAOIs. In Nutt DJ, Ballenger JC, Lépine PD (Eds.), *Panic Disorder: Clinical Diagnosis, Management and Mechanisms* (pp. 125–144) London: Martin Dunitz.

Ross DC, Klein DF, Uhlenhuth EH (2010). Improved statistical analysis of moclobemide dose effects on panic disorder treatment. *European Archives of Psychiatry and Clinical Neuroscience* 260, 243–248.

Ruhe HG, Booij J, Weert HC et al. (2009). Evidence why paroxetine dose escalation is not effective in major depressive disorder: a randomized controlled trial with assessment of serotonin transporter occupancy. *Neuropsychopharmacology* 34, 999–1010.

Saito M, Miyaoka H (2007). Augmentation of paroxetine with clocapramine in panic disorder. *Psychiatry and Clinical Neurosciences* **61**, 449.

Salvador-Carulla L, Segui J, Fernandez-Cano P, Canet J (1995). Costs and offset effect in panic disorders. *British Journal of Psychiatry* **27** (Suppl.), 23–28.

Sareen J, Cox BJ, Afifi TO *et al.* (2005a). Anxiety disorders and risk for suicidal ideation and suicide attempts: a population-based longitudinal study of adults. *Archives of General Psychiatry* **62**, 1249–1257.

Sareen J, Cox BJ, Clara I, Asmundson GJ (2005b). The relationship between anxiety disorders and physical disorders in the U.S. National Comorbidity Survey. *Depression and Anxiety* **21**, 193–202.

Schmidt NB, Wollaway-Bickel K, Trakowski JH *et al.* (2002). Antidepressant discontinuation in the context of cognitive behavioral treatment for panic disorder. *Behaviour Research and Therapy* **40**, 67–73.

Seedat S, van Rheede van Oudtshoorn E, Muller JE *et al.* (2003). Reboxetine and citalopram in panic disorder: a single-blind, cross-over, flexible-dose pilot study. *International Clinical Psychopharmacology* **18**, 279–284.

Sepede G, de Berardis D, Gambi F *et al.* (2006). Olanzapine augmentation in treatment-resistant panic disorder: a 12-week, fixed-dose, open-label trial. *Journal of Clinical Psychopharmacology* **26**, 45–49.

Sheehan DV, Ballenger J, Jacobsen G (1980). Treatment of endogenous anxiety with phobic, hysterical, and hypochondriacal symptoms. *Archives of General Psychiatry* **37**, 51–59.

Sheehan DV, Burnham DB, Iyengar MK, Perera P (2005). Efficacy and tolerability of controlled-release paroxetine in the treatment of panic disorder. *Journal of Clinical Psychiatry* **66**, 34–40.

Simon NM, Hoge EA, Fischmann D *et al.* (2006). An open-label trial of risperidone augmentation for refractory anxiety disorders. *Journal of Clinical Psychiatry* **67**, 381–385.

Simon NM, Kaufman RE, Hoge EA *et al.* (2009a). Open-label support for duloxetine for the treatment of panic disorder. *CNS Neuroscience and Therapeutics* **15**, 19–23.

Simon NM, Otto MW, Worthington JJ *et al.* (2009b). Next-step strategies for panic disorder refractory to initial pharmacotherapy: a 3-phase randomized clinical trial. *Journal of Clinical Psychiatry* **70**, 1563–1570.

Smoller JW, Pollack MH, Wassertheil-Smoller S *et al.* (2007). Panic attacks and risk of incident cardiovascular events among postmenopausal women in the Women's Health Initiative Observational Study. *Archives of General Psychiatry* **64**, 1153–1160.

Spiegel DA, Bruce TJ, Gregg SF, Nuzzarello A (1994). Does cognitive behavior therapy assist slow-taper alprazolam discontinuation in panic disorder? *American Journal of Psychiatry* **151**, 876–881.

Stahl SM, Gergel I, Li D (2003). Escitalopram in the treatment of panic disorder: a randomized, double-blind, placebo-controlled trial. *Journal of Clinical Psychiatry* **64**, 1322–1327.

Stein MB, Cantrell CR, Sokol MC *et al.* (2006). Antidepressant adherence and medical resource use among managed care patients with anxiety disorders. *Psychiatric Services* **57**, 673–680.

Strohle A, Graetz B, Scheel M *et al.* (2009). The acute antipanic and anxiolytic activity of aerobic exercise in patients with panic disorder and healthy control subjects. *Journal of Psychiatric Research* **43**, 1013–1017.

Tiller JW, Bouwer C, Behnke K (1999). Moclobemide and fluoxetine for panic disorder. International Panic Disorder Study Group. *European Archives of Psychiatry and Clinical Neuroscience* **249**, S7–S10.

Toni C, Perugi G, Frare F *et al.* (2004). Spontaneous treatment discontinuation in panic disorder patients treated with antidepressants. *Acta Psychiatrica Scandinavica* **110**, 130–137.

Tyrer P, Candy J, Kelly D (1973). A study of the clinical effects of phenelzine and placebo in the treatment of phobic anxiety. *Psychopharmacologia* **32**, 237–254.

Uhlenhuth EH, Warner TD, Matuzas W (2002). Interactive model of therapeutic response in panic disorder: moclobemide, a case in point. *Journal of Clinical Psychopharmacology* **174**, 205–212.

Van Balkom AJ, Bakker A, Spinhoven P *et al.* (1997). A meta-analysis of the treatment of panic disorder with or without agoraphobia: a comparison of psychopharmacological, cognitive-behavioral, and combination treatments. *Journal of Nervous and Mental Disease* **185**, 510–516.

Van Balkom AJLM, Nauta M, Bakker A (1995). Meta-analysis on the treatment of panic disorder with agoraphobia: review and re-examination. *Clinical Psychology and Psychotherapy* **2**, 1–14.

Versiani M, Cassano G, Benedetti A *et al.* (2002). Reboxetine, a selective norepinephrine reuptake inhibitor, is an effective and well-tolerated treatment for panic disorder. *Journal of Clinical Psychiatry* **63**, 31–37.

Wade AG, Lepola U, Koponen HJ *et al.* (1997). The effect of citalopram in panic disorder. *British Journal of Psychiatry* **170**, 549–553.

Wang PS, Berglund P, Olfson M *et al.* (2005a). Failure and delay in initial treatment contact after first onset of mental disorders in the National Comorbidity Survey Replication. *Archives of General Psychiatry* **62**, 603–613.

Wang PS, Lane M, Olfson M *et al.* (2005b). Twelve-month use of mental health services in the United States: results from the National Comorbidity Survey Replication. *Archives of General Psychiatry* **62**, 629–640.

Watanabe N, Churchill R, Furukawa TA (2007). Combination of psychotherapy and benzodiazepines versus either therapy alone for panic disorder: a systematic review. *BMC Psychiatry* 7, 18.

Wedekind D, Broocks A, Weiss N *et al.* (2010). A randomized, controlled trial of aerobic exercise in combination with paroxetine in the treatment of panic disorder. *World Journal of Biological Psychiatry* **11**, 904–913.

Weissman MM, Klerman GL, Markowitz JS, Ouellette R (1989). Suicidal ideation and suicide attempts in panic disorder and attacks. *New England Journal of Medicine* **321**, 1209–1214.

Whittal ML, Otto MW, Hong JJ (2001). Cognitive-behavior therapy for discontinuation of SSRI treatment of panic disorder: a case series. *Behaviour Research and Therapy* **39**, 939–945.

Wiborg IM, Dahl AA (1996). Does brief dynamic psychotherapy reduce the relapse rate of panic disorder? *Archives of General Psychiatry* **53**, 689–694.

Wittchen HU, Beesdo K, Bittner A, Goodwin RD (2003). Depressive episodes – evidence for a causal role of primary anxiety disorders? *European Psychiatry* **18**, 384–393.

Wittchen HU, Nelson CB, Lachner G (1998). Prevalence of mental disorders and psychosocial impairments in adolescents and young adults. *Psychological Medicine* **28**, 109–126.

Wittchen HU, Nocon A, Beesdo K *et al.* (2008). Agoraphobia and panic. Prospective-longitudinal relations suggest a rethinking of diagnostic concepts. *Psychotherapy and Psychosomatics* **77**, 147–157.

Wright J, Clum GA, Roodman A, Febbraro GA (2000). A bibliotherapy approach to relapse prevention in individuals with panic attacks. *Journal of Anxiety Disorders* **14**, 483–499.

Zwanzger P, Eser D, Nothdurfter C *et al.* (2009a). Effects of the GABA-reuptake inhibitor Tiagabine on panic and anxiety in patients with panic disorder. *Pharmapsychiatry* **42**, 266–269.

Zwanzger P, Fallgatter AJ, Zavorotnyy M, Padberg F (2009b). Anxiolytic effects of transcranial magnetic stimulation – an alternative treatment option in anxiety disorders? *Journal of Neural Transmission* **116**, 767–775.

Zwanzger P, Rupprecht R (2005). Selective GABAergic treatment for panic? Investigations in experimental panic induction and panic disorder. *Journal of Psychiatry and Neuroscience* **30**, 167–175.

Chapter 6

Evidence-based pharmacotherapy of social anxiety disorder

Carlos Blanco, Laura B. Bragdon, Franklin R. Schneier, and Michael R. Liebowitz

Introduction

Social anxiety disorder (SAD) is characterized by a fear of negative evaluation in social or performance situations and a strong tendency for sufferers to avoid feared social interactions or situations. Recent epidemiological studies suggest that the lifetime prevalence of SAD may be as high as 12% (Grant *et al.*, 2005). SAD generally begins in the mid-teens, is associated with substantial impairments in vocational and social functioning (Davidson *et al.*, 1993; Schneier *et al.*, 1992*b*) and often follows a chronic, unremitting course (Amies *et al.*, 1983; Marks, 1970; Öst, 1987). The DSM–IV (American Psychiatric Association, 2000) describes a generalized subtype, characterized by distressing or disabling fears in most social situations. By contrast, individuals with the non-generalized subtype typically fear only a few performance situations, most commonly public speaking.

The current review updates a previous one published in 2003 (Blanco *et al.*, 2003*a*). We first summarize the available evidence for the pharmacological management of SAD, focusing on the published randomized clinical trials, which are summarized in Table 6.1. Because there are few head-to-head comparisons of medication treatments, we rely primarily on meta-analytic reviews to estimate and compare the relative efficacy of different medications.

In order to provide a foundation for identifying evidence-based pharmacological treatments of social anxiety disorder, we conducted a search using electronic databases (MEDLINE, PreMEDLINE, and PsycINFO) for the years 1980–2010 using a search strategy that combined the terms (social adj3 (anxiety or phobi$)) with (control$ or randomized or clinical trial or placebo$ or blind$). To complement the search strategy, we consulted with other colleagues regarding published manuscripts on trials involving medication for the treatment of SAD. In this brief review we attempt to provide evidence-based answers to three main questions: (1) What should be the first-line pharmacological treatment? (2) How long should this treatment last? (3) What strategies can be used if first-line treatments fail? The overwhelming majority of the published work on the pharmacological treatment of SAD is directed at answering the first question, and our review of the literature reflects this fact. However, we also examine the limited available information regarding duration of pharmacological treatment, and suggest strategies for management of treatment-resistant cases. We conclude the review by outlining some future directions.

Essential Evidence-Based Psychopharmacology, Second Edition, ed. Dan J. Stein, Bernard Lerer, and Stephen M. Stahl. Published by Cambridge University Press. © Cambridge University Press.

Table 6.1. Summary of placebo-controlled studies in the acute treatment of social anxiety disorder.

Drug class	Drug	Author	Sample size	Duration	Dose mg/day	Response rates (%) Medication/ Placebo
MAOIs	Phenelzine[a]	Liebowitz et al., 1992	51	8 weeks	45–90	64/23
	Phenelzine[b]	Gelernter et al., 1991	64	12 weeks	30–90	69/20
	Phenelzine[c]	Versiani et al., 1992	52	8 weeks	15–90	81/27
	Phenelzine	Heimberg et al., 1998	64	12 weeks	15–75	52/27
	Phenelzine	Blanco et al., 2010a	128	24 weeks	15–90	49/33
RIMAs	Moclobemide[b]	Versiani et al., 1992	52	8 weeks	100–600	65/20
	Moclobemide	Katschnig et al., 1997	578	12 weeks	300–600	44/32
	Moclobemide	Noyes et al., 1997	506	12 weeks	75–900	35/33
	Moclobemide	Schneier et al., 1998	75	8 weeks	100–400	18/14
	Moclobemide	Stein et al., 2002a	390	12 weeks	450–750	43/30
Benzodiazepines	Clonazepam	Davidson et al., 1993	75	10 weeks	0.5–3	78/20
	Clonazepam	Munjack et al., 1990	23	8 weeks	0.5–6	90/10
	Bromazepam	Versiani et al., 1997a	60	12 weeks	3–27	83/20
	Alprazolam[b]	Gelernter et al., 1991	65	12 weeks	2.1–6.3	38/23
SSRIs	Fluvoxamine	Van Vliet et al., 1994	30	12 weeks	150	46/7
	Fluvoxamine	Stein et al., 1999	86	12 weeks	202, mean dose	43/23
	Fluvoxamine (CR)	Westenberg et al., 2004	300	12 weeks	100–300	48/44
	Fluvoxamine (CR)	Davidson et al., 2004b	279	12 weeks	100–300	34/17
	Paroxetine	Stein et al., 1998	182	12 weeks	10–50	55/22

(cont.)

Table 6.1. (cont.)

Drug class	Drug	Author	Sample size	Duration	Dose mg/day	Response rates (%) Medication/ Placebo
	Paroxetine	Baldwin et al., 1999	290	12 weeks	20–50	66/33
	Paroxetine	Allgulander, 1999		12 weeks	20–50	70/8
	Paroxetine	Liebowitz et al., 2002	384	12 weeks	20–60	66/28
	Paroxetine	Stein et al., 2002c	323	24 weeks	20–50	78/51
	Paroxetine	Seedat & Stein, 2004	28	10 weeks	20–40	79/43
	Paroxetine (CR)	Lepola et al., 2004	370	12 weeks	12.5–37.5	57/30
	Paroxetine	Allgulander et al., 2004	434	12 weeks	20–50	66/36
	Paroxetine	Lader et al., 2004	839	24 weeks	20	80/66
	Paroxetine	Wagner et al., 2003	322	16 weeks	10–50	78/38
	Paroxetine	Liebowitz et al, 2005a	440	12 weeks	25–50	63/36
	Sertraline[d]	Katzelnick et al., 1995	12	10 weeks	50–200	50/9
	Sertraline	Van Ameringen et al., 2001	204	20 weeks	50–200	53/29
	Sertraline	Walker et al., 2000	50	24 weeks	50–200	96/64
	Sertraline	Blomhoff et al., 2001	387	24 weeks	50–150	40/24
	Sertraline	Liebowitz et al., 2003	211	12 weeks	50–200	47/26
	Fluoxetine	Kobak et al., 2002	60	8 weeks	20–60	40/30
	Fluoxetine	Davidson et al., 2004a	295	14 weeks	10–60	51/32
	Fluoxetine	Clark et al., 2003	60	16 weeks	20–60	33/16
	Escitalopram	Lader et al., 2004	839	24 weeks	5–20	54/39
	Escitalopram	Kasper et al., 2005	358	12 weeks	10–20	54/39

Table 6.1. *(cont.)*

Drug class	Drug	Author	Sample size	Duration	Dose mg/day	Response rates (%) Medication/ Placebo
	Escitalopram	Montgomery et al., 2005	371	24 weeks	10–20	78/50
	Venlafaxine (ER)	Rickels et al., 2004	272	12 weeks	75–225	50/34
	Venlafaxine (ER)	Allgulander et al., 2004	434	12 weeks	75–225	69/36
	Venlafaxine (ER)	Liebowitz et al., 2005a	271	12 weeks	75–225	44/30
	Venlafaxine (ER)	Liebowitz et al., 2005b	440	12 weeks	75–225	59/36
	Venlafaxine (ER)	Stein et al., 2005	395	28 weeks	75–225	58/33
Betablocker	Atenolol[a]	Liebowitz et al., 1992	51	8 weeks	50–100	30/23
	Atenolol	Turner et al., 1994	72	12 weeks	25–100	33/6
Other antidepressants	Mirtazapine	Muehlbacher et al., 2005	66	10 weeks	30	26/5.4
	Mirtazapine	Schutters et al., 2010	60	12 weeks	30–45	13/13
	Nefazodone	Van Ameringen et al., 2007	105	14 weeks	300–600	31/24
Anticonvulsants	Gabapentin	Pande et al., 1999	69	14 weeks	900–3600	38/14
	Levetiracetam	Zhang et al., 2005	18	7 weeks	500–3000	22/14
	Pregabalin	Feltner et al., 2011	329	11 weeks	300, 450, 600	29.8/19.7
Atypical antipsychotics	Olanzapine	Barnett et al., 2002	12	8 weeks	5–20	60/0
	Buspirone	Van Vliet et al., 1997	30	12 weeks	15–30	27/13
	Buspirone	Clark & Agras, 1991	34	6 weeks	32 mean dose	57/60

[a] Study had three arms: phenelzine, atenolol, and placebo.
[b] Study had three arms: phenelzine, alprazolam, and placebo.
[c] Study had three arms: phenelzine, moclobemide, and placebo.
[d] Study had a cross-over design.

What is the first-line treatment for social anxiety disorder?

Summary of published clinical trials

Monoamine oxidase inhibitors (MAOIs)

Monoamine oxidase inhibitors (MAOIs) were the first medications to be widely studied as a treatment for SAD. Six double-blind, placebo-controlled trials have consistently demonstrated the efficacy of phenelzine in the treatment of SAD, resulting in symptomatic and functional improvement (Blanco et al., 2010a; Gelernter et al., 1991; Guastella et al., 2008; Heimberg et al., 1998).

Overall, substantial evidence shows that phenelzine and probably other irreversible, non-selective MAOIs are highly effective in the treatment of many patients with SAD. However, concerns regarding side-effects and safety of the non-reversible MAOIs, particularly the risk of hypertensive crisis if a low-tyramine diet and related precautions are not strictly followed, led to the development of the reversible inhibitors of MAOI-A (RIMAs).

Reversible inhibitors of monoamine oxidase-A (RIMAs)

Compared with non-reversible MAOIs, reversible inhibitors of monoamine oxidase-A (RIMAs) have a significantly lower risk of potentiating the dangerous pressor effect of tyramine, which allows for relaxation or total elimination of dietary restrictions. Other MAOI side-effects such as fatigue and hypotension also occur less often with RIMAs. Unfortunately, RIMAs appear to be less effective than MAOIs and are not available in the USA. Moclobemide is currently the only RIMA to have been studied for the treatment of SAD that is still available on the US market.

Moclobemide

Five double-blind placebo-controlled studies of moclobemide have produced mixed results, suggesting modest efficacy in the treatment of SAD. The results of these studies indicate that whereas moclobemide appears better tolerated and safer than phenelzine, it is clearly less efficacious in the treatment of SAD (Versiani et al., 1992).

Selective serotonin reuptake inhibitors (SSRIs) and serotonin norepinephrine reuptake inhibitors (SNRIs)

Selective serotonin reuptake inhibitors (SSRIs) and serotonin norepinephrine reuptake inhibitors (SNRIs) have been studied widely because of their efficacy, safety, and tolerability compared with earlier medications. More than 20 placebo-controlled trials have shown that SSRIs are highly efficacious in the treatment of SAD and a series of meta-analyses have supported their efficacy (Blanco et al., 2003b; Fedoroff & Taylor, 2001; Gould et al., 1997; Hedges et al., 2007; van der Linden et al., 2000). In conjunction with their favorable side-effect profile and their ability to treat comorbid depression, these findings have established them as a first-line medication for SAD. Paroxetine (immediate release and extended release), sertraline, extended-release fluvoxamine and extended-release venlafaxine are the only medications FDA-approved for the treatment of SAD.

Paroxetine

There are 11 published placebo-controlled studies of paroxetine and almost all have found it to be superior to placebo for the treatment of SAD (Allgulander, 1999; Allgulander et al., 2004; Baldwin et al., 1999; Lader et al., 2004; Lepola et al., 2004; Liebowitz et al., 2002, 2005a; Seedat & Stein, 2004; Stein et al., 1998, 2002b; Wagner, 2003).

Fluvoxamine

Four double-blind studies have investigated the efficacy of fluvoxamine in SAD. Results from these studies indicate that fluvoxamine is superior to placebo for reduction of SAD symptoms including anxiety, sensitivity to rejection, and hostility, and for increase in overall functioning (Davidson et al., 2004; Stein et al., 1999; van Vliet et al., 1994; Westenberg et al., 2004).

Sertraline

Five placebo-controlled studies have demonstrated the efficacy of sertraline (Blomhoff et al., 2001; Katzelnick et al., 1995; Liebowitz et al., 2003; Van Ameringen et al., 2001; Walker et al., 2000). Furthermore, sertraline is more effective than placebo in preventing relapse (Walker et al., 2000). A recent reanalysis of the Blomhoff et al. (2001) study suggested that sertraline and exposure therapy may have an additive effect (Blanco et al., 2010a).

Fluoxetine

Early uncontrolled studies of fluoxetine also suggested that it could be efficacious in the treatment of SAD (Black et al., 1992; Schneier et al., 1992a; Sternbach, 1990; Van Ameringen et al., 1993). However, results from more recent studies are mixed (Clark et al., 2003; Davidson et al., 2004; Kobak et al., 2002). Overall, these findings suggest that fluoxetine may have some efficacy in the treatment of SADs, but the results appear less robust that those of other SSRIs.

Escitalopram and citalopram

Results from placebo-controlled trials of escitalopram have found it to be superior to placebo in reducing SAD symptoms and preventing relapse (Kasper et al., 2005; Lader et al., 2004; Montgomery et al., 2005). Only one small, open-label trial of citalopram for the treatment of SAD has been published. Results indicated that citalopram was well tolerated and patients improved significantly on all outcome measures (Simon et al., 2002).

Venlafaxine

Five large placebo-controlled trials have supported the efficacy of venlafaxine, a SNRI, for SAD (Allgulander et al., 2004; Liebowitz et al., 2005a, 2005b; Rickels et al., 2004; Stein et al., 2005). Since at doses typically prescribed, SSRIs and SNRIs have similar pharmacological properties, safety profiles, and efficacy, they share the established role in the treatment of SAD as the first-line pharmacological agents.

Other antidepressants

A placebo-controlled study provided initial support for the efficacy of mirtazapine, a presynaptic adrenoceptor antagonist, in the treatment of SAD (Muehlbacher et al., 2005). However, another recent study (Schutters et al., 2010) failed to confirm that finding. Nefazodone, which has both 5-HT reuptake and 5-HT$_{2A}$ receptor blockade properties, had negative results in the only published placebo-controlled study of this medication (Van Ameringen *et al.*, 2007). Tricyclic antidepressants do not appear particularly useful in the treatment of SAD, either (Simpson *et al.*, 1998; Zitrin *et al.*, 1983).

Benzodiazepines

In the only published placebo-controlled study of alprazolam for SAD, only 38% of patients were considered responders, which did not differ significantly from the response rate with placebo, and symptoms had returned 2 months after discontinuation of alprazolam (Gelernter *et al.*, 1991). Three studies of clonazepam have been more favorable with results indicating significant improvement as compared with placebo (Davidson *et al.*, 1993; Munjack *et al.*, 1990). Davidson *et al.* examined the efficacy of clonazepam in a placebo-controlled study of 75 patients, where 78% of the treatment group were classified as responders *vs.* 20% of the placebo group (Davidson *et al.*, 1993). Use of bromazepam, a benzodiazepine marketed outside the USA, also has been reported to be efficacious for the treatment of SAD (Versiani *et al.*, 1997*b*).

In summary, in double-blind studies, clonazepam and bromazepam, but not alprazolam, have been superior to placebo. Benzodiazepines also may be helpful on an as-needed basis for performance anxiety. The benefit of decreased anxiety must be balanced with the risk of sedation interfering with the quality of performance.

Beta-adrenergic blockers

Studies showing a connection between anxiety, signs and symptoms of peripheral arousal (i.e. tremor, palpitation, and sweating), and increased plasma levels of norepinephrine led to early trials of beta-blockers in non-clinical samples of performers with high levels of anxiety, many of whom would probably be currently diagnosed as having non-generalized SAD. The results of those trials indicate that beta-blockers were successful in decreasing the autonomic manifestations of anxiety.

Anecdotal experience also suggests that β-blockers are effective for non-generalized, circumscribed performance anxiety. However, beta-blockers have not been proven superior to placebo in any controlled clinical trial for the treatment of SAD. Thus, at present, they cannot be considered an evidence-based treatment for SAD.

Other medications

Buspirone

Buspirone is an azapirone that acts as a full agonist on the serotonin 1A ($5HT_{1A}$) autoreceptor and as a partial agonist on the post-synaptic $5\text{-}HT_{1A}$ receptor. Neither of the two controlled trials of buspirone demonstrated efficacy for it as monotherapy for SAD (van Vliet *et al.*, 1997). Additionally, the dosage of buspirone needed seems to be in the upper range (60 mg/day), which may limit its usefulness on the basis of side-effects, such as nausea or headache (Schneier & Saoud, 1993).

Anticonvulsants

Gabapentin is thought to have GABAergic effects, although the exact mechanism of action is unknown. In the only published placebo-controlled trial of gabapentin for SAD, a

Table 6.2. Meta-analysis of Gould et al. (1997).

Drug group	Effect size	Drop-out rate	Number of studies
MAOIs	0.64	13.8%	5
Benzodiazepines	0.72	12%	2
SSRIs	2.73	3%	2
Beta-blockers	−0.08	−22%	3
Buspirone	−0.5	22%	1

significantly higher rate of response was observed among patients on gabapentin than on placebo (Pande et al., 1999).

In a randomized double-blind trial, pregabalin 600 mg/day was superior to placebo (Feltner et al., 2011). Further studies will be needed to define the optimal dose, magnitude of the effect, and long-term effect of pregabalin for SAD.

Levetiracetam is a novel anticonvulsant that modulates voltage-gated calcium channels in the CNS. A small randomized placebo-controlled study by Zhang et al. (2005) found no differences in efficacy as compared with placebo.

Atypical antipsychotics

Some antipsychotics, including olanzapine (Barnett et al., 2002), quetiapine (Schutters et al., 2005), and risperidone have been tested for the treatment of SAD. Some of these studies have shown promise, but larger studies will be needed in order to clarify their effects.

Use of meta-analysis as a basis for evidence-based practice

To date, six meta-analyses have examined the efficacy of medication for the treatment of SAD.

Meta-analysis of Gould and colleagues (1997)

The first meta-analysis to assess the efficacy of medication for SAD was carried out by Gould and colleagues and looked at 24 studies involving a control group (Gould et al., 1997). Effect sizes were found using Glass's delta procedure and heterogeneity of effect sizes across studies were calculated using the chi-square test.

Gould and colleagues found that the mean effect size for pharmacotherapy of SAD was 0.62. The effect size of MAOIs (which included phenelzine and moclobemide) was 0.64, whereas benzodiazepines had an effect size of 0.72. The meta-analysis also included two studies conducted with SSRIs: the first study, conducted with fluvoxamine, had an effect size of 2.73 whereas the second one, a small cross-over of sertraline study had an effect size of 1.05. A linear regression analysis found no gender differences in efficacy. The results of this meta-analysis are summarized in Table 6.2.

Meta-analysis of Van der Linden and colleagues (2000)

Van der Linden and colleagues (Van der Linden et al., 2000) reviewed the efficacy of the SSRIs for SAD using 25 clinical trials, eight of which were placebo-controlled, and used the data of the randomized trials to conduct a formal meta-analysis.

With the exception of two moclobemide studies, all studies showed superiority of drug over placebo. SSRIs ($n = 8$) and clonazepam ($n = 1$) had the largest effect sizes, confirming the initial finding of the Gould meta-analysis.

Meta-analysis of Fedoroff and Taylor (2001)

Fedoroff and Taylor (2001) included both psychological and pharmacological treatment of SAD and examined drug classes (e.g. SSRIs) rather than specific medications. Uncontrolled trials were also included in the meta-analysis.

The authors performed separate meta-analyses for observer-rated and self-report measures. Fedoroff and Taylor found a remarkable homogeneity of effect sizes within each drug class, with only three studies generating heterogeneity according to the chi-square test for heterogeneity. In all three cases the effect sizes of the heterogeneous studies were greater than those of the other studies in their drug classes. Consistent with the findings of Gould and colleagues, the authors found no overall gender differences in treatment efficacy.

Fedoroff and Taylor also found that the confidence intervals of double-blind and non-double-blind trials overlapped with one another, indicating no difference in effect size. They found that the largest mean effect sizes for the acute treatment were for benzodiazepines and SSRIs, which were not significantly different from each other. However, when examining the 95% CI, there was no overlap between the CIs of benzodiazepines and the CIs of MAOIs, cognitive therapy or cognitive therapy with exposure, indicating a greater treatment efficacy for benzodiazepines. The CI of SSRIs, however, did overlap with these treatment conditions, indicating no difference between treatments. Results obtained using the observer-rated measures were in the same direction, but did not show any significant differences across treatment conditions.

Blanco and colleagues (2003b)

Blanco et al. (2003b) conducted a meta-analysis of the placebo-controlled studies of pharmacotherapy for SAD using studies published between January 1980 and June 2001. The Liebowitz Social Anxiety Scale (LSAS; Liebowitz, 1987) was used as the primary outcome measure and proportion of responders (defined as a score of 1 or 2 in the CGI) in each study was used as a secondary measure. Effect sizes were estimated using Hedges g (Hedges & Olkin, 1985) for the LSAS and odds ratio for proportion of responders (Fleiss, 1994).

For trials that included more than one dose of medication in their design (Katschnig et al., 1997; Noyes et al., 1997) a statistical adjustment was used to generate a unique effect size for each study (Glesser & Olkin, 1994).

Quality assessment of the clinical trials was conducted to evaluate whether standard procedures such as randomization of patients had been conducted, blind maintained throughout the trial, and appropriate statistical analyses performed. Overall, the quality of clinical trials was very high. Our analysis found that clonazepam, based on a single study, had the largest mean effect size of all medications. The effect sizes of SSRIs, phenelzine, and clonazepam were not significantly different. Because we found heterogeneity of effect sizes between moclobemide and brofaromine we estimated mean effect sizes for both medications separately. Whereas the effect size of brofaromine was similar to that of SSRIs and MAOIs, the effect size of moclobemide was substantially lower. There were no significant differences between the three SSRIs that had been tested in placebo-controlled studies: paroxetine, sertraline, and fluvoxamine. Gabapentin, which had not been included in previous

Table 6.3. Effect sizes of meta-analysis of Blanco et al. (2003b).

Drug	Number of studies	Effect size based on LSAS[a] (95% CI)	Heterogeneity (LSAS)	Effect size based on the CGI[b] (95% CI)	Heterogeneity based on the CGI
SSRIs	6	0.65 (0.50–0.81)	No	4.1 (2.01–8.41)	Yes
Benzodiazepines	2	1.54 (−0.03–3.32)	Yes	16.61 (10.18–27.39)	Yes
Phenelzine	3	1.02 (0.50–1.02)	Yes	5.53 (2.56–11.94)	Yes
Moclobemide	4	0.30 (0.00–0.6)	Yes	1.84 (0.89–3.82)	Yes
Brofaromine	3	0.66 (0.38–0.94)	No	6.96 (2.39–20.29)	No
Gabapentin[c]	1	0.78 (0.29–1.27)	Not applicable	3.78 (1.88–7.54)	Not applicable
Atenolol	2	0.10 (−0.44–0.64)	No	1.36 (0.87–2.12)	No
Buspirone[c,d]	1	0.02 (−0.70–0.73)	Not applicable	–	Not applicable

[a] LSAS: Liebowitz Social Anxiety Scale.
[b] CGI: Clinical Global Impression Scale.
[c] At least two studies are necessary to test for heterogeneity.
[d] Study did not use the CGI.

meta-analysis, had an effect size similar to that of the SSRIs. The results were consistent across measures, i.e. LSAS and proportion of responders using the CGI. The effect sizes of the Blanco et al. meta-analysis are summarized in Table 6.3.

Hedges and colleagues (2007)

The most recent meta-analyses, conducted by Hedges and colleagues, sought to investigate the efficacy of SSRIs for the treatment of adult SAD and included 15 published randomized double-blind placebo-controlled trials using SSRIs (Hedges et al., 2007).

Effect sizes were measured with Cohen's d. The Q statistic was used to assess heterogeneity across studies, and a funnel-plot analysis was used to examine publication bias.

Results indicated that all SSRIs were significantly more efficacious than placebo. Furthermore, no significant differences were found between LSAS scores for the drugs paroxetine, sertraline, fluvoamine, and fluoxetine.

Choice of medication

The evidence from the reviewed clinical trials and meta-analyses suggests that a number of medications are efficacious in the treatment of SAD. Moreover, based on the meta-analysis of Fedoroff and Taylor, they appear to be superior to psychotherapy, at least in the acute phase of the treatment. Those data are consistent with recent findings from two randomized trials of phenelzine versus cognitive–behavioral psychotherapy (Blanco et al., 2010a; Heimberg et al., 1998). Two direct comparisons of psychotherapy versus fluoxetine have failed to show superiority of medication over psychotherapy (Clark *et al.*, 2003; Davidson *et al.*, 2004). However, as reviewed above, fluoxetine may be less efficacious than other SSRIs in the treatment of SAD. Additional direct comparisons of medication *vs.* psychotherapy would be highly desirable to confirm those findings.

Despite the use of slightly different approaches and inclusion criteria for the clinical trials, the meta-analyses also consistently indicate that benzodiazepines are the medication with the largest effect size for the treatment of SAD. Other medications with moderate to large side-effects included the SSRIs, phenelzine, brofaromine, and gabapentin. Based on those results, what should the practicing clinician do? We believe that choice of medication should be guided by three principles: (1) highest efficacy, based on the effect size of the medication or medication group, and its reproducibility as determined by the number of clinical trials published and overall number of patients in those clinical trials; (2) lowest potential for side-effects of the drug; and, (3) ability to treat commonly comorbid conditions. Furthermore, special considerations pertaining to each individual patient, such as presence of specific comorbidity, contraindications or patient preference should always be taken into account.

Based on those considerations, we believe that at present SSRIs constitute the first-line medication treatment of SAD for most patients. They have been more extensively tested in clinical trials than any other medication for SAD, have a moderate effect size, are generally well tolerated and are efficacious for the treatment of other disorders that are frequently comorbid with SADs, including major depressive disorder and other anxiety disorders. It is important to note, however, that although double-blind studies support the efficacy of paroxetine, sertraline, and fluvoxamine, there are no published placebo-controlled studies of citalopram or duloxetine, and evidence for the efficacy of fluoxetine appears to be weaker than for other SSRIs (Kobak *et al.*, 2002). The SNRI venlafaxine appears to have similar efficacy to SSRIs, although it has been less extensively studied.

Benzodiazepines constitute a reasonable alternative to SSRIs as a first-line treatment for SAD. Clonazepam and bromazepam, considered separately, have shown large effect sizes in the individual randomized trials. However, as shown in our meta-analysis, the results of those two studies show heterogeneity of effect sizes. When combined into a single category, the confidence interval for the effect size of clonazepam and bromazepam included 0, suggesting that the estimates of their effect sizes are unstable. Furthermore, the only published study of alprazolam did not show significant differences from placebo, raising further reservations about the use of benzodiazepines as first-line treatment. Nevertheless it is possible that there may be within-group differences in their efficacy for the treatment of SAD.

Part of the difficulty in assessing the effect size of benzodiazepines is that it is based on only three controlled trials that included a relatively low number of patients. Furthermore, benzodiazepines, in contrast with SSRIs, are not efficacious in the treatment of some of the psychiatric disorders, such as major depressive disorder, that are frequently comorbid with SAD. One additional concern about the use of benzodiazepines is that epidemiological and clinical studies have shown high comorbidity of SAD with alcohol abuse and dependence. However, there is no evidence that use of prescribed benzodiazepines is associated with abuse liability in individuals without a history of substance-abuse disorders. Overall, we think that these considerations make benzodiazepines a less-preferred initial option for most patients.

Another alternative would be the use of phenelzine or another irreversible MAOI. However, results from the meta-analyses suggest that its efficacy is not superior to that of the

SSRIs or clonazepam, and although irreversible MAOIs are often well tolerated the need to follow a low-tyramine diet, and the subsequent risk of hypertensive crisis if the diet is not followed, constitute an important inconvenience for most patients. Furthermore, there is less systematic evidence to support the use of MAOIs than the use of SSRIs as first-line treatment. Gabapentin and pregabalin are also reasonable alternatives in cases when the previous medications fail.

How long should treatment last?

One important question, frequently asked by patients, is how long to continue in treatment once they respond to medication. A number of studies have looked at that question.

Versiani *et al.* (1992) reported 50% loss of treatment gains in the 2 months following discontinuation of phenelzine responders under double-blind conditions after 16 weeks of treatment. Liebowitz *et al.* (1992) also reported relapse in one-third of patients over 2 months following discontinuation after 16 weeks of phenelzine treatment. In our initial collaborative study, responders to 12 weeks of acute treatment were maintained on phenelzine for an additional 6 months, during which there was a 23% relapse (Liebowitz *et al.*, 1999). Continued responders were then discontinued from medication and followed for an additional 6 months, during which time there was an additional 30% relapse. Supporting the concept that concomitant CBT may help maintain the gains following cessation of medication is the finding of Gelernter *et al.* (1991), who reported no loss of phenelzine's effectiveness after 2 months of untreated follow-up.

Stein *et al.* (2002c) treated 437 patients with SAD with paroxetine for 12 weeks. Of those, 323 responded and agreed to continue treatment for an additional 24 weeks. Patients continuing treatment were randomized to paroxetine or placebo. Significantly fewer patients relapsed in the paroxetine group than in the placebo group. Furthermore, at the end of the study, a significantly greater proportion of patients in the paroxetine group showed improvement as shown on the Clinical Global Impression global improvement rating compared with the placebo group.

In another study 203 patients were randomized to sertraline or placebo. Sertraline was superior to placebo with response rates of 53% *vs.* 29% in the intent-to-treat (ITT) sample at the end of 20 weeks (Van Ameringen *et al.*, 2001). Responders to sertraline were entered into a 24-week discontinuation trial, where they were randomized to continue on drug or switch abruptly to placebo (Walker *et al.*, 2000). Relapse rates were 4% for patients continued on sertraline *vs.* 36% for those switched to placebo, a significant difference. An additional 20% of patients switched to placebo were prematurely discontinued due to adverse events *vs.* 0% for those continued on sertraline. Total premature discontinuation by the end of the 24-week follow-up was 60% for patients switched to placebo versus only 12% for those continued on sertraline, a highly significant difference. Thus, these data again suggest that even after 5 months of SSRI treatment, relapse rates are high after discontinuation.

Although data are still limited, the available evidence suggests that discontinuation of medication after 12–20 weeks of treatment results in increased risk for relapse compared with maintenance on medication after that time period. Whether longer treatment periods with medication or the addition of psychotherapy can protect against such relapse is unknown at present. Given the existing data, it appears reasonable to maintain treatment for at least

3–6 months after the patient responds to treatment, with longer periods considered in individual cases, due to the lack of available systematic evidence.

What is the management of treatment-resistant cases?

The first question in the management of treatment-resistant cases is how to define them. Stein *et al.* (2002*b*) recently analyzed pooled data from 3 placebo-controlled studies of paroxetine, including a total of 829 patients to determine predictors of response. Demographic, clinical, baseline disability, duration of treatment, and trial variables were included. After adjusting for the other covariates, only duration of treatment was a predictor of treatment response. The authors found that 46 (27.7%) out of 166 non-responders to paroxetine at week 8 were responders at week 12. The authors concluded that an optimal trial of medications should continue beyond 8 weeks. At present there is no information on the probability of response of patients who have not responded by week 12. It appears reasonable to try a new medication if the patient has not shown any response at that time. If there has been a partial response, it might be preferable to try to augment response using another efficacious medication, such as a benzodiazepine or gabapentin, although no study has systematically tested any of those strategies.

Reasons for treatment resistance

As with any other medical condition, the next step is to identify the sources of non-response. Probably an important source of therapeutic failure is non-adherence to treatment, which may have resulted in sub-optimal medication doses or duration of treatment. If that is the case, the reasons for departures from recommended treatment should be explored and remedied.

A second potential source of treatment resistance is the presence of a comorbid psychiatric disorder. Clinical trials tend to exclude patients with comorbid disorders (Blanco *et al.*, 2008, 2010*b*). Thus, there is a lack of systematic knowledge regarding the influence of comorbidity on treatment response. In an open-label study of citalopram in patients with primary SAD and comorbid depression, 67% of patients completed the study, and the response rate was 67% for SAD and 76% for major depressive disorder (Schneier *et al.*, 2003). In that study, response rates were similar to those found in clinical trials without comorbid depression. Whether presence or absence of other comorbid disorders will result in similar lack of impact is unknown.

Other specific reasons for decreased efficacy may include comorbid medical conditions or individual pharmacokinetic characteristics (such as in rapid metabolizers or drug interactions).

Management strategies

Augmentation with medication

A small number of studies have investigated augmentation strategies, although only one study has specifically examined treatment-resistant cases. In that study, conducted by Van Ameringen *et al.* (1993) ten patients, with generalized SAD who had obtained only partial response to an adequate trial of an SSRI, were studied for 8 weeks after adding buspirone. Seven (70%) patients were considered responders with a CGI of 1 or 2. However, the small sample size and the lack of control condition limit the interpretability of this study.

Stein and colleagues (Stein *et al.*, 2001) conducted a placebo-controlled study of pindolol potentiation of paroxetine for SAD. Pindolol was not superior to placebo when used as an augmenting agent to paroxetine. In this study pindolol was not used in treatment-resistant cases and was started at the same time as paroxetine. However, the fact that it failed to increase response rates in non-resistant patients and that there are no clinical trials supporting the efficacy of beta-blockers in generalized SAD suggests that it might not be a first-line agent for augmentation.

Clonazepam has also been studied as treatment augmentation of paroxetine. Seedat & Stein (2004) randomized 28 patients to paroxetine plus clonazepam or paroxetine plus placebo. More clonazepam patients (79%) than placebo patients (43%) were classified as CGI responders, but the effect only approached significance ($p = 0.06$) in this small sample. Again, an important limitation of this study was its lack of focus on treatment-resistant cases. Nevertheless, clonazepam deserves further study as an augmentation or alternative treatment for patients who do not respond completely to an initial SSRI trial.

Pharmacological alternatives for augmentation include any combination of drugs with demonstrated efficacy for SAD, provided their combined use is not contraindicated. Thus, an SSRI plus clonazepam, gabapentin or pregabalin, or clonazepam plus phenelzine appear as reasonable options. By contrast, the combination of phenelzine and an SSRI is absolutely contraindicated. However, these recommendations are purely based on clinical experience. There are no systematic data to evaluate the efficacy of those combinations.

Psychotherapy

Recent work by our group has suggested that the combination of phenelzine and cognitive–behavioral treatment (CBT) is superior to either treatment alone (Blanco *et al.*, 2010a). Therefore, providing CBT to treatment-resistant cases appears to be a reasonable strategy. However, much more evidence is needed to confirm these initial findings and to see if they extend to other medication groups.

Similarly, preliminary studies have looked at D-cycloserine, a partial agonist at the NMDA receptor, as a possible augmenting agent for fear reduction in exposure therapy (Hofmann *et al.*, 2006). Preliminary evidence has shown D-cycloserine to have a significant effect as compared with placebo in enhancing the effectiveness of attenuated course of exposure therapy for the treatment of SAD (Guastella *et al.*, 2008; Hofmann *et al.*, 2006).

The treatment of non-generalized SAD

This review has focused on the generalized subtype of SAD, which is most impairing and is the most common form among treatment-seeking patients as well as in the general population (Grant *et al.*, 2005). The non-generalized subtype, most commonly characterized by fear of public speaking or other performance situations, has been much less studied. Nearly a dozen small single-dose placebo-controlled cross-over studies in the 1970s and 1980s reported efficacy for propranolol and other beta-blockers for anxious musical performers, public speakers, and students taking a test (Potts & Davidson, 1995). On this basis, beta-blockers are currently widely used on an as-needed basis for persons with non-generalized SAD, since as-needed medication is often preferred by patients who fear predictable and occasional performance situations. Benzodiazepines are also used in this population, and may have the benefit of decreasing the anticipatory anxiety, such as not being able to sleep the night prior to a performance. However, some patients find that benzodiazepine effects of sedation or cognitive slowing may outweigh their anxiolytic benefits. Although SSRIs and MAOIs have not been studied in non-generalized subtype samples, clinical impression suggests that, when used daily, they may also benefit performance anxiety.

Treatment of SAD in children

Although children and adolescents with SAD often have great impairment in their social and family relationships and academic life, this often goes underdiagnosed and undertreated. Few studies of pediatric SAD have examined the efficacy of treatment modalities, making the role of pharmacotherapy for treatment of this disorder less established than for adults. The first group of studies conducted in children included a wide range of anxiety disorders and some of them concentrated on selective mutism, a condition shown to greatly overlap with SAD.

Only two studies have investigated the efficacy of benzodiazepines in this population. In contrast to the scarcity of studies conducted on benzodiazepines, more data are available on the efficacy of SSRIs. Several placebo-controlled trials have been conducted, providing substantial evidence of the efficacy of SSRIs and SNRIs in children 6–17 years of age. However, the increasing concern about studies, most of them in depression, reporting an increased risk of suicidal ideation among adolescents treated with SSRIs or SNRIs led the FDA to add a warning in regard to the use of antidepressants in this population.

Although replication is still needed and long-term effects are still unknown, a growing body of literature supports the efficacy of pharmacological treatments in children and adolescents. SSRIs and SNRIs are the pharmacological treatment of choice in this population, with response rates ranging from 36% to 77%, but concerns regarding the emergence of suicidal ideation suggest the need for close monitoring of these treatments in this population.

Conclusion

There are several medications with substantial evidence of treatment efficacy. Future, cumulative meta-analyses should continue to update our base of knowledge about the relative efficacy of different medications in the treatment of SAD. At the same time, as pointed out in the second section of this review, there are still important gaps in our knowledge. Those gaps constitute important second-generation questions for research in SAD. Another area of future research should be the progressive linkage of biological findings and therapeutic strategies, so that treatment becomes not only evidence-based, but also theory-driven.

Acknowledgements

Supported by grant DA023200 and the New York State Psychiatric Institute.

Statement of interest

Dr. Liebowitz reports the following potential conflict of interests: Equity ownership: Chi-Matrix LLC, electronic data capture and Liebowitz Social Anxiety Scale. Consulting:

AstraZeneca, Wyeth, Pfizer, Takeda, Pherin, Lilly, Otsuka, Eisai. Licensing software or LSAS: GSK, Pfizer, Avera, Tikvah, Endo, Lilly, Indevus, Servier. Recent or Current Clinical trial contracts:

Allergan, Pfizer, GSK, AstraZeneca, Forest, Tikvah, Avera, Eli Lilly, Novartis, Sepracor, Horizon, Johnson and Johnson. Pherin, PGX Health, Abbott, Jazz, MAP, Takeda, Wyeth, Cephalon, Indevus, Endo, Ortho-McNeil, Gruenthal, Otsuka, Gruenthal. All other authors report no conflicts of interests.

References

Allgulander, CI (1999). Paroxetine in social anxiety disorder: a randomized placebo-controlled study. *Acta Psychiatrica Scandinavica* 100, 196–198.

Allgulander CI, Mangano R, Zhang J et al. (2004). Efficacy of venlafaxine ER in patients with social anxiety disorder: a double-blind, placebo-controlled, parallel-group comparison with paroxetine. *Human Psychopharmacology: Clinical and Experimental* 9, 387–396.

American Psychiatric Association (APA) (2000). *Diagnostic and Statistical Manual of Mental Disorders (4th edn) – Text Revision.* Washington, DC: American Psychiatric Association.

Amies PL, Gelder MG, Shaw PM (1983). Social phobia: a comparative clinical study. *British Journal of Psychiatry* 142, 174–179.

Baldwin D, Bobes, J, Stein DJ et al. (1999). Paroxetine in social phobia/social anxiety disorder: randomized, double-blind, placebo-controlled study. *British Journal of Psychiatry* 175, 120–126.

Barnett SD, Kramer ML, Casat CD et al. (2002). Efficacy of olanzapine in social anxiety disorder: a pilot study. *Journal of Psychopharmacology* 16, 365–368.

Black B, Uhde TW, Tancer ME (1992). Fluoxetine for the treatment of social phobia. *Journal of Clinical Psychopharmacology* 12, 293–295.

Blanco C, Heimberg RG, Schneier FR et al. (2010a). A placebo-controlled trial of phenelzine, cognitive behavioral group therapy, and their combination for social anxiety disorder. *Archives of General Psychiatry* 67, 286–295.

Blanco C, Okuda M, Markowitz JC et al. (2010b). The epidemiology of chronic major depressive disorder and dysthymic disorder: results from the National Epidemiologic Survey on Alcohol and Related Conditions. *Journal of Clinical Psychiatry* 71, 1645–1656.

Blanco C, Olfson M, Okuda M et al. (2008). Generalizability of clinical trials for alcohol dependence to community samples. *Drug and Alcohol Dependence* 98, 123–128.

Blanco C, Raza MS, Schneier FR, Liebowitz MR (2003a). The evidence-based pharmacological treatment of social anxiety disorder. *International Journal of Neuropsychopharmacology* 6, 427–442.

Blanco C, Schneier FR, Schmidt AB et al. (2003b). Pharmacological treatment of social anxiety disorder: a meta-analysis. *Depression and Anxiety* 18, 29–40.

Blomhoff, S, Haug TT, Hellstrom K et al. (2001). Randomised controlled general practice trial of sertraline, exposure therapy and combined treatment in generalised social phobia. *British Journal of Psychiatry* 179, 23–30.

Clark D, Agras WS (1991). The assessment and treatment of performance anxiety in musicians. *American Journal of Psychiatry* 148, 598–605.

Clark DM, Ehlers A, McManus F et al. (2003). Cognitive therapy versus fluoxetine in generalized social phobia: a randomized placebo-controlled trial. *Journal of Consulting and Clinical Psychology* 71, 1058–1067.

Davidson JR, Foa EB, Huppert JD et al. (2004a). Fluoxetine, comprehensive cognitive behavioral therapy, and placebo in generalized social phobia. *Archives of General Psychiatry* 61, 1005–1013.

Davidson, JR, Potts N, Richichi E et al. (1993). Treatment of social phobia with clonazepam and placebo. *Journal of Clinical Psychopharmacology* 13, 423–428.

Davidson JR, Yaryura-Tobias J, DuPont R et al. (2004b). Fluvoxamine-controlled release formulation for the treatment of generalized social anxiety disorder. *Journal of Clinical Psychopharmacology* 24, 118–125.

Fedoroff IC, Taylor S. (2001). Psychological and pharmacological treatments of social phobia: a meta-analysis. *Journal of Clinical Psychopharmacology* **21**, 311–323.

Feltner DE, Liu-Dumaw M, Schweizer E, Bielski R (2011). Efficacy of pregabalin in generalized social anxiety disorder: results of a double-blind, placebo-controlled, fixed-dose study. *International Clinical Psychopharmacology* **26**(4), 213–220.

Fleiss JL (1994). Measures of effect size for categorical data. In Cooper H, Hedges L (Eds.), *The Handbook of Research Synthesis* (pp. 245–260). New York, NY: Russell Sage Foundation.

Gelernter CS, Uhde TW, Cimbolic P *et al.* (1991). Cognitive–behavioral and pharmacological treatments of social phobia: A controlled study. *Archives of General Psychiatry*, **48**, 938–945.

Glesser, LJ, Olkin I (1994). Stochastically dependent effect sizes. In Cooper H, Hedges L (Eds.), *The Handbook of Research Synthesis* (pp. 339–356). New York, NY: Russell Sage Foundation.

Gould RA, Buckminister S, Pollack MH *et al.* (1997). Cognitive-behavioral and pharmacological treatments of social phobia: a meta-analysis. *Clinical Psychology: Science and Practice* **4**, 291–306.

Grant BF, Hasin DS, Blanco C, Stinson FS *et al.* (2005). The epidemiology of social anxiety disorder in the United States: Results from the National Epidemiologic Survey on Alcohol and Related Conditions. *Journal of Clinical Psychiatry* **66**, 1351–1361.

Guastella AJ, Richardson R, Lovibond PF *et al.* (2008). A randomized controlled trial of D-cycloserine enhancement of exposure therapy for social anxiety disorder. *Biological Psychiatry* **63**, 544–549.

Hedges DW, Brown BL, Shwalb DA *et al.* (2007). The efficacy of selective serotonin reuptake inhibitors in adult social anxiety disorder: a meta-analysis of double-blind, placebo-controlled trials. *Journal of Psychopharmacology* **21**, 102–111.

Hedges LV, Olkin, I (1985). *Statistical Methods for Meta-analysis*. Orlando, FL: Academic Press.

Heimberg RG, Horner KJ, Juster HR *et al.* (1999). Psychometric properties of the Liebowitz Social Anxiety Scale. *Psychological Medicine* **29**, 199–212.

Heimberg RG, Liebowitz MR, Hope DA *et al.* (1998). Cognitive-behavioral group therapy vs phenelzine therapy for social phobia. *Archives of General Psychiatry* **55**, 1133–1141.

Hofmann SG, Meuret AE, Smits JA *et al.* (2006). Augmentation of exposure therapy with D-cycloserine for social anxiety disorder. *Archives of General Psychiatry* **63**, 298–304.

Kasper S, Stein DJ, Loft H, Nil R (2005). Escitalopram in the treatment of social anxiety disorder: randomised, placebo-controlled, flexible-dosage study. *British Journal of Psychiatry* **186**, 222–226.

Katschnig H, Stein MB, Buller R (1997). Moclobemide in social phobia. A double-blind, placebo-controlled clinical study. *European Archives of Psychiatry and Clinical Neuroscience* **247**, 71–80.

Katzelnick DJ, Kobak KA, Greist JH *et al.* (1995). Sertraline for social phobia: a double-blind, placebo-controlled cross-over study. *American Journal of Psychiatry* **152**, 1368–1371.

Kobak KA, Griest JH, Jefferson JW, Katzelnick DJ (2002). Fluoxetine in social phobia: a double-blind placebo controlled pilot study. *Journal of Clinical Psychopharmacology* **22**, 257–262.

Lader M, Stender K, Burger V, Nil R (2004). Efficacy and tolerability of escitalopram in 12- and 24-week treatment of social anxiety disorder: randomised, double-blind, placebo-controlled, fixed-dose study. *Depression and Anxiety* **19**, 241–248.

Lepola U, Bergtholdt B, St Lambert J *et al.* (2004). Controlled-release paroxetine in the treatment of patients with social anxiety disorder. *Journal of Clinical Psychiatry* **65**, 222–229.

Liebowitz MR (1987). Social phobia. *Modern Problems of Pharmacopsychiatry* **22**, 141–173.

Liebowitz MR, DeMartinis NA, Weihs *et al.* (2003). Efficacy of sertraline in severe generalized social anxiety disorder: results of a double-blind, placebo-controlled study. *Journal of Clinical Psychiatry* **64**, 785–792.

Liebowitz MR, Gelenberg AJ, Munjack D (2005*a*). Venlafaxine extended release vs placebo and paroxetine in social anxiety disorder. *Archives of General Psychiatry* **62**, 190–198.

Liebowitz MR, Heimberg RG, Schneier FR *et al.* (1999). Cognitive-behavioral group therapy versus phenelzine in social phobia: long-term outcome. *Depression and Anxiety* **10**, 89–98.

Liebowitz MR, Mangano RM, Bradwejn J, Asnis G (2005*b*). A randomized controlled trial of venlafaxine extended release in generalized social anxiety disorder. *Journal of Clinical Psychiatry* **66**, 238–247.

Liebowitz MR, Schneier FR, Campeas R *et al.* (1992). Phenelzine *vs.* atenolol in social phobia: a placebo–controlled comparison. *Archives of General Psychiatry* **49**, 290–300.

Liebowitz MR, Stein MB, Tancer M *et al.* (2002). A randomized, double-blind, fixed-dose comparison of paroxetine and placebo in the treatment of generalized social anxiety disorder. *Journal of Clinical Psychiatry* **63**, 66–74.

Marks IM (1970). The classification of phobic disorders. *British Journal of Psychiatry* **116**, 377–386.

Montgomery SA, Nil R, Durr-Pal N *et al.* (2005). A 24-week randomized, double-blind, placebo-controlled study of escitalopram for the prevention of generalized social anxiety disorder. *Journal of Clinical Psychiatry* **66**, 1270–1278.

Muehlbacher M, Nickel MK, Nickel C *et al.* (2005). Mirtazapine treatment of social phobia in women: a randomized, double-blind, placebo-controlled study. *Journal of Clinical Psychopharmacology* **25**, 580–583.

Munjack DJ, Baltazar PL, Bohn PB *et al.* (1990). Clonazepam in the treatment of social phobia: a pilot study. *Journal of Clinical Psychiatry* **51** (Suppl.), 35–53.

Noyes R, Moroz G, Davidson J *et al.* (1997). Moclobemide in social phobia: a controlled dose-response. *Journal of Clinical Psychopharmacology* **17**, 247–254.

Öst LG (1987). Age of onset in different phobias. *Journal of Abnormal Psychology* **96**, 223–229.

Pande AC, Davidson RT, Jefferson JW *et al.* (1999). Treatment of social phobia with gabapentin: a placebo controlled study. *Journal of Clinical Psychopharmacology* **19**, 341–348.

Potts NLS, Davidson JRT (1995). Pharmacological treatments: literature review. In Heimberg RG, Liebowitz MR, Hope DA, Schneier FR (Eds.), *Social Phobia: Diagnosis, Assessment and Treatment* (pp. 334–365) New York, NY: Guilford Press.

Rickels K, Mangano R, Khan A (2004). A double-blind, placebo-controlled study of a flexible dose of venlafaxine ER in adult outpatients with generalized social anxiety disorder. *Journal of Clinical Psychopharmacology* **24**, 488–496.

Schneier FR, Blanco C, Campeas R *et al.* (2003). Citalopram treatment of social anxiety disorder and comorbid major depression. *Depression and Anxiety* **17**, 191–196.

Schneier FR, Chin SJ, Hollander E, Liebowitz MR (1992*a*). Fluoxetine in social phobia. *Journal of Clinical Psychopharmacology* **12**, 62–64.

Schneier FR, Goetz D, Campeas R *et al.* (1998). A placebo-controlled trial of moclobemide in social phobia. *British Journal of Psychiatry* **172**, 70–77.

Schneier FR, Johnson J, Hornig CD *et al.* (1992*b*). Social phobia: comorbidity and morbidity in an epidemiological sample. *Archives of General Psychiatry* **49**, 282–288.

Schneier FR, Saoud JB (1993). Buspirone in social phobia. *Journal of Clinical Psychopharmacology* **13**, 251–256.

Schutters SI, Van Megen HJ, Van Veen JF *et al.* (2010). Mirtazapine in generalized social anxiety disorder: a randomized, double-blind, placebo-controlled study. *International Journal of Clinical Psychopharmacology* **25**, 302–304.

Seedat S, Stein MB (2004). Double-blind, placebo-controlled assessment of combined clonazepam with paroxetine compared with paroxetine monotherapy for generalized social anxiety disorder. *Journal of Clinical Psychiatry* **65**, 244–248.

Simon NM, Korbly NB, Worthington JJ *et al.* (2002). Citalopram for social anxiety disorder: an open-label pilot study in refractory and nonrefractory patients. *CNS Spectrums* **7**, 655–657.

Simpson HB, Schneier FR, Campeas RB *et al.* (1998). Imipramine in the treatment of social phobia. *Journal of Clinical Psychopharmacology* **18**, 132–135.

Stein DJ, Cameron A, Amrein R, Montgomery SA (2002a). Moclobemide is effective and well tolerated in the long-term pharmacotherapy of social anxiety disorder with or without comorbid anxiety disorder. *International Clinical Psychopharmacology* **17**, 161–170.

Stein DJ, Stein MB, Pitts CD et al. (2002b). Predictors of response to pharmacotherapy in social anxiety disorder, an analysis of 3 placebo-controlled paroxetine trials. *Journal of Clinical Psychiatry* **63**, 152–155.

Stein DJ, Versiani M, Hair T, Kumar R (2002c). Efficacy of paroxetine for relapse prevention in social anxiety disorder: a 24-week study. *Archives of General Psychiatry* **59**, 1111–1118.

Stein MB, Fyer AJ, Davidson JRT et al. (1999). Fluvoxamine treatment of social phobia (social anxiety disorder): a double-blind placebo-controlled study. *American Journal of Psychiatry* **156**, 756–760.

Stein MB, Liebowitz MR, Lydiard RB et al. (1998). Paroxetine treatment of generalized social phobia (social anxiety disorder): a randomized, double-blind, placebo-controlled study. *Journal of the American Medical Association* **280**, 708–713.

Stein MB, Pollack MH, Bystritsky A et al. (2005). Efficacy of low and higher dose extended-release venlafaxine in generalized social anxiety disorder: a 6-month randomized controlled trial. *Psychopharmacology* **177**, 280–288.

Stein MB, Sareen J, Hami S, Chao J (2001). Pindolol potentiation of paroxetine for generalized social phobia. A double-blind, placebo-controlled, cross-over study. *American Journal of Psychiatry* **158**, 1725–1727.

Sternbach H (1990). Fluoxetine treatment of social phobia. *Journal of Clinical Psychopharmacology* **10**, 230–231.

Turner SM, Beidel DC, Jacob RG (1994). Social phobia: a comparison of behavior therapy and atenolol. *Journal of Consulting Clinical Psychology* **62**, 350–358.

Van Ameringen MA, Lane RM, Walker JR et al. (2001). Sertraline treatment of generalized social phobia: a 20-week double-blind, placebo-controlled study. *American Journal of Psychiatry*, **158**, 275–281.

Van Ameringen M, Mancini C, Oakman J et al. (2007). Nefazodone in the treatment of generalized social phobia: a randomized, placebo-controlled trial. *Journal of Clinical Psychiatry* **68**, 288–295.

Van Ameringen M, Mancini C, Streiner DL (1993). Fluoxetine efficacy in social phobia. *Journal of Clinical Psychiatry* **54**, 27–32.

Van der Linden GJH, Stein DJ, Van Balkom A (2000). The efficacy of the selective serotonin reuptake inhibitors for social anxiety disorder: a meta-analysis of randomized controlled trials. *International Clinical Psychopharmacology* **15** (Suppl.), S15–S23.

van Vliet IM, den Boer JA, Westenberg HGM (1994). Psychopharmacological treatment of social phobia: a double blind controlled study with fluvoxamine. *Psychopharmacology* **115**, 128–134.

van Vliet IM, den Boer JA, Westenberg HGM, Ho Pian KL (1997) Clinical effects of buspirone in social phobia: a double-blind placebo controlled study. *Journal of Clinical Psychiatry* **58**, 164–168.

Versiani M, Amrein R, Montgomery SA (1997a). Social phobia: long-term treatment outcome and prediction of response – a moclobemide study. *International Clinical Psychopharmacology* **12**, 239–254.

Versiani M, Nardia AE, Figueira I et al. (1997b). Double-blind placebo controlled trials with bromazepam. *Jornal Brasileiro de Psiquiatria* **46**, 167–171.

Versiani M, Nardi AE, Mundim FD et al. (1992). Pharmacotherapy of social phobia: a controlled study with moclobemide and phenelzine. *British Journal of Psychiatry* **161**, 353–360.

Wagner KD (2003). Paroxetine treatment of mood and anxiety disorders in children and adolescents. *Psychopharmacology Bulletin* **37** (Suppl.), 167–175.

Walker JR, Van Ameringen MA, Swinson R et al. (2000). Prevention of relapse in generalized social phobia: results of a 24-week study in responders to 20 weeks of sertraline treatment. *Journal of Clinical Psychopharmacology* **20**, 636–644.

Westenberg HG, Stein DJ, Yang H et al. (2004). A double-blind placebo-controlled study of controlled release fluvoxamine for the treatment of generalized social anxiety disorder. *Journal of Clinical Psychopharmacology* **24**, 49–55.

Wittchen HU, Beloch E (1996). The impact of social phobia on quality of life. *International Clinical Psychopharmacology* **11** (Suppl.), 15–23.

Zhang W, Connor KM, Davidson JR (2005). Levetiracetam in social phobia: a placebo controlled pilot study. *Journal of Psychopharmacology* **19**, 551–553.

Zitrin CM, Klein DF, Woerner MG, Ross DC (1983). Treatment of phobias: a comparison of imipramine hydrochloride and placebo. *Archives of General Psychiatry* **40**, 125–138.

Evidence-based pharmacotherapy of generalized anxiety disorder

David S. Baldwin, Sarah Waldman, and
Christer Allgulander

Introduction

Generalized anxiety disorder (GAD) is characterized by excessive and inappropriate worry-
ing that is persistent (lasting some months in ICD–10, and $\geq$ 6 months in DSM–IV–TR)
and not restricted to particular circumstances. Patients have physical ("somatic") anxiety
symptoms (such as palpitations and tremor) and psychological ("psychic") anxiety symptoms, including restlessness, fatigue, difficulty concentrating, irritability, and disturbed sleep
(Tyrer & Baldwin, 2006).

The disorder is common in both community and clinical settings. A review of epidemiological studies in Europe suggests a 12-month prevalence of 1.2–1.9%, and a lifetime prevalence of 1.7 to 3.4% (Wittchen *et al.*, 2011). "Comorbidity" with major depression or other
anxiety disorders is seen in the majority of cases (Wittchen *et al.*, 2011). The degree of associated functional impairment is similar to that with major depression (Kessler *et al.*, 1999;
Wittchen *et al.*, 2000). Patients with comorbid major depression and GAD tend to have a
more severe and prolonged course of illness and greater functional impairment (Judd *et al.*,
1998; Tyrer *et al.*, 2004). The disorder is more common in women than men, typically with
a gradual evolution (Beesdo *et al.*, 2009) and an onset of the full syndromal disorder later
than that with other anxiety disorders: it is the most common anxiety disorder among the
population aged 55–85 years (Beekman *et al.*, 1998).

GAD is one of the most common mental disorders in primary medical-care settings, and
is associated with increased use of health services. In a study of adult primary-care patients
in Norway, Sweden, Denmark, and Finland, the rates of GAD were 4.1–6.0% among men and
3.7–7.1 among women (Munk-Jorgensen *et al.*, 2006). The proportion of GAD patients recognized by a general practitioner varied from 33% in Denmark to 53% in Norway. A probable
reason for the low detection rate seen in this study is that only a minority of patients present
with anxiety symptoms, and GAD often goes unrecognized as doctors tend to overlook anxiety, unless it is a presenting complaint. Patients with comorbid depression are more likely to
be recognized as having a mental health problem, although not necessarily as having GAD
(Weiller *et al.*, 1998; Wittchen *et al.*, 2002).

Advances in research into anxiety disorders have recently been reviewed (Garner *et al.*,
2009). Anxiety disorders can be regarded as developmental disorders, resulting from gene
and environment interactions that can induce structural and functional changes in amygdala prefrontal circuitry (Leonardo & Hen, 2008). Anxiety disorders are certainly genetically

Essential Evidence-Based Psychopharmacology, Second Edition, ed. Dan J. Stein, Bernard Lerer,
and Stephen M. Stahl. Published by Cambridge University Press. © Cambridge University Press.

complex, and the apparent phenotypes may be the expression of gene–gene as well as gene–environment interactions (Smoller et al., 2009). Current theories on pathological anxiety fit a multifactorial epigenetic model that integrates early stressors, inherited and acquired vulnerabilities, and the risks of developing interrelated or coincidental somatic diseases.

Search strategy

We conducted a computerized literature search of electronic databases for the years 1980–2009 using a strategy which combined the terms (generalized/generalised anxiety disorder) with (randomized/randomised controlled trial). In addition we consulted with colleagues about potential treatment studies not identified through the search and examined recently published systematic reviews and evidence-based guidelines. We also attempted to identify recently completed treatment studies, available only as conference abstracts. It should be noted that not all treatments considered below have a product licence for treatment of patients with GAD across all countries, and it is wise to refer to local prescribing information.

Response rates in acute treatment studies

The findings of randomized placebo-controlled trials show that approximately 40–60% of patients "respond" to placebo and 60–75% to the selective serotonin reuptake inhibitor (SSRI) compounds escitalopram, paroxetine, and sertraline, when using global measures of improvement, most commonly the Clinical Global Impression of Improvement Scale (CGI-I; Guy, 1976). Similar findings are seen in randomized placebo-controlled trials with the serotonin norepinephrine reuptake inhibitors (SNRI) compounds duloxetine and venlafaxine, with the novel anxiolytic drug pregabalin (Baldwin & Ajel, 2007) and with the second-generation antipsychotic drug quetiapine (Table 7.1).

There can be a marked reduction in symptom severity on the primary outcome measure, which is traditionally the Hamilton Rating Scale for Anxiety (HAMA; Hamilton, 1959). For example, a decline from baseline in mean HAMA score of >15 points with the optimal 10 mg/day dosage of escitalopram (Baldwin et al., 2006a), and a decline of almost 16 points with the optimal 150 mg/day dosage of quetiapine (Bandelow et al., 2010). However, many patients remain troubled by significant symptoms at study end-point, despite seemingly making a good overall "response" to treatment, judged by being "much" or "very much" improved on the CGI-I scale.

Benzodiazepine anxiolytic drugs can represent an efficacious and rapid treatment for some patients with GAD (Gould et al., 1997). An early comparison of the benzodiazepine diazepam with the antidepressants trazodone and imipramine found that diazepam-treated patients had the greatest reduction in anxiety symptoms over the first 2 weeks of the trial; however, at the end of the study only imipramine was superior to placebo (Rickels et al., 1993). Furthermore, benzodiazepines have limited effect in relieving comorbid depressive symptoms, and many unwanted side-effects including drowsiness, disturbances of memory, and impaired psychomotor function. These problems can limit their overall effectiveness, particularly as many patients stop treatment before the full anxiolytic effects are seen (Martin et al., 2007). Other potential problems include the development of tolerance and dependence, and some patients describe distressing withdrawal symptoms on stopping treatment (Rickels et al., 1988; Tyrer et al., 1983). Because of these potential difficulties, general guidance has been to prescribe benzodiazepines only in certain circumscribed conditions: for short-term treatment (up to 4 weeks) of anxiety and insomnia; as an initial adjunct to antidepressant

Table 7.1. Generalized anxiety disorder: overall response rates in double-blind placebo-controlled studies of acute treatment with SSRIs, SNRIs, pregabalin, and quetiapine.

Study	Treatment	Dose (mg/day)	Length (weeks)	Efficacy on change in HAMA	Active response (%)	Placebo response (%)
SSRI treatment						
Pollack et al. (2001)	Paroxetine	20–50	8	Yes	62*	47
Hewett et al. (2001)	Paroxetine	20–50	8	No	63 (n.s.)	49.7
Rickels et al. (2003)	Paroxetine	20, 40	8	Yes	61.7*, 68***	45.6
Rynn et al. (2001) (children)	Sertraline	≤50	9	Yes	10	90***
Morris et al. (2003)	Sertraline	50–150	12	Yes	63***	37
Allgulander et al. (2004)	Sertraline	50–150	12	Yes	63***	37
Brawman-Mintzer et al. (2006)	Sertraline	50–200	10	Yes	64.6 (n.s.)	54.3
Davidson et al. (2004)	Escitalopram	10–20	8	Yes	58**	38
Goodman et al. (2005) Pooled analysis, 3 studies	Escitalopram	10–20	8	Yes	52***	37
Baldwin et al. (2006a)	Escitalopram	5, 10, 20	12	Yes (10, 20)	70.9 (n.s.) 78.4**, 74.2*	63
	Paroxetine	20		No	66.2	
Lenze et al. (2009)	Escitalopram	10–20	12	No	69.0***	51.0
SNRI treatment						
Koponen et al. (2007)	Duloxetine	60, 120	9	Yes	63***, 65***	34
Rynn et al. (2008)	Duloxetine	60–120	10	Yes	52*	41[a]
Hartford et al. (2007)	Duloxetine Venlafaxine ER	60–120 75–225	10	Yes Yes	56** 60***	42
Davidson et al. (1999)	Venlafaxine ER Buspirone	75, 150 30	8	No No	62**, 49 (n.s.) 55*	39
Gelenberg et al. (2000)	Venlafaxine ER	75–225	28	Yes	67***	33
Rickels et al. (2000)	Venlafaxine ER	75, 150, 225	8	Yes	n.s., n.s.,* [A]	n.r.

Table 7.1. (cont.)

Study	Treatment	Dose (mg/day)	Length (weeks)	Efficacy on change in HAMA	Active response (%)	Placebo response (%)
Allgulander et al. (2001)	Venlafaxine ER	37.5, 75, 225	24	Yes	63**, 73***, 81*** [b]	47[a]
Lenox-Smith & Reynolds (2003)	Venlafaxine ER	75–225	24	Yes	65**	46
Rynn et al. (2007) Pooled analysis, 2 studies	Venlafaxine ER	Flexible dose in children 6–17 years	8	Yes (1 study)	69**	48
Pregabalin treatment						
Pande et al. (2003)	Pregabalin Lorazepam	150, 600 6	4	Yes Yes	n.r. (n.s.), 47* 57*	28
Pande et al. (2000)	Pregabalin Lorazepam	150, 600 6	4	No	No significant difference in efficacy for any treatment vs. placebo	
Feltner et al. (2003)	Pregabalin Lorazepam	150, 600 6	4	Yes (600) Yes	47.8, 49.2 56.3	42.4
Rickels et al. (2005)	Pregabalin Alprazolam	300, 450, 600 1.5	4	Yes (all) Yes	61***, 44 (n.s.), 51** 45*	31
Montgomery et al. (2006)	Pregabalin Venlafaxine	400, 600 75	6	Yes Yes	56*, 59* 61**	42
Pohl et al. (2005)	Pregabalin	200, 400, 450	6	Yes (all)	56**, 55**, 59**	34
Montgomery et al. (2008) (elderly patients)	Pregabalin	150–600 (mean maximal 270)	8	Yes	58.4 (n.s.)	48.4
Kasper et al. (2009)	Pregabalin Venlafaxine	300–600 75–225	8	Yes No	59≪ 44 (n.s.) [B]	46
Quetiapine treatment						
Bandelow et al. (2010)	Quetiapine ER Paroxetine	50, 150 20	8	Yes Yes	62.6*, 70.8*** 65.9* [B]	52.1
Meredith et al. (2011)	Quetiapine ER	150, 300	8	Yes	65.1	n.s.,

(cont.)

Table 7.1. (cont.)

Study	Treatment	Dose (mg/day)	Length (weeks)	Efficacy on change in HAMA	Active response (%)	Placebo response (%)
57.2	n.s.	51.2				
	Escitalopram	10		Yes	60.6 n.s.	
Khan et al. (2011)	Quetiapine ER	50, 150, 300	8	Yes (50 and 150)	66.2*, 67.3*, 58.0 n.s.	56.9
Eriksson et al. (2008)	Quetiapine ER	50–300	9	Yes	73.4***	24.3

ER, extended release (long-acting formulation); n.r., not reported; n.s., not significantly different from placebo.
Response rates are based on Clinical Global Impression of Improvement (CGI-I) scores of 1 (very much improved) or 2 (much improved) unless otherwise stated.
[a] Response defined as ≥50% reduction in HAMA score.
[b] Estimates from published figure.
[c] $p < 0.05$, vs. venlafaxine; [A], based on distribution of CGI-I scores at study endpoint; [B], based on HAMA response.
(≥50% reduction in symptom severity).
* $p < 0.05$, ** $p < 0.01$, *** $p < 0.001$, advantage for active treatment over placebo.

drugs (Baldwin et al., 2005; Bandelow et al., 2008); and to allow maintenance treatment in patients with severe, distressing, and disabling anxiety symptoms who have not responded to at least two previous treatments, or who have not tolerated other anxiolytic classes of medication (Allgulander & Nutt, in press; Baldwin & Polkinghorn, 2005; Royal College of Psychiatrists, 1997).

Unlike the situation in major depression, there is limited consensus on what constitutes symptom remission in GAD. A post-hoc analysis of randomized placebo-controlled trials with escitalopram (Bandelow et al., 2006) indicates that a HAMA score of ≤9 corresponds to the category of at most "borderline ill" on the CGI-I severity scale (Guy, 1976). Using this cut-off score, 56% of patients treated with the optimal 10 mg/day dosage of escitalopram had remitted at the end of 12 weeks of double-blind treatment (but only 47.9% when using a lower HAMA cut-off score of ≤7) in the dose-finding escitalopram study (Baldwin et al., 2006a). Post-hoc analysis of data from the extensive clinical trial program for paroxetine using this more stringent criterion (HAMA score ≤7) found that only 36% of patients undergoing double-blind treatment with paroxetine had remitted at study end-point (Rickels et al., 2006). Remission rates with quetiapine in the fixed-dose studies which included the optimal150 mg/day dosage range between 37–43% (Baldwin & Waldman, 2009).

Few randomized controlled trials have permitted assessment of the relative efficacy of different treatments, when each is compared with placebo. An analysis of randomized controlled trials of acute treatment found an overall mean effect size of 0.39, with some differences between medication class: pregabalin, 0.50; the antihistamine hydroxyzine, 0.45; SNRIs, 0.42; benzodiazepines, 0.38; SSRIs, 0.36; and the azapirone anxiolytic buspirone, 0.17 (Hidalgo et al., 2007). The mean overall effect size in this analysis is higher than that from a previous meta-analysis (0.33) (Mitte et al., 2005), which may reflect differences in publication selection criteria. A recent mixed treatment comparison suggests that among treatments that are licensed for GAD, duloxetine may be superior in terms of response, escitalopram superior in terms of remission, and pregabalin superior in terms of tolerability (Baldwin et al., 2011a). However, post-hoc analyses such as these are derived from randomized controlled trials which differ in design and are powered for other purposes, and do not take account of tolerability problems, so much caution is needed when viewing relative effect sizes: furthermore, the finding for hydroxyzine is based on limited data, and it is not indicated for the treatment of GAD. What comparisons such as these do demonstrate, however, is that there is much scope for improvement in developing treatments with greater efficacy than is seen with currently available medications.

Tolerability concerns

The tolerability profile of prescribed medication is an important consideration, particularly when long-term treatment is recommended. Whilst adverse effects with SSRIs and SNRIs such as increased nervousness, headache, and nausea, or the drowsiness associated with benzodiazepines and pregabalin, usually resolve after a few weeks of treatment, other side-effects become more important factors in the overall acceptability of treatment in subsequent months. The adverse event profile of different SSRIs and SNRIs is generally rather similar, although significantly fewer patients dropped out due to adverse events in short-term and medium-term randomized controlled trials with escitalopram, than with paroxetine or venlafaxine (Baldwin et al., 2007a).

Common concerns during longer-term treatment with SSRIs or SNRIs include sexual dysfunction, weight gain, and persistent disturbed sleep, and the potential for experiencing discontinuation symptoms on stopping treatment. Treatment-emergent sexual dysfunction is probably the most common complication of SSRI treatment in depressed patients (Baldwin, 2004), although some aspects of sexual function usually improve, as depressive symptoms resolve (Baldwin et al., 2006b, 2008). It is uncertain whether the same pattern applies in the treatment of patients with GAD, in whom the complaint of loss of sexual desire is less common. Treatment-emergent sexual dysfunction has not been reported in studies of pregabalin.

Weight gain may be less troublesome with SSRIs than with many other psychotropic drugs, but the potential for gaining weight can cause concern in many patients. Studies of long-term treatment of depressed patients with SSRIs suggest fluoxetine is not associated with more weight gain than with placebo (Michelson et al., 1999); a review reports that paroxetine is associated with more weight gain than is seen with either fluoxetine or sertraline (Fava, 2000). In a naturalistic study of SSRI-treated patients with obsessive–compulsive disorder, between 4.5% (sertraline) and 14.3% (citalopram, paroxetine) had clinically significant weight gain (i.e. > 7% of baseline body weight) (Maina et al., 2004). Analysis of the pooled clinical trial databases for quetiapine in patients with major depressive disorder or GAD suggests that approximately 15% of patients have experienced clinically significant weight gain (defined as an increase in body mass of ≥ 7) by the end of continuation treatment (Baldwin & Waldman, 2009).

SSRIs and related drugs may have only limited benefit, or even deleterious effects, on sleep disturbance, despite beneficial effects on other depressive and anxiety symptoms (Carney et al., 2007; Cervena et al., 2005). A double-blind, placebo-controlled trial indicates that pregabalin has advantages over venlafaxine in causing less disruption, and greater improvement, of sleep during the acute treatment of patients with GAD (Kasper et al., 2009).

Prediction of response to pharmacological treatment

It is not possible to predict accurately which patients will respond well and which will have only a limited response to treatment. Imaging studies of the neurobiological correlates of symptom improvement with venlafaxine and the glutamate receptor blocker riluzole (which has no proven efficacy in GAD) have produced intriguing findings (Mathew *et al.*, 2008; Nitschke *et al.*, 2009; Whalen *et al.*, 2008) but in clinical practice response prediction rests largely on considering clinical features such as severity of symptoms and duration of illness.

A greater likelihood of response to venlafaxine or the SSRI fluoxetine is associated with a shorter duration of symptoms (Perugi *et al.*, 2002; Simon *et al.*, 2006), and the presence of comorbid dysthymia rather than comorbid major depression (response to venlafaxine) (Perugi *et al.*, 2002). Other predictors of response include absence of psychiatric comorbidity (Rodriguez *et al.*, 2006), a history of depression or panic disorder (response to venlafaxine) (Pollack *et al.*, 2003), and lower severity of psychosocial impairment (Rodriguez *et al.*, 2006). The likelihood of response to escitalopram or placebo is not influenced significantly by baseline symptom severity (Stein *et al.*, 2006), and a history of benzodiazepine use is associated with lower response to venlafaxine (Pollack *et al.*, 2003). Preliminary analysis suggests that greater symptom severity at baseline is associated with greater differential effects of quetiapine *vs.* placebo (Montgomery *et al.*, 2009).

Further investigations of the influence of comorbid depressive symptoms have produced mixed findings, but the majority indicate a lack of negative impact. Comorbid depression was found to delay the response to venlafaxine (Pollack *et al.*, 2003), but it did not substantially reduce overall response rates with escitalopram (Stein *et al.*, 2005) or pregabalin (Stein *et al.*, 2008*a*); nor did comorbid depression affect the degree of reduction in anxiety symptoms with fluoxetine (Olatunji *et al.*, 2008).

There is persisting uncertainty about how long an initial treatment for GAD should continue, before it is reasonable to conclude that the chance of responding is too low to justify continuing with the current approach. In an early study, greater reduction in HAMA score after 1 week of diazepam treatment predicted a higher likelihood of response at 6 weeks (Downing & Rickels, 1985). Limited reduction in symptom severity (i.e. a reduction in total HAMA score of $\leq 25\%$) at 2 weeks of treatment predicted non-response to buspirone or lorazepam at 6 weeks (Laakmann *et al.*, 1998); and the degree of response after 1 or 2 weeks was strongly predictive of response to benzodiazepines or azapirones at 8 weeks (Rynn *et al.*, 2006). Recent post-hoc analyses show that the onset of efficacy (defined as a reduction in HAMA score of $\geq 20\%$) after 2 weeks of treatment is strongly predictive of remission at study end-point for duloxetine (Pollack *et al.*, 2008) or response at study end-point with escitalopram (Baldwin *et al.*, 2009) and response at endpoint with pregabalin, alprazolam and venlafaxine (Baldwin *et al.*, 2011*b*). These analyses imply the likelihood of eventual response is low, if an onset of efficacy is not seen after 4–6 weeks of treatment (Bandelow *et al.*, 2008).

Optimal duration of continuation treatment

GAD has traditionally been regarded as a chronic disorder that waxes and wanes in severity over many years. In a prospective, naturalistic, longitudinal study, the probability of recovering from the index "episode" of GAD was only 58% at the end of 12 years, and $> 40\%$ of those who had recovered experienced a subsequent recurrence of symptoms (Bruce *et al.*, 2005). However, findings from the prospective epidemiological Zurich Study suggest there is rather more longitudinal fluidity in the diagnosis than previously thought (Angst *et al.*, 2009). It is accepted that continuation of antidepressant treatment beyond initial response substantially reduces the risk of early relapse and later recurrence of symptoms in patients with unipolar depressive disorder (Geddes *et al.*, 2003), but the value of long-term treatment in GAD is less well established, due to the smaller number of relapse-prevention studies.

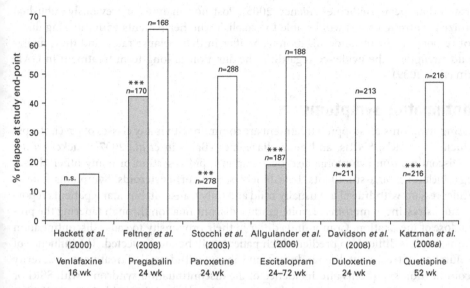

Fig. 7.1. Placebo-controlled relapse-prevention studies in generalized anxiety disorder (***$p < 0.001$ vs. placebo).

Evidence-based guidelines have recommended at least 6 months of continuation treatment after initial response (Baldwin *et al.*, 2005; Ballenger, 1999; Bandelow *et al.*, 2008; Canadian Psychiatric Association, 2006), but more recent data suggest that longer periods of continuation treatment may be preferable (Allgulander *et al.*, 2006; Katzman *et al.*, 2008a; Rickels *et al.* unpublished data).

The potential value of continuation treatment in affective disorders is usually ascertained through double-blind, placebo-controlled relapse-prevention studies, in which patients who have responded well to initial open acute treatment are then randomized, to either continue with active medication or switched to placebo. Five relapse-prevention studies in GAD have been published, of which four demonstrate the value of continuing pharmacological treatment with escitalopram (Allgulander *et al.*, 2006), paroxetine (Stocchi *et al.*, 2003), pregabalin (Feltner *et al.*, 2008), or duloxetine (Davidson *et al.*, 2008). An initial relapse-prevention study with venlafaxine did not reveal efficacy (Hackett *et al.*, 2000), but significantly fewer patients relapsed during venlafaxine treatment in a separate prolonged randomized double-blind, placebo-controlled trial (Montgomery *et al.*, 2002) and a recent extended relapse prevention trial demonstrates that venlafaxine has efficacy in relapse prevention over 12 months (Rickels *et al.*, 2010). In addition, a relapse-prevention study with the second-generation antipsychotic drug quetiapine suggests it is efficacious in long-term treatment (Katzman *et al.*, 2008a) (Fig. 7.1).

The duration of double-blind treatment in the placebo-controlled relapse-prevention study with escitalopram (Allgulander *et al.*, 2006) was for up to 18 months, so it may be reasonable to recommend that treatment should continue for up to 18 months, after an initial response. The United States regulatory body recommends that the double-blind relapse-prevention phase in GAD studies should be preceded by 6 months of unblinded treatment (Food & Drug Administration, 2006). This recommendation is likely to result in the need for larger studies, as the more "stable" patient population prior to randomization is likely to experience fewer relapses during the double-blind phase; and contrasts with the European Union recommendation of between 2 and 6 months "open" treatment, prior to double-blind withdrawal (European Medicines Agency, 2005). Post-hoc analyses of previously published randomized controlled trials will be able to establish whether patients with differing durations of response prior to randomization also differ in their relapse rates, and these analyses could strengthen the evidence regarding the duration of long-term treatment in GAD (Bodkin et al., 2009).

Discontinuation symptoms

Distressing symptoms on stopping treatment are common with many classes of psychotropic drug, including SSRIs, SNRIs, and benzodiazepines (Baldwin et al., 2007b; Rickels et al., 1988). Discontinuation symptoms also occur upon rapid cessation of many other classes of drugs, including beta-stimulants, beta-blockers, and corticosteroids. Symptoms following antidepressant withdrawal are usually mild and only transient, but many patients report severe and distressing symptoms, despite gradual discontinuation through tapering the prescribed dose of medication. Compounds differ in their propensity to cause discontinuation symptoms, but it is difficult to predict which patients will be most affected. The influence of longer duration of treatment, higher dosage, and abrupt withdrawal of treatment on severity of discontinuation symptoms and incidence of the discontinuation syndrome with SSRI or SNRI antidepressants is less established than was previously thought (Baldwin et al., 2007b). Abrupt discontinuation of pregabalin has been found to be associated with discontinuation symptoms in some (Feltner et al., 2003; Pohl et al., 2005) but not all (Pande et al., 2003) studies. After an 8-week study of 50 or 150 mg/day quetiapine, or 20 mg/day paroxetine, or placebo, there were only a few reports of anxiety, insomnia, nausea, or dizziness among those who had been treated with quetiapine (Bandelow et al., 2010).

For all pharmacological treatments, slow stepped withdrawal ("tapering") is probably advisable, in order to minimize the appearance of distressing discontinuation symptoms, but the value of this is not established fully and there is a need for withdrawal studies that adopt a randomized double-blind staggered design, in which both patients and doctors are unsure of whether treatment ends slowly or swiftly, or when dosage reduction occurs.

Management after non-response to initial treatment

Most guidelines recommend a SSRI for first-line pharmacological treatment of GAD, on the balance of efficacy and tolerability, so common second-line drug treatments include a SNRI, pregabalin, the tricyclic antidepressant imipramine, pregabalin, or a benzodiazepine. The azapirone buspirone (a partial agonist at 5-HT_{1A} receptors) is also efficacious in GAD (Chessick et al., 2006) and reasonably well tolerated (Newton et al., 1986). Buspirone is more likely to be effective when patients have not previously been treated with a benzodiazepine: as such it is advisable to consider use of buspirone before prescribing a benzodiazepine anxiolytic (Chessick et al., 2006).

There is little consensus about the optimal next stage in patient management after a poor response to first-line treatment. First, adherence to current treatment should be checked, together with an evaluation of concurrent substance use, persisting stressors, and a check to verify the diagnosis. Potential interventions include increasing the dosage, switching to another evidence-based pharmacological treatment, augmenting with an additional psychotropic drug, and combining medication with a psychological treatment.

There is no published double-blind dosage escalation study in GAD, in which patients either continue with the initial low dose or are switched to a subsequent higher dose. The findings of fixed-dose randomized placebo-controlled studies provide only limited evidence to suggest that higher doses may be preferable. The relative efficacy of paroxetine when compared with placebo is similar for daily dosages of 20 mg or 40 mg (Rickels *et al.*, 2003), and the optimal daily dosage of escitalopram is probably 10 mg rather than 20 mg (Baldwin *et al.*, 2006a). In addition, fixed-dose studies with venlafaxine have produced inconsistent findings, with evidence both for (Rickels *et al.*, 2000) and against (Allgulander *et al.*, 2001) a dose–response relationship. A fixed-dose study with duloxetine provides no evidence to suggest that 120 mg may have greater efficacy compared with placebo, than is seen with a 60 mg/day dosage (Koponen *et al.*, 2007). In addition, the clinical trial database for quetiapine suggests that the efficacy of a 300 mg/day dosage is less certain than the lower 150 mg dosage (Baldwin & Waldman, 2009). Although the lower doses were considered sub-therapeutic on the basis of individual studies, post-hoc analysis of pooled data from randomized controlled trials with pregabalin suggests that higher doses (200–450 mg/day) have greater efficacy than lower doses (150 mg/day), when both are compared with placebo (Bech, 2007).

Despite reservations about potential adverse effects (such as weight gain and metabolic syndrome), an antipsychotic drug may have a role in patient management after non-response to SSRI or SNRI treatment, given the potential for tolerance or dependence with use of benzodiazepines (Gao *et al.*, 2009). Certain conventional neuroleptic drugs have possible efficacy as monotherapy, although design features limit the confidence that can be placed in the findings of some placebo-controlled or comparator-controlled studies (El-Khayat & Baldwin, 1998). Most probably, the adverse event profile and potential long-term risks of antipsychotics will result in their usually being reserved for patients who have not responded to earlier SSRI treatment, perhaps followed by SNRI treatment. In small and probably underpowered studies, there was some evidence that risperidone and olanzapine can enhance the efficacy of SSRI treatment (Brawman-Mintzer *et al.*, 2005; Pollack *et al.*, 2006), but currently the evidence for augmentation with quetiapine is only limited (Baldwin & Waldman, 2009; Katzman *et al.*, 2008b; Simon *et al.*, 2008).

Preliminary findings of a large placebo-controlled pregabalin augmentation study, in patients who have made a limited response to previous SSRI or SNRI treatment, suggests it is efficacious, with 50% responding, compared with 37% with placebo (Weaver *et al.*, 2009). Other potential augmentation approaches may include use of the novel antidepressant drug agomelatine, which has been found efficacious in acute treatment in GAD (Stein *et al.*, 2008a, 2008b), or the novel anticonvulsant drug zonisamide, following limited response to treatment with a SSRI or clonazepam (Kinrys *et al.*, 2007).

Psychological interventions may be suitable in some patients, particularly the young and especially motivated (Allgulander, 2010; Hoyer & Gloster, 2009). Cognitive–behavior therapy has been the most studied form of psychological treatment, but although superior to "treatment as usual" or waiting-list control, it is not clearly superior to other psychological approaches in adequately controlled studies (Hunot *et al.*, 2007). Whilst combining pharmacological and psychological approaches is often advocated in the overall management of patients with anxiety disorders, in GAD it is uncertain whether combination treatment is superior to psychological or drug treatment given alone (Bandelow *et al.*, 2007).

Late-life GAD

Partly due to previous restrictions regarding the inclusion of elderly patients in phase III studies, we are ill informed for dealing with the oncoming demographic shift in anxiety disorders in the developed world (Allgulander, 2009). Late-life GAD poses new research questions. GAD symptoms may result from stroke, from social isolation, immobilization and institutionalization, and from bereavement. The condition may be aggravated by increasing physical ill-health and by the prospects of impending death: in addition, GAD may worsen the outcome of cardiovascular disease (Martens *et al.*, 2010). Reliance on extrapolating experiences from treatment studies in younger adult patients into more elderly populations may be ill-judged, due to the influence of concurrent medications, chronic and multiple physical illnesses, and increasing disability.

Pregnancy and breastfeeding

It is important to consider the potential for teratogenicity and any behavioral effects both acutely and long-term, on the developing child (Hallberg & Sjöblom, 2005), for any psychotropic drug given to women of reproductive age. According to the Swedish Medical Birth Registry of 4000 mothers exposed to SSRIs or SNRIs during pregnancy, and according to 15 studies in another 2600 mothers, there is no apparent risk of teratogenic effects of these drugs in therapeutic doses. Cases of acute adaptation disturbances in newborn infants, probably due to serotonin over-activity, have been reported, and it is advisable that a fetus exposed to SSRIs/SNRIs *in utero* should be monitored for 48 h for such symptoms, including increased muscle tone, irritability, jitteriness, hypothermia, abnormal breathing, and petechia (Levinson-Castiel *et al.*, 2006).

All SSRIs and SNRIs are excreted in breast milk, but no adverse reactions in the baby have been reported. According to a prospective long-term study of children exposed *in utero* to psychotropic medications, levels of depression, anxiety, and social withdrawal did not differ significantly between exposed children and those who were not exposed (Misri *et al.*, 2006). On the other hand, maternal anxiety during pregnancy can adversely affect both maternal and fetal well-being. A number of studies conclude that pregnant mothers with anxiety and depression should be vigorously screened and treated to reduce the risks to both the mother and child (Pinheiro *et al.*, 2005; Rondo *et al.*, 2003; Weissman *et al.*, 2006).

Conclusions

There are many psychotropic drugs and psychotherapies available for the treatment of patients with GAD. Randomized double-blind placebo-controlled trials provide good evidence for the efficacy of certain SSRIs, SNRIs, pregabalin, and quetiapine, but in wider clinical practice overall outcomes can be poor in many patients. The "ideal" treatment for GAD does not yet exist, as existing treatments have insufficient overall efficacy in short-term and long-term treatments, and some can have troublesome adverse effects when prescribed for long periods. The particular choice of treatment should be determined by the clinical features of the patients (such as the presence of comorbid depression and a history of a good response to previous treatment), patients' preferences for one approach over another, and by the availability of services. Doctors should counsel patients that they will not respond immediately, that sometimes symptoms can worsen in the early stage of treatment, and that long-term treatment is often needed to maintain an initial response. There is clearly room for improvement in the development of more efficacious and more acceptable pharmacological approaches to the management of this common, distressing, typically disabling, and often persistent anxiety disorder.

Acknowledgements

This manuscript is an update of a previous review of the drug treatment of GAD (Baldwin & Polkinghorn, *International Journal of Neuropsychopharmacology* 2005; 8: 293–302). We are grateful to the Series Editor, Professor Dan Stein, for giving us the opportunity to submit an updated version. We received secretarial and administrative help in preparing this manuscript from Catherine Carr.

Statement of interest

David Baldwin has acted as a consultant to Asahi, AstraZeneca, Cephalon, Eli Lilly, GSK, Lundbeck, Organon, Pharmacia, Pierre Fabre, Pfizer, Roche, Servier, Sumitomo, and Wyeth; holds or has held research grants (on behalf of his employer) from Cephalon, Eli Lilly, GSK, Lundbeck, Organon, Pfizer, Pharmacia, Roche, and Wyeth. Christer Allgulander has been a speaker for AstraZeneca, Eli Lilly and Pfizer; and has acted as a consultant to Pfizer.

References

Allgulander C (2009). Generalized anxiety disorder (GAD): from now to DSM-V. *Psychiatric Clinics of North America* 32, 611–628.

Allgulander C (2010). Novel approaches to treatment of generalised anxiety disorder. *Current Opinion in Psychiatry* 23, 37–42.

Allgulander C, Dahl AA, Austin C et al. (2004). Efficacy of sertraline in a 12-week trial for generalized anxiety disorder. *American Journal of Psychiatry* 161, 1642–1649.

Allgulander C, Florea I, Huusom AK (2006). Prevention of relapse in generalized anxiety disorder by escitalopram treatment. *International Journal of Neuropsychopharmacology* 9, 495–505.

Allgulander C, Hackett D, Salinas E (2001). Venlafaxine extended release (ER) in the treatment of generalised anxiety disorder: twenty-four-week placebo-controlled dose-ranging study. *British Journal of Psychiatry* 179, 15–22.

Angst J, Gamma A, Baldwin DS et al. (2009). The generalized anxiety spectrum: prevalence, onset, course and outcome. *European Archives of Pyschiatry and Clinical Neuroscience* 259, 37–45.

Baldwin DS (2004). Sexual dysfunction associated with antidepressant drugs. *Expert Opinion on Drug Safety* 3, 457–470.

Baldwin DS, Ajel K (2007). The role of pregabalin in the treatment of generalized anxiety disorder. *Neuropsychiatric Disease and Treatment* 3, 185–191.

Baldwin DS, Anderson IM, Nutt DJ et al. (2005). Evidence-based guidelines for the pharmacological treatment of anxiety disorders: recommendations from the British Association for Psychopharmacology.

Journal of Psychopharmacology 19, 567–596.

Baldwin DS, Bridgman K, Buis C (2006b). Resolution of sexual dysfunction during double-blind treatment of major depression with reboxetine or paroxetine. *Journal of Psychopharmacology* 20, 91–96.

Baldwin DS, Huusom AKT, Maehlum E (2006a). Escitalopram and paroxetine in the treatment of generalised anxiety disorder. Randomised, double-blind, placebo-controlled study. *British Journal of Psychiatry* 189, 264–272.

Baldwin DS, Lawson R, Wood R, Taylor D (2011a). Systematic review and meta-analysis of the efficacy of drug therapies for generalised anxiety disorder. *British Medical Journal* 342, d1199 (pico version 342; 637).

Baldwin DS, Montgomery SA, Nil R, Lader M (2007b). Discontinuation symptoms in depression and anxiety disorders. *International Journal of Neuropsychopharmacology* 10, 73–84.

Baldwin DS, Moreno R, Briley M (2008). Resolution of sexual dysfunction during acute treatment of major depression with milnacipran. *Human Psychopharmacology* 23, 527–532.

Baldwin DS, Polkinghorn C (2005). Evidence-based pharmacotherapy of generalized anxiety disorder. *International Journal of Neuropsychopharmacology* 8, 293–302.

Baldwin DS, Reines EH, Guiton C, Weiller E (2007a). Escitalopram therapy for major depression and anxiety disorders. *Annals of Pharmacotherapy* 41, 1583–1592.

Baldwin DS, Schweizer E, Xu Y, Lyndon G (2011b). Does early improvement predict endpoint response in patients with generalized anxiety disorder (GAD) treated with pregabalin or venlafaxine XR? *European Neuropsychopharmacology.* E-pub ahead of print.

Baldwin DS, Stein DJ, Dolberg OT, Bandelow B (2009). How long should a trial of escitalopram treatment be in patients with major depressive disorder, generalised anxiety disorder or social anxiety disorder? An exploration of the randomised controlled trial database. *Human Psychopharmacology* **24**, 269–275.

Baldwin DS, Waldman S (2009). Antipsychotic drugs in the treatment of generalized anxiety disorder. *International Journal of Psychiatry in Clinical Practice* **13** (Suppl. 1), Sll.

Ballenger JC (1999). Clinical guidelines for establishing remission in patients with depression and anxiety. *Journal of Clinical Psychiatry* **60** (Suppl. 22), 29–34.

Bandelow B, Baldwin DS, Dolberg OT *et al.* (2006). What is the threshold for symptomatic response and remission for major depressive disorder, panic disorder, social anxiety disorder, and generalized anxiety disorder? *Journal of Clinical Psychiatry* **67**, 1428–1434.

Bandelow B, Chouinard G, Bobes J *et al.* (2010). Extended-release quetiapine fumarate (quetiapine XR): a once-daily monotherapy effective in generalized anxiety disorder. Data from a randomized, double-blind, placebo- and active-controlled study. *International Journal of Neuropsychopharmacology* **13**, 305–320.

Bandelow B, Seidler-Brandler U, Becker A *et al.* (2007). Meta-analysis of randomized controlled comparisons of psychopharmacological and psychological treatments for anxiety disorders. *World Journal of Biological Psychiatry* **8**, 175–187.

Bandelow B, Zohar J, Hollander E *et al.* (2008). World Federation of Societies of Biological Psychiatry (WFSBP) guidelines for the pharmacological treatment of anxiety, obsessive-compulsive and post-traumatic stress disorders – first revision. *World Journal of Biological Psychiatry* **9**, 248–312.

Bech P (2007). Dose-response relationship of pregabalin in patients with generalized anxiety disorder. A pooled analysis of four placebo-controlled trials. *Pharmacopsychiatry* **40**, 163–168.

Beekman AT, Bremmer MA, Deeg DJ *et al.* (1998). Anxiety disorders in later life: a report from the longitudinal Aging Study Amsterdam. *International Journal of Geriatric Psychiatry* **13**, 717–726.

Beesdo K, Knappe S, Pine DS (2009). Anxiety and anxiety disorders in children and adolescents: developmental issues and implications for DSM-V. *Psychiatric Clinics of North America* **32**, 483–524.

Bodkin JA, Allgulander C, Llorca PM *et al.* (2009). Predictors of relapse in a study of duloxetine treatment for patients with generalized anxiety disorder. ACNP 4th Annual Meeting Final Programme, 6–10 December 2009, Hollywood, Florida (www.acnp.org/ asset.axd?id = a55d7404–334e-43df-a40c-9cda68719743).

Brawman-Mintzer O, Knapp RG, Nietert PJ (2005). Adjunctive risperidone in generalized anxiety disorder: a double-blind, placebo-controlled study. *Journal of Clinical Psychiatry* **66**, 1321–1325.

Brawman-Mintzer O, Knapp RG, Rynn M *et al.* (2006). Sertraline treatment for generalized anxiety disorder: a randomized, double-blind, placebo-controlled study. *Journal of Clinical Psychiatry* **67**, 874–881.

Bruce SE, Yonkers KA, Otto MW *et al.* (2005). Influence of psychiatric comorbidity on recovery and recurrence in generalized anxiety disorder, social phobia, and panic disorder: a 12-year prospective study. *American Journal of Psychiatry* **162**, 1179–1187.

Canadian Psychiatric Association (2006). Clinical practice guidelines. Management of anxiety disorders. *Canadian Journal of Psychiatry* **51**, 9S–91S.

Carney CE, Segal ZV, Edinger JD, Krystal AD (2007). A comparison of rates of residual insomnia symptoms following pharmacotherapy or cognitive-behavioral therapy for major depressive disorder. *Journal of Clinical Psychiatry* **68**, 254–260.

Cervena K, Matousek M, Prasko J *et al.* (2005). Sleep disturbances in patients treated for panic disorder. *Sleep Medicine* **6**, 149–153.

Chessick CA, Allen MH, Thase M *et al.* (2006). Azapirones for generalized anxiety disorder.

Cochrane Database of Systematic Reviews 3, CD006115.

Davidson JR, Bose A, Korotzer A, Zheng H (2004). Escitalopram in the treatment of generalized anxiety disorder: double-blind, placebo controlled, flexible-dose study. *Depression and Anxiety* 19, 234–240.

Davidson JR, DuPont RL, Hedges D, Haskins JT (1999). Efficacy, safety, and tolerability of venlafaxine extended release and buspirone in outpatients with generalized anxiety disorder. *Journal of Clinical Psychiatry* 60, 528–535.

Davidson JRT, Wittchen H-U, Llorca P-M *et al.* (2008). Duloxetine treatment for relapse prevention in adults with generalized anxiety disorder: a double-blind placebo-controlled trial. *European Neuropsychopharmacology* 18, 673–681.

Downing RW, Rickels K (1985). Early treatment response in anxious outpatients treated with diazepam. *Acta Psychiatrica Scandinavica* 72, 522–528.

El-Khayat R, Baldwin DS (1998). Antipsychotic drugs for non-psychotic patients: assessment of the benefit/risk ratio in generalized anxiety disorder. *Journal of Psychopharmacology* 12, 323–329.

Eriksson H, Mezhebovsky I, Magi K *et al.* (2008). Double-blind, randomised study of extended release quetiapine fumarate (quetiapine XR) monotherapy in elderly patients with generalized anxiety disorder. *International Journal of Psychiatry in Clinical Practice* 12, 322–333.

European Medicines Agency (2005). Committee for Medicinal products for Human Use (CHMP). Guideline on the clinical investigation of medicinal products indicated for generalised anxiety disorder. CPMP/EWP/4284/02, London, January 2005.

Fava M (2000). Weight gain and antidepressants. *Journal of Clinical Psychiatry* 61 (Suppl. 11), 37–41.

Feltner D, Wittchen HU, Kavoussi R *et al.* (2008). Long-term efficacy of pregabalin in generalized anxiety disorder. *International Clinical Psychopharmacology* 23, 18–28.

Feltner DE, Crockatt JG, Dobovsky SJ *et al.* (2003). A randomized, double-blind, placebo-controlled, fixed-dose, multicenter study of pregabalin in patients with generalized anxiety disorder. *Journal of Clinical Psychopharmacology* 23, 240–249.

Food and Drug Administration (FDA) (2006). New controversial clinical trial design gives better long-term data. *FDA Week*, 10 May 2006.

Gao K, Sheehan DV, Calabrese JR (2009). Atypical antipsychotics in primary generalized anxiety disorder or comorbid with mood disorders. *Expert Reviews in Neurotherapeutics* 9, 1147–1158.

Garner M, Möhler H, Stein DJ, Mueggler T, Baldwin DS. (2009). Research in anxiety disorders: from the bench to the bedside. *European Neuropsychopharmacology* 19, 381–390.

Geddes JR, Carney SM, Davies C *et al.* (2003). Relapse prevention with antidepressant drug treatment in depressive disorders: a systematic review. *Lancet* 361, 653–661.

Gelenberg AJ, Lydiard B, Rudolph RL *et al.* (2000). Efficacy of venlafaxine extended-release capsules in nondepressed outpatients with generalized anxiety disorder. *Journal of the American Medical Association* 283, 3082–3088.

Goodman WK, Bose A, Wang Q (2005). Treatment of generalized anxiety disorder with escitalopram: pooled results from double-blind, placebo-controlled trials. *Journal of Affective Disorders* 87, 161–167.

Gould RA, Otto MW, Pollack MH, Yap L (1997). Cognitive behavioural and pharmacological treatment of generalised anxiety disorder: a preliminary meta-analysis. *Behaviour Therapy* 28, 285–305.

Guy W (1976). The clinical global impression severity and impression scales. In *ECDEU Assessment Manual for Psychopathology* (pp. 218–222). Rockville, MD: US Department of Health, Education and Welfare.

Hackett D, White C, Salinas E (2000). Relapse prevention in patients with generalised anxiety disorder (GAD) by treatment with venlafaxine ER. Poster presented at 1st International Forum on Mood and Anxiety Disorders, Monte Carlo, November 2000 (www.aimgroup.it/2000/ifmad/POSTER20.htm). Accessed 6 July 2010.

Hallberg P, Sjoblom V (2005). The use of selective serotonin inhibitors during pregnancy and breast-feeding: a review and clinical aspects. *Journal of Clinical Psychopharmacology* 25, 59–73.

Hamilton M (1959). The assessment of anxiety states by rating. *British Journal of Medical Psychology* 32, 50–55.

Hartford J, Kornstein S, Liebowitz M *et al.* (2007). Duloxetine as an SNRI treatment for generalized anxiety disorder: results from a placebo and active-controlled trial. *International Clinical Psychopharmacology* 22,167–174.

Hewett K, Adams A, Bryson H *et al.* (2001). Generalized anxiety disorder: efficacy of paroxetine. Paper presented at the 7th World Congress of Biological Psychiatry, Berlin, Germany.

Hidalgo RB, Tupler LA, Davidson JRT (2007). An effect-size analysis of pharmacologic treatments for generalized anxiety disorder. *Journal of Psychopharmacology* 21, 864–872.

Hoyer J, Gloster AT (2009). Psychotherapy for generalized anxiety disorder: don't worry, it works! *Psychiatric Clinics of North America* 32, 629–640.

Hunot V, Churchill R, Silva de Lima M *et al.* (2007). Psychological therapies for generalized anxiety disorder [Review]. *Cochrane Database of Systematic Reviews* 24, CD001848.

Judd LL, Kessler RC, Paulus MP *et al.* (1998). Comorbidity as a fundamental feature of generalized anxiety disorders: results from the National Comorbidity Survey (NCS). *Acta Psychiatrica Scandinavica* 98 (Suppl. 393), 6–11.

Kasper S, Herman B, Nivoli G *et al.* (2009). Efficacy of pregabalin and venlafaxine-XR in generalized anxiety disorder: results of a double-blind, placebo-controlled 8-week trial. *International Clinical Psychopharmacology*. Published online: January 2009. doi:10.1097/YIC.0b013e 32831d7980.

Katzman M, Brawman-Mintzer O, Reyes E *et al.* (2008*a*). Extended release quetiapine fumarate (quetiapine XR) monotherapy in long-term treatment of generalized anxiety disorder (GAD): efficacy and tolerability results from a randomized, placebo-controlled trial. *Biological Psychiatry* 63 (Suppl.), 141S.

Katzman MA, Vermani M, Jacobs L *et al.* (2008*b*). Quetiapine as an adjunctive

pharmacotherapy for the treatment of non-remitting generalized anxiety disorder: a flexible-dose, open-label pilot trial. *Journal of Anxiety Disorders* 22, 1480–1486.

Kessler RC, DuPont RL, Berglund P (1999). Impairment in pure and comorbid generalized anxiety disorder and major depression at 12 months in two national surveys. *American Journal of Psychiatry* 156, 1915–1923.

Khan A, Joyce M, Atkinson S *et al.* (2011). A randomized, double-blind study of once-daily extended release quetiapine fumarate (quetiapine XR) monotherapy in patients with generalized anxiety disorder. *Journal of Clinical Psychopharmacology* 31, 418–428.

Kinrys G, Vasconcelos e Sa D, Nery F (2007). Adjunctive zonisamide for treatment refractory anxiety. *International Journal of Clinical Practice* 61, 1050–1053.

Koponen H, Allgulander C, Erickson J *et al.* (2007). Efficacy of duloxetine for the treatment of generalized anxiety disorder: implications for primary care physicians. *Primary Care Companion Journal of Clinical Psychiatry* 9, 100–107.

Laakmann G, Schtile C, Lorkowski G *et al.* (1998). Buspirone and lorazepam in the treatment of generalized anxiety disorder in outpatients. *Psychopharmacology* 136, 357–366.

Lenox-Smith AJ, Reynolds A (2003). A double-blind, randomised, placebo controlled study of venlafaxine XL in patients with generalised anxiety disorder in primary care. *British Journal of General Practice* 53, 772–777.

Lenze EJ, Rollman BL, Shear MK *et al.* (2009). Escitalopram for older adults with generalised anxiety disorder: a randomized controlled trial. *Journal of the American Medical Association* 301, 295–303.

Leonardo ED, Hen R (2008). Anxiety as a developmental disorder. *Neuropsychopharmacology* 33, 134–140.

Levinson-Castiel R, Merlob P, Linder N *et al.* (2006). Neonatal abstinence syndrome after in utero exposure to selective serotonin reuptake inhibitors in term infants. *Archives of Paediatric and Adolescent Medicine* 160, 173–176.

Maina G, Albert U, Salvi V, Bogetto F (2004). Weight gain during long-term treatment of obsessive-compulsive disorder: a prospective comparison between serotonin reuptake inhibitors. *Journal of Clinical Psychiatry*, 63, 391–395.

Martens EJ, de Jonge P, Na B *et al.* (2010). Scared to death? Generalized anxiety disorder and cardiovascular events in patients with stable coronary heart disease. *Archives of General Psychiatry* 67, 750–758.

Martin JLR, Sainz-Pardo M, Furukawa TA *et al.* (2007). Benzodiazepines in generalized anxiety disorder: heterogeneity of outcomes based on a systematic review and meta-analysis of clinical trials. *Journal of Psychopharmacology* 21, 774–782.

Mathew SJ, Price RB, Mao X *et al.* (2008). Hippocampal N-acetylaspartate concentration and response to riluzole in generalized anxiety disorder. *Biological Psychiatry* 63, 891–898.

Meredith C, Cutler AJ, She F, Eriksson H (2011). Efficacy and tolerability of extended release quetiapine fumarate monotherapy in the acute treatment of generalized anxiety disorder: a randomized, placebo controlled and active-controlled study. *International Clinical Psychopharmacology* 27(1), 40–54.

Michelson D, Amsterdam JD, Quitkin FM *et al.* (1999). Changes in weight during a 1-year trial of fluoxetine. *American Journal of Psychiatry* 156, 1170–1176.

Misri S, Reebye P, Kendrick K *et al.* (2006). Internalizing behaviors in 4-year-old children exposed in utero to psychotropic medications. *American Journal of Psychiatry* 163, 1026–1032.

Mitte K, Noack P, Steil R, Hautzinger M (2005). A meta-analytic review of the efficacy of drug treatment in generalized anxiety disorder. *Journal of Clinical Psychopharmacology* 25, 141–150.

Montgomery S, Chatamra K, Pauer L *et al.* (2008). Efficacy and safety of pregabalin in elderly people with generalised anxiety disorder. *British Journal of Psychiatry* 193, 389–394.

Montgomery SA, McIntyre RS, Szamosi J *et al.* (2009). Extended release quetiapine fumarate monotherapy in patients with MDD: a pooled analysis of sustained response data from studies D1448C00001 and D1448C00002. *International Journal of Psychiatry in Clinical Practice* 13 (Suppl. 1), S39.

Montgomery SA, Sheehan DV, Meoni P *et al.* (2002). Characterization of the longitudinal course of improvement in generalized anxiety disorder during long-term treatment with venlafaxine XR. *Journal of Psychiatric Research* 36, 209–217.

Montgomery SA, Tobias K, Zornberg GL *et al.* (2006). Efficacy and safety of pregabalin in the treatment of generalized anxiety disorder: a 6-week, multicenter, randomized, double-blind, placebo-controlled comparison of pregabalin and venlafaxine. *Journal of Clinical Psychiatry* 67, 771–782.

Morris PLP, Dahl AA, Kutcher S *et al.* (2003). Efficacy of sertraline for the acute treatment of generalized anxiety disorder. *European Neuropsychopharmacology* 13, S375.

Munk-Jorgensen P, Allgulander C, Dahl AA *et al.* (2006). Prevalence of generalized anxiety disorder in general practice in Denmark, Finland, Norway, and Sweden. *Psychiatric Services* 57, 1738–1744.

Newton RE, Marunycz JD, Alderdice MT, Napoliello MJ (1986). Review of the side-effect profile of buspirone. *American Journal of Medicine* 31, 17–21.

Nitschke JB, Sarinopoulos I, Oathes DJ *et al.* (2009). Anticipatory activation in the amygdala and anterior cingulate in generalized anxiety disorder and prediction of treatment response. *American Journal of Psychiatry* 166, 302–310.

Olatunji BO, Feldman G, Smits JAJ *et al.* (2008). Examination of the decline in symptoms of anxiety and depression in generalized anxiety disorder: impact of anxiety sensitivity on response to pharmacotherapy. *Depression and Anxiety* 25, 167–171.

Pande AC, Crockatt JG, Feltner DE *et al.* (2003). Pregabalin in generalized anxiety disorder: a placebo-controlled trial. *American Journal of Psychiatry* 160, 533–540.

Pande AC, Crockatt MA, Janne C, Feltner DE (2000). Pregabalin treatment of GAD. Presented at the 153rd Annual Meeting of the American Psychiatric Association, Chicago, IL, 13–18 May (Abstract NR244) (http://www. psych.org/edu/other_res/ lib_archives/archives/meetings/2000nra).

Perugi G, Frare F, Toni C et al. (2002). Open-label evaluation of venlafaxine sustained release in outpatients with generalized anxiety disorder with comorbid depression or dysthymia: effectiveness, tolerability and predictors of response. *Neuropsychobiology* **46**, 145–149.

Pinheiro SN, Laprega MR, Furtado EF (2005). Psychiatric morbidity and alcohol use by pregnant women in a public obstetric service. *Revista Saude Publica* **39**, 593–598.

Pohl RB, Feltner DE, Fieve RR, Pande AC (2005). Efficacy of pregabalin in the treatment of generalized anxiety disorder: double-blind, placebo-controlled comparison of BID versus TID dosing. *Journal of Clinical Psychopharmacology* **25**, 151–158.

Pollack MH, Kornstein SG, Spann ME et al. (2008). Early improvement during duloxetine treatment of generalized anxiety disorder predicts response and remission at endpoint. *Journal of Psychiatric Research* **42**, 1176–1184.

Pollack MH, Meoni P, Otto MW et al. (2003). Predictors of outcome following venlafaxine extended-release treatment of DSM–IV generalized anxiety disorder: a pooled analysis of short- and long-term studies. *Journal of Clinical Psychopharmacology* **23**, 250–259.

Pollack MH, Simon NM, Zalta AK et al. (2006). Olanzapine augmentation of fluoxetine for refractory generalized anxiety disorder: a placebo controlled study. *Biological Psychiatry* **59**, 211–215.

Pollack MH, Zaninelli R, Goddard A et al. (2001). Paroxetine in the treatment of generalized anxiety disorder: results of a placebo-controlled, flexible-dosage trial. *Journal of Clinical Psychiatry* **62**, 350–357.

Rickels K, Downing R, Schweizer E, Hassman H (1993). Antidepressants for the treatment of generalized anxiety disorder. A placebo-controlled comparison of imipramine, trazodone, and diazepam. *Archives of General Psychiatry* **50**, 884–895.

Rickels K, Etemad B, Khalid-Khan S et al. (2010). Time to relapse after 6 and 12 months' treatment of generalized anxiety disorder with venlafaxine extended release. *Archives of General Psychiatry* **67**, 1274–1281.

Rickels K, Pollack MH, Feltner DE et al. (2005). Pregabalin for treatment of generalized anxiety disorder: a 4-week, multicenter, double-blind, placebo-controlled trial of pregabalin and alprazolam. *Archives of General Psychiatry* **62**, 1022–1030.

Rickels K, Pollack MH, Sheehan DV, Haskins JT (2000). Efficacy of extended-release venlafaxine in non-depressed outpatients with generalized anxiety disorder. *American Journal of Psychiatry* **157**, 968–974.

Rickels K, Rynn M, Iyengar M, Duff D (2006). Remission of generalized anxiety disorder: a review of the paroxetine clinical trials database. *Journal of Clinical Psychiatry* **67**, 41–47.

Rickels K, Schweizer E, Csanalosi I et al. (1988). Long-term treatment of anxiety and risk of withdrawal: prospective study of clorazepate and buspirone. *Archives of General Psychiatry* **45**, 444–450.

Rickels K, Zaninelli R, McCafferty J et al. (2003). Paroxetine treatment of generalized anxiety disorder: a double-blind, placebo-controlled study. *American Journal of Psychiatry* **160**, 749–756.

Rodriguez BF, Weisberg RB, Pagano ME et al. (2006). Characteristics and predictors of full and partial recovery from generalized anxiety disorder in primary care patients. *Journal of Nervous and Mental Disease* **194**, 91–97.

Rondo PHC, Ferreira RF, Nogueira F et al. (2003). Maternal psychological stress and distress as predictors of low birth weight, prematurity and intrauterine growth retardation. *European Journal of Clinical Nutrition* **57**, 266–272.

Royal College of Psychiatrists (1997). *Benzodiazepines: Risks, Benefits or Dependence. A Re-evaluation*. Council Report CR59. London: Royal College of Psychiatrists.

Rynn M, Khalid-Khan S, Garcia-Espana F (2006). Early response and 8-week treatment outcome in GAD. *Depression and Anxiety* **23**, 461–465.

Rynn MA, Riddle MA, Yeung PP, Kunz NR. (2007). Efficacy and safety of extended-release venlafaxine in the treatment of generalized anxiety disorder in children and adolescents: two placebo-controlled trials. http://www.ncbi.nlm.nih.gov/pubmed/17267793

Rynn MA, Russell J, Erickson J et al. (2008). Efficacy and safety of duloxetine in the treatment of generalized anxiety disorder: a flexible-dose, progressive titration, placebo-controlled trial. *Depression and Anxiety* 25, 182–189.

Rynn MA, Siqueland L, Rickels K (2001). Placebo-controlled trial of sertraline in the treatment of children with generalized anxiety disorder. *American Journal of Psychiatry* 158, 2008–2014.

Simon NM, Connor KM, LeBeau RT et al. (2008). Quetiapine augmentation of paroxetine CR for the treatment of generalized anxiety disorder: preliminary findings. *Psychopharmacology (Berlin)* 197, 675–681.

Simon NM, Zalta AK, Worthington III JJ et al. (2006). Preliminary support for gender differences in response to fluoxetine for generalized anxiety disorder. *Depression and Anxiety* 23, 373–376.

Smoller JW, Block SR, Young MM (2009). Genetics of anxiety disorders: the complex road from DSM to DNA. *Depression and Anxiety* 26, 965–975.

Stein DJ, Ahokas AA, de Bodinat C (2008b). Agomelatine in generalized anxiety disorder: a randomized, placebo-controlled study. *Journal of Clinical Psychopharmacology* 28, 561–566.

Stein DJ, Andersen HF, Goodman WK (2005). Escitalopram for the treatment of GAD: efficacy across different subgroups and outcomes. *Annals of Clinical Psychiatry* 17, 71–75.

Stein DJ, Baldwin DS, Baldinetti F, Mandel F (2008a). Efficacy of pregabalin in depressive symptoms associated with generalized anxiety disorder: a pooled analysis of 6 studies. *European Neuropsychopharmacology* 18, 422–430.

Stein DJ, Baldwin DS, Dolberg OT et al. (2006). Which factors predict placebo response in anxiety disorders and major depression? An analysis of placebo-controlled studies of escitalopram. *Journal of Clinical Psychiatry* 67, 1741–1746.

Stocchi F, Nordera G, Jokinen RH et al. (2003). Efficacy and tolerability of paroxetine for the long-term treatment of generalized anxiety disorder. *Journal of Clinical Psychiatry* 64, 250–258.

Tyrer P, Baldwin DS (2006). Generalised anxiety disorder. *Lancet* 368, 2156–2166.

Tyrer P, Owen R, Dawling S (1983). Gradual withdrawal of diazepam after long-term therapy. *Lancet* 321, 1402–1406.

Tyrer P, Seivewright H, Johnson T (2004). The Nottingham Study of Neurotic Disorder: predictors of 12 year outcome of dysthymic, panic and generalised anxiety disorder. *Psychological Medicine* 34, 385–394.

Weaver J, Miceli J, Shiovitz T et al. (2009). Adjunctive pregabalin after partial response to SSRI or SNRI in GAD: results of a double-blind, placebo-controlled trial. *European Neuropsychopharmacology* 19 (Suppl. 3), S593–S594.

Weiller E, Bisserbe JC, Maier W, Lecrubier Y (1998). Prevalence and recognition of anxiety syndromes in five European primary care settings. A report from the WHO Study on Psychological Problems in General Health Care. *British Journal of Psychiatry* 173 (Suppl. 34), 18–23.

Weissman MM, Pilowsky DJ, Wickramaratne PJ et al. (2006). Remissions in maternal depression and child psychopathology. A STAR*D-Child report. *Journal of the American Medical Association* 295, 1389–1398.

Whalen PJ, Johnstone T, Somerville LH et al. (2008). A functional magnetic resonance imaging predictor of treatment response to venlafaxine in generalized anxiety disorder. *Biological Psychiatry* 63, 858–863.

Wittchen H-U, Carter RM, Pfisster H et al. (2000). Disabilities and quality of life in pure and comorbid generalized anxiety disorder and major depression in a national survey. *International Clinical Psychopharmacology* 15, 319–328.

Wittchen H-U, Jacobi F (2005). Size and burden of mental disorders in Europe: a critical review and appraisal of 27 studies. *European Neuropsychopharmacology* 15, 357–376.

Wittchen H-U, Kessler RC, Beesdo K et al. (2002). Generalized anxiety disorder and depression in primary care: prevalence, recognition, and management. *Journal of Clinical Psychiatry* 63 (Suppl. 8), 24–34.

Chapter 8

Evidence-based pharmacotherapy of obsessive–compulsive disorder

Naomi A. Fineberg, Angus Brown, and Ilenia Pampaloni

Introduction

Obsessive–compulsive disorder (OCD), with its own distinctive pathophysiology and pharmacology, is an enduring, lifespan illness and was considered untreatable prior to the 1960s. Epidemiological surveys using DSM–III, DSM–III–R, and DSM–IV criteria have shown lifetime prevalence to range between 1% and 3% of the worldwide population (Robins *et al.*, 1984; Weissman *et al.*, 1994; Wittchen & Jacobi, 2005). Despite this relatively high prevalence, only a fraction of those with OCD present for treatment and the diagnosis is often missed. OCD is less common in men than women (1 : 1.5). The mean age of onset is 20 years with peaks at 12–14 years and 20–22 years (Rasmussen & Eisen, 1990). Rare in the very young, it increases to adult rates at puberty and affects around 1% of children and adolescents overall (Heyman *et al.*, 2001). Untreated OCD pursues an unremitting and fluctuating course with the highest prevalence in the early years of middle adult life. Major comorbidity with Axis I and Axis II disorders has been identified (Hollander *et al.*, 1998), including depression in about two-thirds of clinical cases, simple phobia (22%), social phobia (18%), eating disorder (17%), alcohol dependence (14%), panic disorder (12%), and Tourette's syndrome (7%) (Pigott *et al.*, 1994), as well as increased rates of suicidal behavior. Individuals with OCD report substantial impairment in health-related quality of life and social functioning (Hollander *et al.*, 2010) and children with early onset OCD are particularly badly affected (Piacentini & Langley, 2004). The cost to society, in terms of human suffering, diminished individual potential, and lost revenue as a consequence of OCD, is high (Hollander & Wong, 1998). Severe, chronic OCD is associated with high levels of hospitalization (Drummond, 1993).

OCD remains poorly recognized and under-treated. Although surveys suggest that the time between the onset of symptoms and diagnosis may be decreasing, it is often only when depressive symptoms emerge that treatment is started. The average duration of untreated illness has been estimated at 17 years (Hollander & Wong, 1998). The success of treatment to a large extent depends on the condition not being overlooked and better recognition of the disorder has been cited as a public health priority (NICE, 2006). OCD responds preferentially to drugs which powerfully inhibit the reuptake of serotonin at the synapse, i.e. clomipramine and the selective serotonin reuptake inhibitors (SSRIs). Drugs without potent serotonin reuptake inhibitor (SRI) activity, when used as monotherapy, have been shown to be ineffective in controlled trials. This selective pharmacological response has generated

Essential Evidence-Based Psychopharmacology, Second Edition, ed. Dan J. Stein, Bernard Lerer, and Stephen M. Stahl. Published by Cambridge University Press. © Cambridge University Press.

hypotheses about the role of serotonin in the etiology of OCD but, so far, no unifying theory has emerged and the mechanisms by which SSRIs exert anti-obsessional benefits remain poorly understood. Indeed, it is widely believed that OCD encompasses a heterogeneous group of illnesses, and that other neurotransmitters such as dopamine, noradrenaline, and glutamate (Fineberg *et al.*, 2010) are involved in its pathophysiology.

Methods

This paper represents a revision and update of the original published in 2005 (Fineberg & Gale, 2005). Our narrative review is based, wherever possible, on randomized controlled trials (RCTs). We present the evidence supporting the pharmacological treatment of OCD and aim to address key clinical issues including (1) What are the first-line treatments? (2) Does pharmacotherapy improve health-related quality of life? (3) How do we evaluate clinical response and relapse? (4) How long should treatment continue? (5) Can we predict treatment outcomes? (6) What is the management of treatment-refractory OCD? In addition, we draw attention to important aspects of the methodology or outcome of some of the studies under review, that we consider may enlighten clinical practice or advance future trial design in this field. Uncontrolled studies are cited where systematic data are lacking and meta-analyses are also cited, for example where adequate head-to-head comparator studies do not exist. Expert consensus guidelines are considered and practical recommendations made for the clinical setting. A systematic search of electronic databases [EMBase (1974–date), MEDLINE (1966–date), PsycINFO (1987–date)] was run using a combination of the terms obsessive compulsive (randomized or control$ or clinical trial$ or placebo$ or blind$) and (systematic or review$ or meta-analysis), as well as individual drug names. This was complemented by consulting with colleagues in the field and reviewing data presented at international, peer-reviewed symposia. There is a shortage of long-term and relapse-prevention studies in OCD and the majority of published studies present short-term data. OCD is a lifespan disorder, and effective treatment early on may prevent the problems of long-term chronicity. Available data suggest children may respond rather like adults. In this paper we include an analysis of the limited studies that have been conducted in children with OCD. Unfortunately there is almost no research into the pharmacotherapy of OCD in the elderly.

First-line treatments for OCD: Clomipramine

Uncontrolled case series demonstrating successful treatment with clomipramine first appeared in the 1960s (Fernandez & Lopez-Ibor, 1967; Reynghe de Voxrie, 1968). By 1990, several double-blind placebo-controlled trials had suggested that clomipramine may be an effective treatment for OCD (Flament *et al.*, 1985; Insel *et al.*, 1983; Jenike *et al.*, 1989; Marks *et al.*, 1980; Mavissakalian *et al.*, 1985; Thoren *et al.*, 1980). However, the inclusion of cases with comorbid depression in these studies, together with reports of the beneficial effect of clomipramine on obsessional symptoms within depression, led to uncertainty as to whether this was a specific effect on OCD or a more general antidepressant effect. Therefore, studies were performed in which patients with clinically relevant depression were specifically excluded (Clomipramine Collaborative Study Group, 1991; de Veaugh-Geiss *et al.*, 1989; Greist *et al.*, 1990; Marks *et al.*, 1988; Montgomery, 1980) or where patients were stratified (Katz *et al.*, 1990), on the basis of scores on the Hamilton Depression Scale (Hamilton, 1960). These also showed clear evidence of efficacy for clomipramine, thereby demonstrating that the anti-obsessional effect is independent of depression. The treatment effect was slow to develop and gains on clomipramine accrued for several weeks. Moreover, in some of the studies investigating OCD subjects with comorbid depression, an active, non-serotonergic comparator antidepressant was included (de Veaugh-Geiss *et al.*, 1992; Flament *et al.*, 1985; Insel *et al.*, 1983; Jenike *et al.*, 1989; Marks *et al.*, 1980; Mavissakalian *et al.*, 1985; Thoren *et al.*, 1980) and in these, clomipramine was consistently demonstrated to be superior to the comparator control. For example, in the study by Thoren *et al.* (1980), clomipramine out-performed the noradrenergic antidepressant nortriptyline as well as placebo. In addition, clomipramine was superior to the monoamine oxidase inhibitor (MAOI) clorgyline in a small (*n* = 12) cross-over study (Insel *et al.*, 1983). The placebo-controlled cross-over study by Flament *et al.* (1985) was the first to demonstrate the efficacy of a pharmacological treatment in OCD in children (6–18 years). Irrespective of baseline depression, a significant improvement in obsessional symptoms was seen for clomipramine (mean dose 141 mg) compared with placebo. Significant post-baseline improvements were also observed in the placebo group, suggesting that children may be susceptible to non-specific treatment effects. However, another study of children and adolescents by de Veaugh-Geiss *et al.* (1992) reported improvement of only 8% in the placebo group (*n* = 29) at the 8-week end-point, compared with 37% in the clomipramine group (*n* = 31), with a significant difference evident from week 3.

Most of these studies are considered small by current standards but the pattern of results is highly consistent, which is rare in psychopharmacological research. Together, the results provide unequivocal support for the efficacy of clomipramine in adults and children with OCD. They also reflect the special qualities of the patients under investigation at that time. There were few treatment-refractory cases and most had long histories of stable, severe, untreated illness. The studies' power also depended on low placebo-response rates and these distinguish OCD from depression and other anxiety disorders where placebo-response rates are higher.

SRIs compared with other antidepressants lacking strong serotonergic activity

Clomipramine differs from other tricyclics due to its more powerful SRI activity, though its effects are not entirely serotonergic. The poor performance of the noradrenergic tricyclic desipramine, relative to clomipramine, was apparent in a placebo-controlled cross-over study (Insel *et al.*, 1985) and in two cross-over studies in children (Leonard *et al.*, 1988, 1991). Later studies showed an inferiority for desipramine compared with SSRIs such as fluvoxamine (Goodman *et al.*, 1990) and sertraline (Hoehn-Saric *et al.*, 2000). Similarly, comparisons of imipramine with clomipramine demonstrated superiority for clomipramine (Foa *et al.*, 1987; Volavka *et al.*, 1985) though in one of these studies imipramine produced antidepressant but not anti-obsessional effects (Foa *et al.*, 1987). Thoren *et al.* (1980) demonstrated clomipramine but not nortriptyline was superior to placebo and there was a significant within-group advantage for clomipramine but not amitriptyline in a small study by Ananth *et al.* (1981). There has been no study thus far demonstrating a convincing advantage for an MAOI over placebo in OCD. Clomipramine was found to be superior to clorgyline in a small (*n* = 13) placebo-controlled study (Insel *et al.*, 1983) and Jenike *et al.* (1997) demonstrated a significant advantage for fluoxetine over phenelzine which did not distinguish from placebo.

Thus, in some studies, anti-obsessional benefit has been shown by comparator agents, but the effect is consistently weaker that that of SRIs. Large sample sizes are usually required to demonstrate a significant difference between active treatments, so the fact that several small studies show superiority for SRIs strongly suggests that non-SRIs have little, if any, efficacy in OCD.

SSRIs

In addition to clomipramine's powerful SRI activity, its active metabolite has strong nor-adrenergic properties. Given that the more highly selective SSRIs are also beneficial (see below), and show a similar slow, incremental effect on OCD symptoms, it would appear that their anti-obsessional actions are related to SRI activity. Early promising reports suggesting efficacy for zimelidine were curtailed by its withdrawal for safety reasons.

Placebo-controlled studies of fluvoxamine

In a double-blind cross-over study of fluvoxamine ($n = 20$) by Perse et al. (1987), efficacy was evident after 8 weeks, based on 16 completers. Cottraux et al. (1990) emphasized the strength of drug effect relative to psychotherapy by demonstrating the superiority of fluvoxamine over placebo in spite of concurrent exposure therapy in the placebo group. However, the study was criticized for not including an intention-to-treat (ITT) analysis and for relying on behavioral ratings for the OCD. Similar response profiles in depressed and non-depressed OCD patients were demonstrated by Goodman et al. (1989c), with significant placebo-referenced improvement in the fluvoxamine-treated group seen from week 2 onwards using the Yale–Brown Obsessive Compulsive Scale (YBOCS; Goodman et al., 1989a) – a scale that has become the pivotal rating measure for clinical treatment trials. Jenike et al. (1990a) also reported efficacy for fluvoxamine compared with placebo, although significant between-group differences did not appear until week 10. The 10-week, multi-center study by Goodman et al. (1996) examined two groups of 78 patients who received fluvoxamine (100–300 mg) or placebo. Fluvoxamine was superior on all outcome measures from week 4 onwards. Only 10 cases discontinued because of side-effects. Obsessions and compulsions both improved with a possible earlier benefit for obsessions. The multi-center study by Hollander et al. (2003a) investigated flexible, once-daily doses of controlled-release (CR) fluvoxamine (100–300 mg), which was superior to placebo in decreasing YBOCS scores from week 2 onwards. By the 12-week end-point, fluvoxamine CR ($n = 127$) produced a 32% YBOCS improvement, compared with 21% for placebo ($n = 126$). Remission rates for fluvoxamine CR were 44% and 18% respectively, with remission defined as either a YBOCS total score <16, or an obsessive or compulsive subscale score <8. Withdrawal due to adverse effects (mainly nausea, insomnia, somnolence, dizziness, and diarrhoea) occurred in 19% in the fluvoxamine-treated group compared with 6% in the placebo group.

Riddle et al. (2001) examined fluvoxamine (50–200 mg) in 120 children aged 8–17 years. From weeks 1–6 and at the 10-week end-point, there was significant improvement on the Children's Yale-Brown Obsessive-Compulsive Scale (C-YBOCS; Scahill et al., 1997). Only three patients on fluvoxamine and one on placebo withdrew through adverse effects. This finding supports the rapid efficacy and tolerability of fluvoxamine in childhood OCD. However, Harris et al. (2010) published a retrospective case-note review suggesting that three out of 17 cases of pediatric OCD treated with fluvoxamine in their outpatient clinic developed behavioral disinhibition including physical and verbal aggression and risk-taking behavior.

Two cases had pre-existing symptoms of other 'impulsive' forms of illness including tic disorder and attention deficit hyperactivity disorder. These findings hint that young OCD patients with impulsive or tic disorders may be at risk of behavioral disinhibition following the initiation of SRI medication.

Placebo-controlled studies of sertraline

In a study of flexible doses of sertraline (20–200 mg), Chouinard et al. (1990) demonstrated superiority over placebo on the YBOCS and NIMH-Global OC scale, but not on the Maudsley Obsessive–Compulsive Inventory (Hodgson & Rachman, 1977), suggesting that the latter scale lacks sensitivity for detecting clinical change. An arguably under-powered study comparing sertraline ($n = 10$) and placebo ($n = 9$) by Jenike et al. (1990b) found no differences between groups. However, a larger study by Kronig et al. (1999) demonstrated superiority for sertraline (50–200 mg, $n = 86$) over placebo ($n = 81$) as early as week 3. Discontinuation rates due to side-effects were 10% in the sertraline group and 5% in the placebo group. The multicenter fixed-dose study by Greist et al. (1995a), showed efficacy on the YBOCS for pooled sertraline (50–200 mg, $n = 240$) at week 2 onwards compared with placebo ($n = 84$). However, at the 12-week end-point, almost as many in the placebo group (30%) were much or very much improved compared with those on sertraline (39%).

In a cohort of 107 children and 80 adolescents, March et al. (1998) found a significant advantage for sertraline, titrated up to 200 mg, over placebo on the C-YBOCS as early as week 3. Insomnia, agitation and tremor were over-represented in the drug-treated condition and 13% of sertraline-treated patients discontinued early because of adverse effects (3% in the placebo group). No clinically meaningful adverse effects were detected, suggesting that, in doses up to 200 mg, sertraline is safe in children (Wilens et al., 1999). The Paediatric OCD Treatment Study (POTS 2004) in children and adolescents examined sertraline alone, CBT alone, combined sertraline and CBT, or pill placebo. Participants tolerated the active treatments well but conclusions about efficacy were limited by the absence of a matched control treatment for CBT. Sertraline, either alone or in combination with CBT, was efficacious when compared with pill placebo. A post-hoc review of the POTS data by Garcia et al. (2010) identified that children with lower severity of OCD, less OCD-related functional impairment, fewer comorbid symptoms, lower levels of family accommodation and better insight, showed a better improvement than their counterparts. It was also reported that children with a family history of OCD were more likely to respond to CBT in combination with SRI than CBT alone.

Placebo-controlled studies of fluoxetine

Two multicenter studies were designed to compare the efficacy of different fixed doses of fluoxetine. Montgomery et al. (1993), in an 8-week study, showed the 20 mg dose ($n = 52$) did no better than placebo ($n = 56$), while the 40 mg dose ($n = 52$) was superior on the responder analysis and the 60 mg dose ($n = 54$) was superior both on reduction of YBOCS scores and on measures of "responder" rates. There were few side-effects and fewer than 6% subjects withdrew early as a result. In the longer and larger study by Tollefson et al. (1994), all fixed doses (20, 40, 60 mg) of fluoxetine were superior to placebo by the 13-week end-point; however the 60 mg dose showed a trend towards superiority over the 20 mg and 40 mg doses on the YBOCS analysis. Side-effects included nausea, dry mouth, tremor, and sexual problems. No association between fluoxetine and emergent suicidality in OCD was seen in a meta-analysis (Beasley et al., 1992). Jenike et al. (1997) compared fluoxetine (up to 80 mg), phenelzine, and placebo. Fluoxetine ($n = 23$) was superior to placebo ($n = 21$) and phenelzine ($n = 20$), which did not differentiate from placebo.

Studies of fluoxetine in childhood OCD have also shown superiority over placebo. Fixed 20 mg doses were used in a cross-over study on 14 children (Riddle et al., 1992). A significant advantage was observed on the CGI (44% improvement after 8 weeks of treatment compared with 27% on placebo) but not C-YBOCS. "Behavioral activation" occurred as an adverse effect in a few children, and one left the study early because of suicidal ideation. The authors considered these side-effects to be dose related, and advocated initiating treatment at low doses. Geller et al. (2001) examined a larger cohort of children ($n = 103$; age 7–17), titrating fluoxetine doses upwards from 10 to 60 mg over 13 weeks, depending on clinical response. Fluoxetine was well tolerated across all doses and superior to placebo on the C-YBOCS from week 6. There were similar drop-out rates from adverse events on drug (8.5%) and placebo. In a 16-week, placebo-controlled trial ($n = 43$; age 6–18) of children and adolescents spanning 7 years, Leibowitz et al. (2002) extended the dose range to 80 mg for 2 weeks after an initial 6 weeks (doses up to 60 mg/day). Responders continued for a further 8 weeks in a double-blind manner. At the 16-week end-point 57% of the fluoxetine group compared with 27% of the placebo group were much or very much improved on CGI. No patient withdrew because of adverse effects.

Placebo-controlled studies of paroxetine

Positive results were reported in a multinational study by Zohar & Judge (1996), using clomipramine as an additional active comparator. Paroxetine ($n = 201$) in doses of up to 60 mg was significantly more effective than placebo ($n = 99$) on all a-priori efficacy measures (including YBOCS), and of comparable efficacy to clomipramine (50–200 mg, $n = 99$). Only 9% of paroxetine-treated patients withdrew because of side-effects (mainly asthenia, headache, dry mouth, and nausea) compared with 6% given placebo and 17% on clomipramine (see below). Hollander et al. (2003b) compared paroxetine in fixed doses (20, 40, 60 mg) with placebo in a 12-week, multicenter trial of 348 patients. Respectively, post-baseline reductions in YBOCS scores of 16%, 25%, 29%, and 13% were reported. Both higher doses (40 mg and 60 mg) were significantly superior to the 20 mg dose (which did not separate from placebo). Paroxetine was well tolerated at all doses.

Placebo-controlled studies of citalopram

In a multinational, placebo-controlled study, Montgomery et al. (2001) showed efficacy for fixed doses of 20 mg ($n = 102$), 40 mg ($n = 98$) and 60 mg citalopram ($n = 100$) compared with placebo ($n = 101$). A significant reduction in baseline YBOCS score was seen earlier i.e. from week 3 for the 60 mg group, and from week 7–12 for other doses. Citalopram was well tolerated (4% withdrew through adverse effects; mainly nausea, headache, fatigue, insomnia) and improved psychosocial disability on the Sheehan Disability Scale (Sheehan et al., 1996).*

Placebo-controlled studies of escitalopram

Escitalopram was investigated in a 24-week, active-referenced (paroxetine), placebo-controlled multicenter study (Stein et al., 2007). Patients received either 10 mg ($n = 112$)

---

* See new MHRA guidance, p. 136.

Table 8.1. Rate of clinical response in placebo-controlled studies of SSRIs for patients with OCD.

Drug (duration, weeks)	Much or very much improved on CGI-I (Criterion A)	>25% improved on baseline Y-BOCS (Criterion B)	>35% improved on baseline Y-BOCS	Criteria A & B	Study
Citalopram 20 mg (12)	57.4%				Montgomery et al. (2001)
Citalopram 40 mg (12)	52%				
Citalopram 60 mg (12)*	65%				
Escitalopram 10 mg (24)	40%	75%			Stein et al. (2007)
Escitalopram 20 mg (24)	38%	78%			
Fluvoxamine (8)	9/21				Goodman et al. (1989c)
Fluvoxamine (10)	33.3%				Goodman et al. (1996)
Fluvoxamine CR (12)	34% from graph	53%			Hollander et al. (2003a)
Fluvoxamine (10)		42% (C-Y-BOCS)	45%		Riddle et al. (2001)
Fluoxetine 20 mg (8)				36%	Montgomery et al. (1993)
Fluoxetine 40 mg (8)				48%	
Fluoxetine 60 mg (8)				47%	
Fluoxetine 20 mg (13)			32%		Tollefson et al. (1994)
Fluoxetine 40 mg (13)			34%		
Fluoxetine 60 mg (13)			35%		
Fluoxetine (13)	55%				Geller et al. (2001)
Fluoxetine (16)	57%				Leibowitz et al. (2002)
Paroxetine (12)	55.1%				Zohar & Judge (1996)
Paroxetine 40 mg (24)	31%	69%			Stein et al. (2007)
Sertraline (12)	41%				Kronig et al. (1999)
Sertraline (12)	38.9%				Greist et al. (1995a)
Sertraline (12)	42%				March et al. (1998)

Definition of clinical response

* See new MHRA guidance, p. 136.

20 mg ($n = 114$) escitalopram, 40 mg ($n = 116$) paroxetine, or placebo ($n = 113$). The primary end-point was 12 weeks, and the study continued for a further 12 weeks under double-blind conditions. Escitalopram 20 mg and paroxetine were superior to placebo at 12 weeks and all three active treatments were superior to placebo at 24 weeks. When compared with placebo, the 20 mg escitalopram dose produced an earlier onset of action and was more effective than the 10 mg dose across the duration of the trial. This study demonstrates the importance of continuing treatment for an adequate duration (in this case, 24 weeks). Escitalopram was well tolerated.* A post-hoc factor analysis by Stein *et al.* (2008) showed escitalopram to be effective for most symptom dimensions of OCD, but the hoarding/symmetry subtype was associated with a relatively poor response.

Have changes in study populations affected treatment trial design?

The magnitude of the observed treatment effect has diminished from 40–50% average reduction in baseline scores in the clomipramine studies, to around 30% in some of the later SSRI studies. The reasons for this may to some extent lie with changes in the characteristics of the patients entering the trials over time. Based upon the efficacy data, SSRIs and clomipramine were rapidly accepted as first-line pharmacological treatments for OCD (NICE, 2006). Consequently, it has become increasingly challenging for research centers to recruit treatment-naive patients into clinical trials. Thus, greater numbers of treatment-refractory individuals may have been included in the more recent studies. At the same time, rigorous attempts to exclude comorbid illness, such as depression, may have led to the inclusion of milder cases with less capacity for symptomatic improvement. Indeed, the application of increasingly stringent inclusion criteria in recent studies, often driven by regulatory authority requirements, may contribute to the changing pattern of response rates, since treatment groups are less heterogeneous. Table 8.1 summarizes the rates of clinical response in those studies that report them. Between 32% and 78% of the SSRI-treated study participants showed a clinically meaningful improvement using the various recognized criteria for clinical response. Increased placebo-response rates, in some cases exceeding 20% improvement in baseline scores, have also been observed in the more recent studies. The reasons for this are also likely to be complex, including changes in patient expectation of improvement, as well as a shift toward the inclusion of milder, atypical cases, some of whom undergo spontaneous remission. In addition, in the face of recruitment difficulties, baseline severity scores may be artificially inflated to fulfill entry criteria, and if they subsequently diminish to their real values after study entry, this may contribute towards seemingly increased response rates on drug or placebo, further reducing the discriminatory power of the studies. The rise in the placebo response rate cautions against drawing conclusions about efficacy from open, naturalistic reporting, and emphasizes the crucial importance of controlled investigation (Fineberg *et al.*, 2006b). The net effect of these changes has been to reduce the statistical power of studies, so that larger numbers are now needed to test efficacy of new treatments. Meta-analyses of existing studies can, to some extent, compensate by pooling data, but if they fail to take these changes into account they may be misleading.

---

* See new MHRA guidance, p. 136.

Direct head-to-head comparisons of SRIs in OCD

SSRI vs. SSRI

SSRIs differ from one another in terms of the selectivity and potency of effect at the serotonin transporter and their secondary pharmacological actions (Stahl, 2008) and consequently one might predict differences in clinical efficacy in OCD. So far, three controlled studies of the relative efficacy of different SSRIs have been conducted. An arguably under-powered single-blind study by Mundo *et al.* (1997*a*) did not detect differences between fluvoxamine, paroxetine, or citalopram with 10 patients per group. In addition, in the double-blind comparison of sertraline ($n = 77$) and fluoxetine ($n = 73$) (Bergeron *et al.*, 2001) no significant difference was seen at the 24-week end-point on any of the primary efficacy measures. However there was a non-significant trend towards an earlier effect in the sertraline group, and a greater number of sertraline patients reached remission, defined as a CGI-I score of ≤ 2 and a YBOCS score of ≤ 11. Stein *et al.* (2007) compared escitalopram (10 mg and 20 mg) with paroxetine (40 mg) and placebo. Whereas symptomatic improvements on escitalopram 20 mg and paroxetine 40 mg appeared similar from the 12-week primary end-point onwards, improvement in YBOCS score was significantly better than placebo as early as week 6 in the escitalopram 20 mg group only. These results are not strong enough to support the superior efficacy or tolerability of any one SSRI, even in conjunction with meta-analysis data (see below). Therefore, treatment selection should take into account other factors, such as potential drug–drug interactions with co-administered compounds. It should be borne in mind that fluoxetine, paroxetine, and to a much lesser extent sertraline, inhibit the P450 isoenzyme CYP2D6 which metabolizes tricyclic antidepressants, antipsychotics, anti-arrhythmics and beta-blockers, and fluvoxamine inhibits both CYP1A2 and CYP3A4, which eliminate warfarin, tricyclics, benzodiazepines, and some anti-arrhythmics. Citalopram and escitalopram are relatively free from hepatic interactions (Culpepper, 2002). According to recent guidance (Medicines and Healthcare Products Regulatory Authority (MHRA): *Drug Safety Update Vol 5, Issue 5, Dec 2011*) citalopram and escitalopram are associated with dose-dependent QT interval prolongation and should be avoided in those with established pre-existing QT interval prolongation or in combination with other medicines that prolong the QT interval. ECG measurements should be considered for patients with cardiac disease, and electrolyte disturbances corrected before starting treatment. For citalopram, new restrictions on the maximum daily doses now apply: 40 mg for adults; 20 mg for patients older then 65 years; and 20 mg for those with hepatic impairment. For escitalopram, the maximum daily dose for patients older than 65 years is now reduced to 10 mg/day; other doses remain unchanged. Fluoxetine has a long half-life, and has fewer discontinuation effects, which can be of benefit in patients who forget to take their medication, whereas paroxetine is generally associated with adverse activation effects during treatment initiation as well as discontinuation effects (Greenblatt *et al.*, 1998), though these effects have not been particularly evident in OCD treatment trials.

SSRI vs. clomipramine

While meta-analyses report a smaller effect-size for SSRIs relative to clomipramine (see below), head-to-head studies tend to demonstrate equivalent efficacy. While some individual trials were small and therefore subject to type II error (Montgomery *et al.*, 1990), the study by Bisserbe *et al.* (1997) was sufficiently powered and demonstrated a significant advantage for sertraline over clomipramine, however the advantage, apparent for certain efficacy measures in the ITT analysis, was not clear-cut. In contrast, another small study by Lopez-Ibor et al. (1996) detected an advantage for clomipramine over fluoxetine (40 mg) on secondary but not primary outcome measures. Rouillon (1998; also see Mundo et al., 2001) in a larger study showed equivalent efficacy for clomipramine and SSRI at all visits and on all outcome measures. Zohar & Judge (1996) compared paroxetine and clomipramine and at weeks 6, 8, and 12 showed similar placebo-referenced efficacy on OCD symptom scores, though paroxetine was superior to placebo on depression ratings whereas clomipramine was not. Response was defined as ≥25% improvement in baseline YBOCS scores. At the end-point, 55% of both paroxetine- and clomipramine-treated patients met this criterion, compared with 35% in the placebo group.

Improved tolerability favors SSRIs

SSRIs, compared with clomipramine, have better overall acceptability and tolerability. Zohar & Judge (1996) demonstrated the drop-out rate from adverse effects in the clomipramine group (approximately 17%) was considerably higher than for the paroxetine group (9%). Rouillon (1998) reported that, compared with fluvoxamine, clomipramine was associated with significantly more side-effect related early withdrawals. Moreover, the ITT analysis by Bisserbe et al. (1997) concluded that the greater benefit of sertraline could have been explained by its superior tolerability over clomipramine. The risk of dangerous side-effects occurring such as convulsions (up to 2% on clomipramine, compared to 0.1–0.5% on high-dose SSRI; Clomipramine Collaborative Study Group, 1991), cardiotoxicity, and cognitive impairment is substantially lower with SSRIs. Clomipramine shares anticholinergic side-effects associated with tricyclics and is lethal in overdose. According to a meta analysis of published and unpublished trials, clomipramine was associated with higher rates of adverse-event related premature trial discontinuations when compared with SSRIs (NICE, 2006; see below). All SRIs are associated with impaired sexual performance (up to 30% of cases) but clomipramine (up to 80% cases; Monteiro et al., 1987) appears more problematic. SSRIs may be responsible for more asthenia, insomnia, and nausea (Bisserbe et al., 1997). Maina et al. (2003a) reported clinically relevant weight gain in approximately 14.5% of cases (mainly females), with clomipramine producing more weight gain than sertraline and fluoxetine.

Meta-analyses of relative effectiveness of SRIs in OCD

Meta-analyses may provide a more objective and quantifiable measure of treatment effect than narrative reviews such as this. However, problems arise in controlling for between-study differences such as dose, duration, blinding, method of assessment, and population changes, so results must be viewed cautiously (Pigott & Seay, 1999). Moreover, the large numbers that result from conflation of multiple studies may produce results that are statistically significant but are actually spurious. In short, meta-analyses cannot substitute for high-quality head-to-head comparator trials. Early meta-analyses comparing clomipramine, SSRIs, and placebo (Greist et al., 1995c; Jenike et al., 1990c; Piccinelli et al., 1995; Stein et al., 1995) showed that clomipramine and SSRIs are more effective than placebo and that clomipramine was associated with a significantly greater mean change in YBOCS scores, as well as a larger premature drop-out rate than SSRIs. However, bias favoring clomipramine may develop as a consequence of variation between the studies; such as year of publication, severity of OCD, pre-randomization period duration, trial duration, clomipramine-related adverse effects leading to unblinding and rising placebo-response rates. Subsequent meta-analyses comparing RCTs of SRI and psychological interventions (Abramowitz, 1997; Kobak et al., 1998) also reported an apparent superiority in efficacy for clomipramine over SSRIs, other than fluoxetine or fluvoxamine, even when certain of these potentially confounding variables were controlled for; and superiority tolerability for SSRIs. However, it was suggested that "unblinding" by the more obvious adverse effects of clomipramine may have amplified its apparent efficacy and poorer tolerability. The more recent UK National Institute for Health and Clinical Excellence report (NICE, 2006) systematically accessed all available published and unpublished RCTs. In terms of efficacy, clomipramine and SSRIs were indistinguishable. However, clomipramine was associated with higher rates of adverse-event related premature trial discontinuations when compared with SSRIs. The meta-analysis of SSRI versus placebo by Soomro et al. (2008) that included 17 studies (3097 participants), unequivocally demonstrated the efficacy of SSRIs in OCD. Analysis of 13 studies (2697 participants) indicated that SSRIs are nearly twice as likely as placebo to produce a clinical response ($\geq 25\%$ reduction in YBOCS from baseline).

Geller et al. (2003a) performed the first meta-analysis on pharmacotherapy for childhood OCD. The results of 12 trials showed modest but significant advantages for all SRIs over placebo and superiority for clomipramine over SSRIs. SSRIs were more or less comparable and the findings were not dependent on publication date or placebo-response rate. However, the authors expressed caution because of the absence of head-to-head active comparator studies and recommended that, because of its side-effect profile, clomipramine should not generally be used first-line in children. Watson & Rees (2008) performed a meta-analysis of 13 RCTs in young people aged ≤ 19 with a diagnosis of OCD. Ten contained comparisons of pharmacotherapy and control while five compared CBT with control. They found that pharmacotherapy and CBT are significantly more effective than placebo in controlling OCD symptoms in young people. The strength of this study is limited, however, by the search strategy employed – there was no search for unpublished or non-English material nor was the validity of the included studies formally assessed.

In summary, according to the current evidence from head-to-head trials and meta-analyses, we consider the concept of a "gold-standard" drug for OCD to be misleading. The combined evidence from head-to-head trials and meta-analyses does not appear to back up the superiority of clomipramine over SSRIs and SRIs appear equally effective at relieving obsessional thoughts and compulsive rituals. However, the improved safety and tolerability of SSRIs offer considerable advantages for the long-term treatment of OCD, and indicate that the SSRIs should usually be considered the treatment of choice, with clomipramine reserved for those who cannot tolerate or who have failed to respond to them.

Suicide in children on SSRIs

A meta-analysis conducted by Bridge et al. (2007) examined the effects of SSRIs in children aged 6–18 years following warnings from the American Food and Drug Administration that SSRIs in the young may increase the risk of suicidal thoughts and behaviors compared with placebo (4% vs. 2%). They identified 27 randomized controlled trials of SSRIs used in major depressive disorder (MDD, $n = 15$), OCD ($n = 6$) and non-OCD anxiety disorders ($n = 6$). There were no completed suicides during any of the studies; pooled absolute rates of either suicidal ideation/suicide attempt (treatment vs. placebo) in MDD (3% vs. 2%), OCD (1% vs. 0.3%) and non-OCD anxiety disorders (1% vs. 0.2 %) compare favorably with pooled absolute clinical response rates (treatment vs. placebo; MDD (61% vs. 50%); OCD (52% vs. 32%) and non-OCD anxiety disorders (69% vs. 39%). For patients with OCD, the data suggest a number needed to treat (NNT) of six compared with a number needed to harm (NNH) of 200. The authors concluded that the benefits of SSRI medication probably outweigh the risks in the OCD pediatric population. March *et al.* (2006) calculated the NNT and NNH for multi-center trials of sertraline in children and adolescents with MDD and OCD. NNT ranged from 2 to 10 with no apparent age effect in OCD. No patients reported suicidality in the two OCD trials giving a NNH approaching infinity. The authors concluded a positive benefit to risk ratio for sertraline in pediatric OCD, with the doctor–patient relationship playing an important role.

CBT *vs.* pharmacotherapy

In a multidimensional meta-analysis of psychological and pharmacological therapy (Eddy *et al.*, 2004), the authors report findings consistent with the literature that psychological and pharmacological therapy produce substantial improvement, reflected by pre- and post-treatment effect sizes. Behaviorally inclined psychological approaches were more efficacious than cognitively focussed approaches. The effect sizes for combination (drug plus CBT) treatment were higher than for pharmacotherapy alone. However, shortcomings of contributing studies that limit the validity and clinical utility of the analysis include the frequent absence of placebo CBT in the trial design, poor reporting of screening criteria, high exclusion rates secondary to co-morbidity, restricted focus on few outcomes and limited data on long-term maintenance of treatment gains. For example, only three of the 15 studies included in the analysis reported exclusion rates. Reporting of improvement and recovery rates was inconsistent as was reporting of effect size and few of the studies reported long-term follow-up. NICE (2006) identified that there is limited evidence for the superior efficacy of exposure and response prevention therapy over clomipramine and that evidence for other comparisons between CBT and pharmacotherapy were inconclusive.

What is the most effective dose?

Traditionally it has been thought that OCD requires treatment with higher doses of medication than depression or anxiety. Indeed, controlled studies demonstrate efficacy and tolerability for doses as high as 80 mg fluoxetine (Jenike *et al.*, 1997; Leibowitz *et al.*, 2002) and 300 mg clomipramine (de Veaugh-Geiss *et al.*, 1989). However to address this issue, studies comparing different fixed doses of active drug head-to-head with placebo are required. Clomipramine has not been tested in this way. Single-dose studies have shown efficacy compared with placebo for relatively low fixed clomipramine doses (75 mg and 125 mg), but most studies examined flexible doses titrated up to the upper end of the range (200–300 mg). Fluvoxamine has similarly been shown to be effective in doses ranging from 150–300 mg.

Fluoxetine, paroxetine, sertraline, citalopram, and escitalopram have each been investigated in a series of multiple, fixed-dose studies (see Fineberg & Gale, 2005). A positive dose–response relationship was demonstrated for 40 mg and 60 mg of paroxetine (Hollander *et al.*, 2003b; Wheadon *et al.*, 1993). Similar results were reported for fluoxetine, with the greatest benefit seen in those patients receiving the 60 mg dose (Montgomery *et al.*, 1993; Tollefson *et al.*, 1994) which was additionally shown to be significantly more effective than the 20 mg dose in a meta-analysis (Wood *et al.*, 1993). In the case of paroxetine, the 60 mg dose was significantly superior to the 20 mg dose which did not separate from placebo (Hollander *et al.*, 2003b). The dose–response relationship is less clear-cut for sertraline and citalopram (Greist *et al.*, 1995b; Montgomery *et al.*, 2001; Ushijima *et al.*, 1997). However, Stein *et al.* (2007)

Table 8.2. Placebo-controlled comparator studies of fixed-doses of SSRI.

Drug	Duration (weeks)	n	Fixed dose	Positive dose–response relationship	Study
RCTs					
Citalopram	12	352	20/40/60 mg*	No	Montgomery et al. (2001)
Fluoxetine	8	214	20/40/60 mg	Yes[a]	Montgomery et al. (1993)
Fluoxetine	13	355	20/40/60 mg	No	Tollefson et al. (1994)
Paroxetine	12	348	20/40/60 mg	Yes	Wheadon et al. (1993)
Paroxetine	12	348	20/40/60 mg	Yes	Hollander et al. (2003b)
Sertraline	12	324	50/100/200 mg	No	Greist et al. (1995b)
Meta-analysis				Yes	Bloch et al. (2010)

[a] Marginally significant benefit for medium and higher doses on primary analysis (total Y-BOCS, $p = 0.059$); significant on "responder" analysis ($p < 0.05$).
* See new MHRA guidance, p. 136.

demonstrated a clear and sustained advantage for 20 mg escitalopram, over the 10 mg dose, which continued until the 24-week end-point. Escitalopram 20 mg was superior to placebo on the YBOCS from 6 weeks onwards, and on secondary end-points including remission, whereas escitalopram 10 mg separated from placebo only at 16 weeks on secondary outcome measures only. Bloch et al. (2010) conducted a meta-analysis of nine SSRI studies to determine dose-related differences in efficacy and tolerability using a fixed-effects model. Higher doses of SSRI were associated with improved treatment efficacy than low or medium doses using YBOCS score or proportion of responders as outcome measures. Higher SSRI dose was not associated with "all cause" dropout rates but was associated with higher rates of dropouts "due to side-effects."

Table 8.2. summarizes these results, which suggest that while lower doses may be efficacious, despite poorer tolerability, better anti-obsessional efficacy is usually produced by higher doses.

Strategies for dose titration in OCD

Exacerbation of anxiety in the early stages of treatment appears to be rare in OCD, as demonstrated in acute studies of SRIs which show a slow, gradual treatment effect. Irrespective of dose, it can take several weeks for improvements to become established and patients should be informed about this from the outset. Early signs of improvement may be noticed by an informant before individuals with OCD, who are poor at recognizing their own progress. The use of observer-rated scales such as the YBOCS may be helpful to detect small improvements in a clinical setting, although in some cases observable benefits may not appear for several months. In these circumstances, clinicians can feel pressured to change treatments or increase SSRI doses prematurely. A balance must be struck between tolerability and rate of dose-increase. A significant difference in favor of rapid dose escalation was seen at weeks 4 and 6 of a single-blind study comparing dose escalation with sertraline to 150 mg over 5 days, with slower dose escalation over 15 days, but this advantage disappeared thereafter (Bogetto et al., 2002). The study was too small to discern differences in tolerability. Koran et al. (1997) demonstrated that pulse loading with intravenous clomipramine produced a large and rapid decrease in obsessive symptoms, but oral pulse loading did not, though the early advantages were not sustained. The arguments for slower dose increases may be more persuasive, particularly in children and the elderly. Slow titration over weeks or months can ameliorate early SSRI-related adverse events such as nausea and agitation. Longer-term, dose-related side-effects such as sleep disturbance and headache also need to be monitored. Sexual dysfunction is a common cause of drug discontinuation, and, if necessary, strategies such as dose reduction, short drug-holidays or use of drugs with restorative potency (e.g. mirtazapine, Lee *et al.*, 2010; viagra, Farre *et al.*, 2004; agomelatine, Eser *et al.*, 2010; mianserin, Aizenberg *et al.*, 1999) can be considered in stable cases.

The British Association for Psychopharmacology Expert Consensus Guidelines (Baldwin *et al.*, 2005) suggest waiting for 12 weeks before assessing efficacy and upwards dose titration in the face of insufficient clinical response.

Do SSRIs improve health-related quality of life?

Several published, peer-reviewed studies measured the impact of OCD on health-related quality of life (HR-QoL) of which a small number were treatment trials (for a review see Hollander *et al.*, 2010). The relationship between HR-QoL and symptom severity in OCD appears complex. Whilst one study suggested a linear correlation between QoL and YBOCS (Goodman *et al.*, 1989*a*, 1989*b*) others found no correlation, indicating that QoL and symptom changes represent independent variables and emphasizing the importance of their separate evaluation in OCD-treatment trials. Moreover, there is a differential impact of obsessions, compulsions, and comorbid depression on QoL, correlations with QoL being most pronounced for depression severity and the number of OCD symptoms (World Health Organization, 1999). These findings imply that OCD-related HR-QoL may be most meaningfully assessed in patient samples where depression is not strictly excluded. Amongst the several measures used, the 36-Item Short-Form Health Survey (SF-36; Koran *et al.*, 1996) was applied most frequently (Bobes *et al.*, 2001; Eisen *et al.*, 2006; Koran *et al.*, 1996; Moritz *et al.*, 2005; Rodriguez-Salgado *et al.*, 2006).

Hollander *et al.* (2010) analyzed function- and health-related quality of life measures (Sheehan Disability Scale, SDS; and Medical Outcome Study Short Form, SF-36 respectively) in two prospective, randomized, placebo-controlled trials of escitalopram (fixed dose, paroxetine referenced, Stein *et al.*, 2007; relapse prevention, Fineberg *et al.*, 2007*b*). In the study by Stein *et al.*, by week 12 there were statistically significant improvements on the social life and family life subscales of the SDS in all the active treatment groups and by 24 weeks there were statistically significant improvements in all three subscales. The escitalopram 20 mg group showed significant improvements in the work subscale from week 6 onwards. Further, statistically significant improvements in all four of the mental health domains of the SF-36 were seen for escitalopram and paroxetine at 12 weeks and were sustained through to 24 weeks. There was a less pronounced effect on the physical health domains. In the fixed dose study 224 of the 342 receiving active treatment were classified as responders ($\geq$25% improvement in YBOCS from baseline) by the primary end-point (12 weeks). There was a statistically significant and clinically relevant distinction between responders and non-responders based on mean scores for SDS and all domains of SF-36 (with the exception of bodily pain). Responders reported significantly less disability and had significantly higher HR-QoL scores than non-responders. In addition, there were significant correlations between the YBOCS total score and SDS total score as well as the four mental health domains of the SF-36 at the 12-week end-point, implying a direct relationship between OCD symptom-severity, function, and quality of life. These results suggest that SSRI is associated with clinically relevant improvements in health-related quality of life in OCD.

Criteria for treatment response and relapse

Substantial improvement can be achieved in many patients but for approximately 50% the treatment response is incomplete (Table 8.1). The problem of partial response is beset with a lack of universally agreed definition and is an area that has received little controlled investigation. Different trials have used different criteria to define response (Tables 8.1 and 8.5) Pallanti *et al.* (2002*a*) advocated the use of standardized operational criteria across treatment trials, proposing that meaningful clinical response could be represented by an improvement of 25–35% in baseline YBOCS score, or "much" or "very much improved" on the Clinical Global Impression of Improvement Scale (CGI-I; Guy, 1976), while "remission" necessitated a total YBOCS score of <16. Partial response was defined as an improvement in YBOCS between 25% and 35% and relapse as a worsening of 25% (or a CGI-I score of 6), following a period of remission. Levels of non-response were also defined according to the numbers of failed treatments (Pallanti *et al.*, 2002*a*). The term "treatment refractory" was reserved for those who do not respond to "all available treatments." Stein *et al.* (2007) proposed a more stringent remission criterion, needing a YBOCS score of 10 or less. Storch *et al.* (2010*b*) have proposed criteria for treatment response and remission in children with OCD, arguing that a C-YBOCS reduction of 25% constitutes treatment response and a reduction of 45% to 50% constitutes symptom remission, and a C-YBOCS raw score of 14 best reflects remission after treatment. However, the definition of a meaningful clinical response and the concept of "relapse" continue to spark debate and can be difficult to apply to an illness which naturally runs a chronic, fluctuating course and shows partial response to longer-term treatment. Other proposed relapse criteria include a worsening of post-baseline YBOCS of ≥50%, a 5-point worsening of YBOCS, total YBOCS score ≥19, CGI-I scores of "much" or "very much worse" (Fineberg *et al.*, 2007*a*, 2007*b*).

Hollander *et al.* (2010) attempted to validate the otherwise empirical responder and relapse criteria by correlating functional disability and health-related quality of life with YBOCS changes. They found a statistically significant and clinically relevant distinction between responders and non-responders based on mean scores for SDS and SF-36 when response was defined as at least 25% improvement in YBOCS score relative to baseline. This indicates that a 25% improvement in YBOCS is clinically relevant and represents at least a partial response. Likewise, relapse defined as a 5-point worsening of YBOCS correlated with deterioration in HR-QoL and social function; patients who relapsed had statistically significantly worse outcomes on SDS and SF-36 than those who did not.

Other pharmacological treatments

Of theoretical value are preliminary reports hinting at benefits for a variety of agents acting on serotonin, such as mianserin (Visänen *et al.*, 1977) and the serotonin precursor L-tryptophan (Montgomery *et al.*, 1992). Mirtazapine monotherapy was evaluated in a small double-blind, placebo-controlled discontinuation study (Koran *et al.*, 2005). Thirty patients (15 treatment naive and 15 treatment experienced) were enrolled into the 12-week open-label mirtazapine 30–60 mg phase. At 12 weeks, 15 of 16 responders (reduction in YBOCS of >25% from baseline) were randomly allocated to receive either ongoing mirtazapine or placebo. The mean YBOCS score in the mirtazapine group fell by 2.6 and in the placebo group rose by 9.1 indicating mirtazapine's potential in treating OCD. The role of venlafaxine has generated particular interest in OCD. In low doses, it acts mainly as a SSRI, but in doses exceeding 225 mg combines this activity with norepinephrine reuptake inhibition. Yaryura-Tobias & Neziroglu (1996) conducted a small, placebo-controlled trial ($n = 30$) which failed to separate venlafaxine from placebo. Venlafaxine was also compared with paroxetine in a non-placebo, double-blind study of non-depressed OCD cases (Denys et al., 2003). Seventy-five individuals received paroxetine (60 mg) and 75 venlafaxine (300 mg), with both treatments appearing equally effective at reducing YBOCS scores. The study also showed equivalent improvements in an evaluation of quality-of-life measures (Tenney et al., 2003). Venlafaxine compared unfavorably with clomipramine in a smaller single-blind study which failed to reach significance, in which 42.6% (20/47) of the clomipramine group were responders compared with 34.6% (9/26) on venlafaxine in the ITT analysis (Albert et al., 2002). Further investigation into the relative efficacy and tolerability of venlafaxine is warranted before it can be accepted as an effective treatment for OCD.

How long should treatment be continued?

Long-term efficacy studies

Given its usually protracted course, we must ascertain whether treatments maintain anti-obsessional efficacy in the longer term. Treatment responders, on uncontrolled SRI, from acute-phase studies have been followed for up to 2 years, without tolerance developing (Cottraux et al., 1990; Greist et al., 1995a; Katz et al., 1990; Rasmussen et al., 1997; Tollefson et al., 1994; Wagner et al., 1999). However, evidence from controlled studies would be more convincing (see Fineberg & Gale, 2005).

The study by Stein et al. (2007) continued for up to 24 weeks. Patients received either placebo ($n = 113$), paroxetine 40 mg ($n = 116$) or escitalopram 10 mg ($n = 112$) or 20 mg ($n = 114$). The 20 mg escitalopram dose and paroxetine were superior to placebo at the primary, 12-week rating point and by 24 weeks all three active treatments were superior. At 24 weeks, the 20 mg escitalopram dose was more effective than the 10 mg dose when compared with placebo. This study highlights the importance of continuing treatment for a sufficient period of time and shows that whereas both doses of escitalopram can be effective, the 20 mg dose has an earlier onset of action and better long-term efficacy than the 10 mg dose.

Relapse prevention studies

Discontinuation studies that compare outcomes for patients randomized to continuing drug treatment or discontinuation provide important information on the ability of continuation treatment to protect against relapse. However, planning and interpretation of these studies is not always straightforward. The population under test are usually selected to be treatment-responders, and therefore may not be representative of all treatment-receiving patients. Overly rigorous relapse criteria have been imposed with some studies requiring more than two criteria to be present at any one time (Romano et al., 2001), or to persist over several visits (Koran et al., 2002). This stringency has compromised the sensitivity to detect outcome differences. Studies also need to be able to differentiate between gradual re-emergence of OCD and early "discontinuation effects" occurring soon after drug termination, which are related to the pharmacological properties of the compound, and are believed to complicate clomipramine and paroxetine more than fluoxetine (Rosenbaum et al., 1998).

Table 8.3. Double-blind discontinuation studies of relapse prevention in OCD.

Drug	Duration prior drug treatment	Follow-up after discontin-uation (wk)	No. in discontin-uation phase	Study	Outcome
Escitalopram	24 weeks	8	320	Fineberg et al. (2007)[b]	Relapse on placebo > escitalopram
Fluoxetine	20 weeks	52	71	Romano et al. (2001)[b]	Relapse rate on placebo = pooled fluoxetine Relapse rate on placebo > fluoxetine 60 mg
Paroxetine	12 weeks	36	105	Hollander et al. (2003b)[b]	Relapse rate on placebo > paroxetine
Paroxetine	16 weeks	16	193	Geller et al. (2003b)[a]	Relapse rate on placebo = paroxetine
Paroxetine	9 months	36	104	Dunbar et al. (1995)[b]	Relapse rate on placebo > paroxetine
Sertraline	52 weeks	28	223	Koran et al. (2002)[b]	Relapse rate on placebo = sertraline Acute exacerbation of OCD on placebo > sertraline Drop-outs due to relapse on placebo > sertraline

[a] In children and adolescents.
[b] Survival analysis performed.

A series of controlled studies has shown that irrespective of duration of treatment (up to 2 years) discontinuation is usually positively associated with symptomatic relapse (Table 8.3). The relatively high early relapse rates which were seen in the clomipramine studies were possibly related to discontinuation effects (Leonard et al., 1988; Pato et al., 1988). In almost every case, symptoms re-emerged within a few weeks of stopping medication, whereas improvement to a level near to that prior to discontinuation was achieved by reinstatement of clomipramine. In contrast, studies with fluoxetine (Romano et al., 2001) and sertraline (Koran et al., 2002) did not differentiate between continuation of active drug or placebo, though patients remaining on higher (60 mg) fluoxetine doses showed significantly lower relapse rates than placebo. Moreover, continued improvement in YBOCS, NIMH-OC, CGI-I scores and quality-of-life measures was associated with ongoing sertraline as opposed to discontinuation.

Clearer advantages for staying on active treatment were shown in paroxetine discontinuation studies in adults (Dunbar et al., 1995; Hollander et al., 2003b) and children and adolescents (Geller et al., 2003b). The authors found that patients with comorbidity are at increased risk of relapse following discontinuation and studies that too rigorously exclude comorbid disorders may underestimate relapse rates in clinical samples of OCD (Geller et al., 2003b). Fineberg et al. (2007b) assessed the efficacy and tolerability of escitalopram in the prevention of relapse in patients with non-comorbid OCD. Patients were first treated with open-label escitalopram (10 mg or 20 mg). Of the 468 entrants 320 were classified as responders (YBOCS total score decrease $\geq$ 25%) and were entered into the relapse prevention phase (24 weeks). Patients were randomized to escitalopram at the assigned dose or to placebo.

Escitalopram was well tolerated and group improvements in symptoms were sustained throughout the extension phase. Relapse was defined as a worsening from baseline of ≥ 5 YBOCS points. Patients randomized to placebo relapsed more quickly than those remaining on escitalopram. Moreover, 52% of the placebo group compared with 23% of the escitalopram group relapsed overall; this difference was statistically significant. Relapse also correlated with deterioration in function; patients who relapsed had statistically significantly worse outcomes that those who did not on SDS and SF-36 (Hollander et al., 2010). These results illustrate the damaging effect of symptomatic relapse associated with treatment discontinuation on quality of life.

In summary, the relapse prevention studies have produced mixed results. At least some of the negative studies appear to reflect design flaws. Indeed, a meta-analysis detected overall superiority of SSRIs to placebo in preventing relapse amongst adult treatment-responders (Fineberg et al., 2007a). Worsening by five YBOCS points holds credibility as a threshold for relapse. Viewed collectively, these results suggest that medication, as long as it is continued, probably confers protection against relapse, SSRIs are effective long-term treatments, and relapse–prevention represents a rational treatment target for OCD. Recent guidelines (Greist et al., 2003) recommend continuation of pharmacotherapy for a minimum of 1–2 years in treatment-responsive individuals and emphasize the importance of long-term treatment from the outset. Prior to discontinuation, patients should be warned to look out for the early signs of relapse so that pharmacotherapy can be reinstated; hopefully achieving the same level of improvement though this cannot be guaranteed (Ravizza et al., 1998). Discontinuation should be gradual to minimize discontinuation effects. In many cases life-long medication may be the best option until clear predictors of relapse are available.

What is the best dose for long-term treatment?

Other than results from one small study by Mundo et al. (1997b) there is little evidence to support dose reduction as a strategy in the long-term management of OCD. In this study, 30 patients successfully treated with either clomipramine or fluvoxamine were randomly assigned to receive either no reduction in dose, 33–40% reduction in dose or 60–66% reduction in dose. The criterion for withdrawal from the study was arbitrarily set as >5% worsening from base line in YBOCS score on two successive measurements and deterioration in CGI. Differences in the proportion of patients withdrawing from the study were not statistically significant; possibly due to the withdrawal criterion being too sensitive. In contrast, the study by Romano et al. (2001), in which a 60 mg dose of fluoxetine appeared the most effective over the 24-week placebo-controlled extension phase, supports the continuation of treatment at higher dose levels. On the basis of the limited data available, most experts recommend resisting the urge to reduce the dose level and continuing treatment at the effective dose for optimal relapse prevention.

Predictors of treatment response

OCD is a heterogeneous condition and roughly half of patients fail to make a good response to SSRI treatment (Table 8.1). The literature on pharmacological response predictors is sparse and inconsistent. One small study identified better responses in females (Mundo et al., 1999). A factor analysis by Mataix-Cols et al. (1999) suggested poor response to clomipramine and SSRIs in adults with compulsive rituals, young onset, longer duration, chronic course, comorbid tics and personality disorders; a better response for SRI-naïve and poorer response for patients with subclinical depression was reported in analyses of large databases for clomipramine and fluoxetine. Earlier age of onset predicted poor response to clomipramine but not to fluoxetine (Ackerman & Greenland, 2002). Analysis of data from a large trial of citalopram reported a poorer response to active drug in patients with a longer duration of illness, previous SSRI treatment or greater illness severity (Stein *et al.*, 2001). A 9-year follow-up study of 142 children and adolescents with OCD (Micali *et al.*, 2010) also found that the main predictor for persistent OCD was the duration of illness at assessment. Garcia *et al.* (2010) reported that youth with lesser symptom severity and OCD-related functional impairment, greater insight, fewer comorbid externalizing symptoms, and poorer family accommodation showed greater improvement across treatment conditions than their counterparts after acute POTS treatment (March, 2004). In the studies by Geller *et al.* (2003*b*) and Storch *et al.* (2008*b*), children with comorbid illnesses such as ADHD, tic disorder and oppositional defiant disorder showed a less favorable response.

In a small follow-up study by Bloch *et al.* (2009) female gender, earlier age at childhood assessment, later age of OCD onset, more-severe childhood OCD symptoms, and comorbid oppositional defiant disorder were associated with persistence of OCD symptoms into adulthood.

A long-term follow-up study of treatment non-responders (Reddy *et al.*, 2010) also reported that poor outcome was predicted by later age of onset, as well as poorer quality of life at onset, shorter duration of follow-up and not receiving CBT during the interval period.

The identification of symptom "dimensions" attempts to produce more homogeneous OCD subgroups that might aid prediction of treatment response and outcome. Stein *et al.* (2008) analyzed data on 466 patients from a randomized, double-blind, placebo-controlled trial of escitalopram. Five factors (contamination/cleaning, harm/checking, hoarding/symmetry, religious/sexual, and somatic/hypochondriacal) were identified in an exploratory factor analysis of individual YBOCS items. The hoarding/symmetry dimension was associated with a poorer response to escitalopram. In the study by Bloch *et al.* (2009) the presence of prominent hoarding symptoms was associated with the persistence of OCD symptoms. Landeros-Weisenberger *et al.* (2010) found that 60% of OCD patients with predominant symptoms in the harm/checking dimension were much or very much improved in response to SRI treatment, particularly if treated with fluoxetine and fluvoxamine. Too few patients reported symptoms of hoarding for reliable conclusions to be drawn. The ordering/symmetry dimension was associated with poor response to SRI and with comorbid tic disorder which may itself be associated with poor response to treatment (Leckman *et al.*, 1994) (though not according to Bloch *et al.*, 2009).

In summary, we do not have reliable response predictors derived from demographic or clinical factors, though there is a growing consensus that the hoarding dimension may predict a poorer response to SSRI. Research into potential OCD biomarkers, such as genes or neurocognitive changes, may provide new scope for optimizing treatment strategies for individual patients on a more personalized basis.

Preferred options if poor response to first-line treatment

Switch the SSRI

The American Psychiatric Association Practice Guideline (Koran *et al.*, 2007) recommends a variety of approaches for partial, little, or no response to initial SSRI therapy. Switching from one SSRI to another remains the preferred option for most clinicians given its acceptability and the limited data supporting alternative strategies. However, it may sometimes be appropriate to persist for longer with a given SSRI even in patients who show little sign of improvement, since delayed response may occur after 6 months or more. This is illustrated in the study by Miguel *et al.* (2009) in which patients who did not respond to at least 8 weeks of fluoxetine were randomized to remain on 12 weeks fluoxetine 80 mg ($n = 18$) and outperformed those randomized to receive other forms of treatment such as adjunctive clomipramine ($n = 18$) or adjunctive quetiapine ($n = 18$). March *et al.* (1997) recommended changing SSRI if the clinical effect was incomplete after 8–12 weeks on the maximum dose. They estimated the chance of responding to a second SSRI at 40%, and to a third at even less, and proposed switching to clomipramine after two to three failed trials on SSRI. Denys *et al.* (2003) demonstrated no significant difference between venlafaxine 300 mg compared with paroxetine 60 mg and a response rate of 40% in both groups. Further study revealed a less favorable response in treatment-resistant cases switched from paroxetine to venlafaxine than vice versa, generating less certainty for the efficacy of venlafaxine in OCD. Patients who failed to respond to at least two trials of SSRI (excluding citalopram) were examined in an unpublished report by Ravizza *et al.* (2001). They were randomized to 12-weeks treatment with clomipramine, venlafaxine, or citalopram; 37.5% responded to clomipramine, 42% to venlafaxine and 14% to citalopram. These results hint that switching to an agent with a different mode of action may benefit patients who have failed to respond to at least two SSRIs. Practice guidelines produced by the American Psychiatric Association (Koran *et al.*, 2007) recommend continuing with SSRI for 8 to 12 weeks, of which 6 should be at maximum tolerated dose, before augmentation or switching is considered.

Increase the SSRI dose

Results from uncontrolled case studies suggest that increasing SSRI doses beyond formulary limits can produce better effects in some patients (Bejerot & Bodlund, 1998; Byerly *et al.*, 1996). Ninan *et al.* (2006) evaluated the efficacy and safety of high-dose (400 mg) sertraline in patients with OCD who had failed to respond to 16-weeks treatment with standard dose (200 mg) sertraline. Patients ($n = 66$) were randomized to increase the dose of sertraline (to 250–400 mg) or to continue at 200 mg for a further 12 weeks. Efficacy measures including YBOCS and CGI-I scales showed significantly greater improvements in the 400 mg (mean 357 mg) sertraline group compared with the 200 mg group. However, possibly as a result of a type II error, responder rates were not significantly different between the groups on completer (52% *vs.* 34%) or end-point (40% *vs.* 33%) analyses. There were similar adverse event rates in each group indicating that high-dose sertraline is well tolerated. Pampaloni *et al.* (2009) assessed long-term high-dose SSRI prescribing in a specialist OCD outpatient service by conducting a systematic, retrospective case-note survey. Of 192 cases identified, 26 received high doses of SSRI (above the UK SPC recommendations or SPC maximum daily dose of one SSRI plus another SSRI or clomipramine). All fulfilled criteria for treatment-resistance and the average duration of treatment in the high-dose group was 1.5 years. Control patients taking normal doses of SSRI were selected from the same population and matched for duration of treatment. There was no statistically significant difference in the frequency of adverse events between the two groups though 50% of the high-dose group reported clinically relevant side-effects. The high-dose group appeared to constitute a more treatment-refractory cohort and made comparatively less improvement than the controls.

Table 8.4. Dosing of SRIs in OCD (adapted from Koran et al., 2007).

Drug	Citalopram	Clomipramine	Escitalopram	Fluoxetine	Fluvoxamine	Paroxetine	Sertraline[c]
Initial dose (mg/day)[a]							
Child (under 18)	10	–	–	10	25	–	25
Adult (18–65)	20	10	10	20	50	20	50
Over 65	20	10	5	20	50	20	50
Maintenance dose (mg/day)							
Child (under 18)	10–20	–	–	10–20	25–200	–	25–200
Adult (18–65)	40–60[e]	30–150	10–20	40–60	100–300	40–60	200
Over 65	20–40	30–75	5–10	20–60	100–300	20–40	200
British National Formulary maximum dose (mg/day)[b]							
Child (under 18)	60[e]	–	–	20	200	–	200
Adult (18–65)	60[e]	250	20	60	300	60	200
Over 65 years	40	–	20	60	300	40	200
Occasional maximum dose[b]	120[e]	–[d]	60[e]	120	450	100	400

[a] Lower doses may be required to avoid side-effects.
[b] Used for rapid metabolizers, patients with no or mild side effects or inadequate clinical response following treatment at the usual maximum dose.
[c] Better absorbed with food.
[d] Combined plasma level of clomipramine and desmethylclomipramine 12 hours after the dose should be kept below 500 ng/mL to minimize the risk of seizures and cardiac conduction delay.
[e] See new MHRA guidance, page 136.

The American Psychiatric Association Practice Guideline on the treatment of patients with OCD (Koran *et al.*, 2007) contains a table of recommended starting, usual, maximum, and occasionally prescribed doses of SSRIs (Table 8.4). Though doses of clomipramine up to 300 mg have been systematically investigated and found to be acceptable, doses exceeding this should be generally avoided due to the associated risks of seizures and cardiotoxicity and the maximum recommended dose is 250 mg.

Altering mode of delivery

Altering the mode of administration is impractical in many cases. Fallon *et al.* (1998) demonstrated that intravenous clomipramine is more effective than placebo in a double-blind study investigating refractory OCD. Six of the 29 patients randomized to clomipramine were classed as responders following 14 daily infusions, compared with none in the placebo group. The authors hypothesized that the greater bioavailability of the more scrotonergic parent compound clomipramine compared with the more noradrenergic metabolite desmethyl-clomipramine, as a consequence of the IV preparation bypassing the first-pass hepatoenteric metabolism, accounts for its greater efficacy. Pallanti *et al.* (2002*b*) reported a positive open study of 21 daily intravenous citalopram infusions.

Combining SSRIs and drugs exerting antidepressant or anxiolytic properties

Based mainly on the results of small studies and open-case series, the evidence supporting adjunctive antidepressant or anxiolytic drugs is rather limited. For children or adults unresponsive to monotherapy with an SSRI, the combination of clomipramine with SSRI has been proposed. This strategy should be approached cautiously, with ECG and plasma-level monitoring being advisable, given the pharmacokinetic interactions on the hepatic cytochrome P450 isoenzymes that could lead to a dangerous build up of clomipramine. Citalopram/escitalopram and to a lesser extent sertraline may be less likely to interact with clomipramine than other SSRIs. Small, uncontrolled case series have shown positive results (Szegedi *et al.*, 1996), though ECG changes were reported in some cases of the fluoxetine-clomipramine combination. In a randomized open-label trial by Pallanti *et al.* (1999), nine treatment-refractory patients were given citalopram with clomipramine and seven were treated with citalopram alone. Significantly larger improvements in YBOCS ratings were reported for those given the combination, all of whom experienced decreases ≥35% from baseline. This combination was well tolerated and did not alter the metabolism of clomipramine. However in a study by Diniz *et al.* (2010), combining fluoxetine with clomipramine was less effective that ongoing fluoxetine. No controlled studies of the co-administration of different SSRIs have been published.

Pallanti *et al.* (2004) conducted a randomized, controlled, single-blind trial of mirtazapine augmentation of citalopram in OCD. Forty-nine OCD patients without comorbid depression were allocated to receive citalopram (40–80 mg/day) plus placebo, or citalopram plus mirtazapine (15–30 mg/day). At 4 weeks there was a statistically significant difference between the two groups. However at 12 weeks there was no significant difference between the two groups indicating that any benefit of augmenting with mirtazapine may be short-lived.

Lithium augmentation has been demonstrated in controlled studies to be ineffective in the management of OCD (McDougle *et al.*, 1991; Pigott *et al.*, 1991). Buspirone has also been shown to provide no additional benefit in three double-blind, placebo-controlled studies (Grady *et al.*, 1993; McDougle *et al.*, 1993; Pigott *et al.*, 1992*a*). Clonazepam is a benzodiazepine with putative effects on serotonin neurotransmission; while it may help with associated anxiety, as monotherapy it has little impact on the core symptoms of OCD (Hollander *et al.*, 2003c). However, in a placebo-controlled study, Pigott *et al.* (1992b) reported some benefit for clonazepam administered with fluoxetine or clomipramine. In addition, Hewlett *et al.* (1992) reported that 40% of 28 subjects failing to respond to clomipramine had clinically significant response to clonazepam in a trial comparing clomipramine, clonazepam, and clonidine to diphenhydramine. Pindolol is a beta-blocker which also acts as an antagonist at pre-synaptic $5-HT_{1A}$ auto-receptors. In a double-blind, placebo-controlled study of 14 treatment-resistant cases, Dannon *et al.* (2000) demonstrated efficacy for pindolol when combined with paroxetine, however another study combining pindolol with fluvoxamine did not (Mundo *et al.*, 1998). A beneficial effect for pindolol when L-tryptophan was openly added to the combination was found by Blier & Bergeron (1996). Investigators have re-examined the role of noradrenergic agents in resistant OCD in light of the limitations of adding drugs acting on serotonin. Barr *et al.* (1997), in a double-blind, placebo-controlled study, investigated the addition of desipramine to 20 patients who had failed SSRI monotherapy and found no added benefit.

Combining SSRIs with drugs with antipsychotic properties

First-generation antipsychotics

No positive studies of antipsychotic monotherapy in OCD meet today's standards, and OCD is not recognized as responding to these drugs on their own. McDougle *et al.* (1995) reported a trial of clozapine monotherapy in subjects that were arguably too refractory. Twelve treatment-refractory OCD subjects, who had not improved following treatment with clomipramine, fluoxetine or combination clomipramine, fluoxetine, or fluvoxamine with a typical neuroleptic such as haloperidol and a trial of behavior therapy, were selected. Open-label clozapine was titrated to a maximum of 600 mg, over 6 weeks. There was no significant change from baseline measures in any of the 10 patients who completed the study.

McDougle *et al.* (1990) reported benefit from adding open-label pimozide (6.5 mg) in 17 patients unresponsive to fluvoxamine. Patients with comorbid chronic tics or schizotypal disorder were the most responsive. A subsequent double-blind, placebo-controlled study by the same author demonstrated a significant improvement with haloperidol (mean dose 6.2 mg) added to fluvoxamine. Eleven out of 17 patients receiving the active drug achieved "responder" status by as early as 4 weeks, compared with none on placebo. Again, a preferential response was seen in patients with comorbid tics (McDougle *et al.*, 1994). Antipsychotics such as haloperidol and sulpiride are first-line treatments for Tourette's syndrome, so this finding supports a theoretical link between these disorders. However, this combination notably increases the side-effect burden, including extra-pyramidal effects. It is therefore wise to start treatment with very low doses, and increase cautiously subject to tolerability (e.g. 0.25–0.5 mg haloperidol, titrated slowly to 2–4 mg; McDougle & Walsh, 2001).

Second-generation antipsychotics (Table 8.5)

Adjunctive risperidone

Newer second-generation antipsychotics that modulate serotonin and dopamine neurotransmission, also offer promise and constitute a lower risk for adverse effects. Positive reports

Table 8.5. Adjunctive second-generation antipsychotics.

Drug	Study	n	Dose (mg/day) [mean dose]	Definition of clinical response		
				Response criteria	Response rate on active drug	Placebo response rate
Risperidone	McDougle et al. (2000)	36	1 titratec to 6 as tolerated [2.2]	Marked = 3 of a, c, e; Partial = 2 of a, c, e	4/18 (22%); 5/18 (28%)	0/15 (0%)
Risperidone	Hollander et al. (2003d)	16	0.5–3.0	b, d	4/10 (40%)	0/6 (0%)
Risperidone	Li et al. (2005)	16	1	not defined	not reported	not reported
Olanzapine	Bystritsky et al. (2004)	26	up to 20 [11.2]	b	6/13 (46%)	0/13 (0%)
Olanzapine	Shapira et al. (2004)	44	5–10 [6.1]	not defined	5/22 (23%)[a]; 9/22 (41%)[b]	4/22 (18%)[a]; 9/22 (41%)[b]
Quetiapine	Denys et al. (2004)	40	300	a, d	8/20 (40%)	2/20 (10%)
Quetiapine	Carey et al. (2005)	41	300	b, d	8/20 (40%)	10/21 (47%)
Quetiapine	Fineberg et al. (2005)	21	400 [215]	b	3/11 (27%)	1/10 (10%)
Quetiapine	Kordon et al. (2008)	40	400–600	a	5/20 (33%)	3/20 (15%)
Aripiprazole	Muscatello et al. (2011)[f]	40	15	a, b	4/16 (25%)[a]; 11/16 (68.7%)[b]	0/14 (0%)

[a] ≥35% improvement in Y-BOCS.
[b] ≥25% improvement in Y-BOCS.
[c] Final Y-BOCS score <16.
[d] CGI of "much improved" or "very much improved."
[e] Consensus opinion of investigators.
[f] Completer analysis.

from case-series were confirmed by McDougle *et al.* (2000) in the first double-blind, placebo-controlled study showing efficacy for risperidone augmentation in 36 patients unresponsive to 12 weeks SSRI. Risperidone (2.2 mg) was superior to placebo in reducing YBOCS scores as well as anxiety and depression, was well tolerated and there was no difference between those with and without comorbid tics or schizotypy. A smaller double-blind study by Hollander *et al.* (2003*d*) examined patients failing to respond to at least two trials of SSRI. Four out of 16 patients randomized to risperidone (0.5–3 mg) were responders at the 8-week end-point, compared with none of the six patients randomized to placebo. In an 8-week, double-blind, placebo-controlled study, Li *et al.* (2005) compared the benefits of 2-weeks adjunctive risperidone (1 mg), haloperidol (2 mg), and placebo in 16 SSRI-resistant OCD patients. Risperidone and haloperidol were both significantly superior to placebo in reducing obsessions and anxiety. In addition, risperidone but not haloperidol improved depressed mood.

Adjunctive olanzapine

Encouraging results from a small number of open-label studies of adjunctive olanzapine (D'Amico *et al.*, 2003, Marazziti *et al.*, 2005) suggested that this drug may also be helpful. Bystritsky *et al.* (2004) conducted a 6-week, double-blind, placebo-controlled study of adjunctive olanzapine in 26 OCD patients who had failed to respond to SSRI monotherapy. The olanzapine group (mean dose 11.2 mg) showed a mean improvement in YBOCS of 4.2 points, compared with a mean increase of 0.54 points in the placebo group. Six of the 13 patients in the olanzapine group met response criteria compared with none in the placebo group. Olanzapine was well tolerated with only two patients dropping out because of side-effects. Shapira *et al.* (2004) conducted a similar study in 44 patients with OCD who had failed to respond to 8-weeks open-label fluoxetine (mainly 40 mg). It is possible that these subjects were not truly resistant since both groups showed significant improvement from baseline with no significant difference between them.

Adjunctive quetiapine

In addition to published case reports and open-label studies, there have been four randomized, double-blind, placebo-controlled trials of quetiapine therapy in OCD and one meta-analysis.

In a double-blind, randomized, parallel-group, flexible-dose, placebo-controlled study in subjects who had responded inadequately to 12-weeks open-label SSRI, adjunctive quetiapine failed to show superiority to placebo after 6 weeks (Carey *et al.*, 2005). Eight (40%) of the quetiapine group and 10 (47.6%) of the placebo group were classed as responders. Once again, the high placebo response rate seen in this study may reflect the fact that patients were not truly SSRI-resistant at the point of study entry. However, the double-blind, placebo-controlled study by Denys *et al.* (2004), showed clear evidence of efficacy for 8-weeks quetiapine (<300 mg) augmentation in 20 SSRI-refractory patients, producing a mean decrease of 31% on baseline YBOCS, compared with 20 patients on adjunctive placebo who showed only 6% improvement. Fineberg *et al.* (2006*a*) enrolled 21 patients who had failed to respond to SSRI monotherapy over the preceding 6 months. Eleven were randomized to adjunctive quetiapine treatment and ten to placebo. Quetiapine (mean 215 mg) produced a mean reduction in YBOCS scores of 3.4 points (14%) compared with 1.4 (6%) for placebo and three of the quetiapine-treated subjects achieved a response compared with one on placebo. These differences did not reach statistical significance. Neither was there any significant difference in adverse event reporting. Kordon *et al.* (2008) conducted a 12 week, double-blind, randomized, placebo-controlled study of adjunctive quetiapine in 40 patients with severe OCD who had not responded to treatment with 12-weeks SSRI. Between weeks 6 and 12, the dose of quetiapine was titrated to between 400 mg and 600 mg. The reduction in mean YBOCS from baseline was not significantly different between the groups (5.2 for quetiapine and 3.9 for placebo). The latter two studies may have been compromised by small size.

In a meta-analysis (Fineberg *et al.*, 2006a) the authors analyzed data from three qualifying double-blind, randomized, placebo-controlled quetiapine trials. Results were limited by between-study heterogeneity but showed evidence of efficacy for quetiapine (<400 mg/day) on the primary efficacy criterion (changes from baseline in total YBOCS). Denys *et al.* (2007) assessed the impact of type and dose of SSRI when augmenting with quetiapine. Pooled data from all available double-blind, placebo-controlled quetiapine addition studies were analyzed. Quetiapine was found to be superior to placebo on mean reduction in YBOCS (6.8 *vs.* 3.9) and the benefit of quetiapine was seen mainly in patients taking the lowest SSRI doses when compared with those on the median and highest doses. This may suggest that both SSRI and antipsychotic share the same mechanism for their clinical effect. The best responses for quetiapine were achieved in combination with clomipramine, fluoxetine, and fluvoxamine.

Another double-blind, randomized placebo-controlled study has investigated the efficacy of quetiapine (300–450 mg/day) in combination with citalopram (60 mg/day) in 76 OCD patients who were treatment naïve or medication-free (Vulink *et al.*, 2009). Thirty-one received quetiapine and 35 placebo. When compared with placebo, quetiapine showed a significantly greater reduction on the YBOCS (11.9 *vs.* 7.8) and CGI-I (2.1 *vs.* 1.4) scales. However, more of the quetiapine-treated patients withdrew due to adverse effects. If replicated, this result would suggest that adjunctive quetiapine may be a more efficacious first-line treatment than SSRI monotherapy.

Adjunctive aripiprazole

In a small, open-label 12-week study, Pessina *et al.* (2009) showed a significant improvement from baseline in 12 SSRI-resistant OCD patients co-administered flexible doses of aripiprazole (up to 20 mg). More recently, Muscatello *et al.* (2011) reported a highly significant advantage for adjunctive aripiprazole (15 mg) in a 16-week, randomized, double-blind, placebo-controlled study involving 40 patients with treatment-resistant OCD (YBOCS total score; $p < 0.001$). Patients randomized to aripiprazole showed a mean reduction from baseline YBOCS of nearly 7 points, whereas the placebo group barely changed. Of the 16 aripiprazole completers, 11 met response criteria of 25%, seven met criteria between 25 and 34% and four >35% reduction from baseline.

Which antipsychotic?

In summary, despite the number of studies of small size, there is at least one positive randomized controlled trial of adjunctive haloperidol, risperidone, olanzapine, and quetiapine in resistant OCD. Skapinakis *et al.* (2007) conducted a meta-analysis of antipsychotic augmentation of SSRI therapy in OCD, concluding that patients randomized to take part in the antipsychotic arm of trials were more likely (up to three times) to respond than those randomized to receive placebo. Taken together, there is now convincing evidence supporting the efficacy of antipsychotic agents as adjunctive treatments in OCD. However, there are insufficient data upon which to determine the most effective choice of agent. The small study by Li *et al.* (2005) suggested a stronger antidepressant effect for risperidone compared with haloperidol, which may be relevant in treatment-resistant cases for whom depression is common. An 8-week, single-blind, randomized trial (Maina *et al.*, 2008) compared adjunctive risperidone (1–3 mg) with olanzapine (2.5–10 mg) in 50 treatment-resistant OCD patients. Other than reports of adverse effects, the two groups did not significantly differ in outcome and both responded significantly to augmentation, with 44% (11/25) of the risperidone group and 48% (12/25) in the olanzapine group achieving responder status. Risperidone was associated with amenorrhea and olanzapine with weight gain. In a small, retrospective comparator study (Savas *et al.*, 2008) adjunctive quetiapine was evaluated against ziprasidone. Clinical improvement was seen in 80% of the quetiapine group ($n = 15$) and 44% of the ziprasidone group ($n = 9$) suggesting superiority of quetiapine to ziprasidone. In a recent randomized, open-label trial (Diniz *et al.*, 2010), the effectiveness of adjunctive quetiapine (up to 200 mg) was compared with that of adjunctive clomipramine (up to 75 mg) in 21 patients who failed to respond to 12 weeks of SSRI. Though the difference between the mean initial and final YBOCS in the quetiapine group was significant (22 *vs.* 18) it was not significantly different from the clomipramine group (21.9 *vs.* 21.5). However, four (36%) patients in the quetiapine group showed a clinical response, compared with just one (10%) in the clomipramine group, suggesting possible superiority for adjunctive quetiapine.

Long-term adjunctive antipsychotics

We do not have controlled studies to allow an evaluation of the long-term effectiveness of adjunctive antipsychotics in OCD. In a naturalistic study, Marazziti *et al.* (2005) assessed the long-term efficacy of adjunctive olanzapine (2.5–10 mg) in 26 patients with treatment-resistant OCD. At one year, 17 patients (68%) showed a reduction in YBOCS of at least 35%. In another long-term trial of antipsychotic augmentation, Matsunaga *et al.* (2009) randomly allocated 44 patients who had failed to respond to 12 weeks SSRI monotherapy to treatment with adjunctive olanzapine, quetiapine, or risperidone plus CBT for 1 year. Patients who had initially responded to SSRI monotherapy ($n = 46$) continued on SSRI and CBT for 1 year. Compared with the non-responder group, the responder group had lower YBOCS scores both at the start and the end of the study (25.8–13.7 *vs.* 29.3–19.3). The authors concluded that this does not support the long-term effectiveness of augmentation of SSRIs with atypical antipsychotics in OCD. However, the uncontrolled nature of the study renders these results open to question and evaluation under randomized, double-blind conditions is warranted.

Some authors report emergent obsessions during treatment of schizophrenia with second-generation antipsychotics (Kim *et al.*, 2009) and this may be particularly evident for clozapine (Sa *et al.*, 2009), though there have also been reports of obsessive symptoms in patients with schizophrenia improving with clozapine treatment (Kumar *et al.*, 2003) or with the addition of aripiprazole (Englisch *et al.*, 2009). These effects may be related to the mixed receptor profile of the drugs, combined with the neurological changes associated with schizophrenia, and are hard to reconcile with the evidence of efficacy for the same drugs when used to treat OCD. New evidence is emerging from association and pharmacogenetic studies that variants of the glutamate transporter gene, SLC1A1, are associated with transmission of OCD traits, particularly in males (Arnold *et al.*, 2006), and that these variants may be associated with susceptibility to the emergence of atypical antipsychotic-induced OCD (Kwon *et al.*, 2009).

Altogether, these results favor the use of adjunctive risperidone, quetiapine, olanzapine, and haloperidol and to a lesser extent aripiprazole as an important strategy for resistant OCD. In view of the long-term adverse effects associated with these drugs, despite their evident efficacy, it remains controversial as to whether they should be used in preference to dose increase or augmenting with another agent such as clomipramine. Head-to-head studies comparing the relative efficacy and tolerability of these interventions, over the long-term, as well as relapse prevention trials are badly needed in this area. For example, it remains uncertain as to how long patients need to remain on augmented treatment. A small retrospective study by Maina et al. (2003b) showed that the majority of patients (15 of 18; 83.3%), who had responded to the addition of an antipsychotic to their SSRI, subsequently relapsed when the antipsychotic was withdrawn.

Combining SSRIs with other agents

Augmentation with the 5-HT$_3$ receptor antagonist ondansetron has been explored in an open-label study by Pallanti et al. (2009), showing a clinical response and good tolerability in treatment-resistant patients. In addition, in an 8-week double-blind, placebo-controlled pilot study ($n = 42$; Soltani et al., 2010) patients were randomized to receive either fluoxetine (20 mg/day) and ondansetron (4 mg/day) or fluoxetine (20 mg/day) and placebo. Mean YBOCS score reduced in both groups and by week 8 the mean YBOCS score in the ondansetron group was significantly lower (5 vs. 15; baseline in both groups was 35) suggesting possible efficacy in OCD.

Preliminary findings of Pasquini & Biondi (2006), reporting an immediate beneficial effect of augmentation with the glutamatergic compound memantine, in one of two cases, led to the exploration of adjunctive memantine in a number of small uncontrolled studies that have shown promising results. In a 12-week open-label trial (Aboujaoude et al., 2009), adjunctive memantine (5–20 mg) was given to 15 patients who had failed to respond adequately to 12 weeks SSRI. Almost half the subjects had a meaningful improvement in symptoms. Memantine was well tolerated and no patient left the study early because of an adverse event. In the study by Feusner et al. (2009) 10 OCD and seven GAD subjects received 12 weeks of open-label memantine 10 mg twice daily, as either monotherapy or augmentation of their existing medication. The results suggested that memantine may have preferential efficacy in the treatment of OCD vs. GAD. The OCD group experienced a significant mean 40.6% reduction in YBOCS scores at end-point. Three of 10 of OCD subjects were classified as responders, whereas none of the GAD subjects were responders. Again, memantine was well tolerated and there were no serious adverse effects. Stewart et al. (2010) conducted a further single-blind case-control study of memantine in inpatients with severe OCD. Twenty-two subjects receiving memantine in addition to standard care were matched with 22 OCD inpatient controls. The mean reduction in the YBOCS was 7.2 (27%) for memantine and 4.6 (16.5%) for standard care providing further evidence for the possible efficacy of memantine in OCD.

Riluzole, another glutamate-modulating agent, was used as an adjunctive agent in a small ($n = 13$) open-label trial (Coric et al., 2005). It was associated with an improvement of OCD symptoms in seven patients and five of them were classified as "recovered." These results are supported by two further small open-label studies of riluzole in children with OCD which reported improvement on the C-YBOCS without major adverse effects

(Grant *et al.*, 2007; Pittenger *et al.*, 2008*a*, 2008*b*). These findings were supported by preliminary results of an ongoing trial (Grant *et al.*, 2010), despite the occurrence of two cases of pancreatitis.

D-cycloserine is a partial agonist of the N-methyl-D-aspartate (NMDA) receptor and has been used as an augmentation agent to enhance exposure therapy outcome in pediatric OCD in a randomized, double-blind, placebo-controlled augmentation trial (Storch *et al.*, 2010*a*). Though not statistically significant, the active treatment arm showed small-to-moderate treatment effects. There have been mixed results with d-cycloserine augmentation of exposure and response prevention (ERP) therapy in adults. Three small studies (Storch *et al.*, 2008*a*; Kushner *et al.*, 2007; Wilhelm *et al.* 2008) each used different doses (100 mg, 125 mg, and 250 mg) and different timings (1 hour, 2 hours, and 4 hours before ERP). Only the study by Wilhelm *et al.* (2008) yielded positive results, though these were at the mid- rather than the end-point of the study. Overall the results are not convincing.

Treatment with glycine, another NMDA receptor modulator, over a 5-year period in a patient with OCD and body dysmorphic disorder (BDD) led to robust reduction of BDD and OCD symptoms apart from partial relapses during treatment cessation (Cleveland *et al.*, 2009). In a 12-week randomized, double-blind, placebo-controlled trial of adjunctive glycine (up to 60 mg; Greenberg *et al.*, 2009) patients completing glycine treatment ($n = 5$) experienced a statistically insignificant mean reduction in YBOCS of 6 points compared with 1 point in the placebo group ($n = 9$). Two patients taking glycine were classed as responders, however, the compound was poorly tolerated and 10 dropped out mainly because of its aversive taste or nausea.

Antiepileptics such as topiramate have been explored as augmenting agents; in a retrospective, open-label case series in 16 patients who were non-responsive or partially responsive to SSRI or to a combination of SSRI and antipsychotics, 11 patients prescribed adjunctive topiramate (up to 400 mg/day; mean dose 253 mg) were found to be much improved or very much improved in their CGI-I scores (Van Ameringen *et al.*, 2006). However, a small, 12-week, double-blind, placebo-controlled, parallel-group trial, in which topiramate was poorly tolerated, produced negative results, suggesting that at best SSRI augmentation with topiramate may be beneficial for compulsions, but not obsessions (Berlin *et al.*, 2010).A single case report suggests a possible role for adjunctive lamotrigine titrated up to 150 mg/day (Uzun, 2010).

Initially positive results for inositol (an experimental compound acting through intracellular messenger systems) were subsequently not confirmed (Fux *et al.*, 1999). Sumatriptan (a 5-HT$_{1D}$ agonist used in the treatment of migraine) was found to make OCD symptoms worse (Koran *et al.*, 2001). An interesting case report in which 4 mg of nicotine added to clomipramine and valproate produced a clinical response may merit further attention (Pasquini *et al.*, 2005).

Adjunctive behavior therapy

CBT that includes ERP, given in combination with an SSRI, is often considered superior to either treatment given alone; however, there have been few controlled studies addressing this and better studies are required. One difficulty of assessing CBT in such trials is the frequent absence of placebo CBT. Cottraux *et al.* (1990) demonstrated that fluvoxamine enhances the efficacy of exposure therapy. Hohagen *et al.* (1998) showed that there was a significantly higher response rate (87.5% *vs.* 60%) and greater reduction in obsessions (13.8 to 6.1 *vs.* 13.3 to 8.3) and total YBOCS scores (27.9 to 12.4 *vs.* 28.4 to 15.9) in patients treated with fluvoxamine and multi-modal CBT ($n = 30$) when compared with those treated with placebo and CBT ($n = 30$). In a controlled trial that randomized relatively SSRI-resistant patients to continued SRI therapy plus either 17 sessions of ERP ($n = 54$) or stress management ($n = 54$), 94 of the 108 entrants completed the course of therapy with no significant group difference in dropouts (Simpson *et al.*, 2008). Significantly more patients receiving ERP showed a clinical response and the mean reduction in YBOCS was 44% in the BT group and 14% in the placebo group. Taken together, the evidence suggests that augmenting behavioral forms of psychotherapy with SSRI is likely to be an effective first-line strategy, and conversely that augmenting SSRI pharmacotherapy with ERP is effective in reducing OCD symptoms in partial or non-responders to SSRI monotherapy.

Conclusions

The pharmacological evidence base for the treatment of OCD is developing apace. Treatment with SSRIs and clomipramine remains uncontroversial and improvements are sustained over time. SSRIs are usually preferred over clomipramine, in view of their improved tolerability, and relapse-prevention, achieved through sustained treatment, is now a realistic goal for the majority of SSRI-responders. Moreover, SSRIs are associated with improved health-related quality of life, which is lost if symptomatic relapse occurs. On the other hand, SSRI-response is often incomplete and a substantial proportion of cases fail to make a satisfactory recovery. Better predictors of treatment outcome, that could be used to plan personalized care, are needed. Treatment-resistant OCD is now receiving systematic evaluation. Evidence-based options include continuing the SSRI at maximal dose levels for a longer period, increasing the dose beyond formulary limits, or augmenting the SSRI with a first- or second-generation antipsychotic, while novel treatments such as compounds acting on serotonin or glutamate neurotransmission are under evaluation.

Acknowledgments

The authors would like to thank Christine Lawes, Vivienne Eldridge and Lesley Gibbon of the Postgraduate Medical Centre Library, and Kiri Jefferies, research assistant in the Research and Development Department, Hertfordshire Partnership Foundation Trust for their tireless support in locating and obtaining papers on our behalf. Without their help this project would have taken twice as long and been half as interesting to the reader.

Statement of interest

Naomi Fineberg has consulted for Lundbeck, Glaxo-Smith Kline, Servier, Transept and Bristol Myers Squibb and has received research support from Lundbeck, Glaxo-Smith Kline, AstraZeneca, Wellcome, Cephalon, Servier and ENCP and has received honoraria for lecturing at scientific meetings from Janssen, Jazz, Lundbeck, Servier, AstraZeneca and Wyeth. Financial support to attend scientific meetings has been received from Janssen, Bristol Myers Squibb, Jazz, Lundbeck, Servier, AstraZeneca, Wyeth, Cephalon and the International College of OC Spectrum Disorders.

Between 2001 and 2006 Angus Brown was co-investigator at Roche Products Ltd. Phase I Clinical Pharmacology Unit in Welwyn Garden City and has subsequently participated in research sponsored by Servier.

Ilenia Pampaloni has consulted for Lundbeck. Financial support to attend scientific meetings has been received from Eli-Lilly and Pfizer.

References

Aboujaoude E, Barry JJ, Gamel N (2009). Memantine augmentation in treatment-resistant obsessive-compulsive disorder: an open-label trial. *Journal of Clinical Psychopharmacology* 29, 51–55.

Abramowitz JS (1997). Effectiveness of psychological and pharmacological treatments for obsessive compulsive disorder: a quantitative review. *Journal of Consulting and Clinical Psychology* 65, 44–52.

Ackerman DL, Greenland S (2002). Multivariate meta-analysis of controlled drug studies for obsessive compulsive disorder. *Journal of Clinical Psychopharmacology* 22, 309–317.

Aizenberg D, Naor S, Zemishlany Z, Weizman A (1999). The serotonin antagonist mianserin for treatment of serotonin-reuptake inhibitor-induced sexual dysfunction: an open-label study. *Clinical Neuropharmacology* 22, 347–350.

Albert U, Aguglia E, Maina G, Bogetto F (2002). Venlafaxine versus clomipramine in the treatment of obsessive compulsive disorder: a preliminary, single-blind 12-week controlled study. *Journal of Clinical Psychiatry* 63, 1004–1009.

Ananth J, Pecknold JC, Van Den Steen N, Engelsmann F (1981). Double-blind comparative study of clomipramine and amitriptyline in obsessional neurosis. *Progress in Neuro-Psychopharmacology* 5, 257–262.

Arnold PD, Sicard T, Burroughs E, Richter MA, Kennedy JL (2006). Glutamate transporter gene SLC1A1 associated with obsessive-compulsive disorder. *Archives of General Psychiatry* 63, 769–776.

Baldwin SD, Anderson IM, Nutt DJ et al. (2005). Evidence-based guidelines for the pharmacological treatment of anxiety disorders: recommendations from the British Association for Psychopharmacology. *Journal of Psychopharmacology* 19, 567–596.

Barr LC, Goodman WK, Anand A, McDougle CJ, Price LH (1997). Addition of desipramine to serotonin reuptake inhibitors in treatment-resistant obsessive-compulsive disorder. *American Journal of Psychiatry* 154, 1293–1295.

Beasley CM, Potvin JH, Masica DN et al. (1992). Fluoxetine: no association with suicidality in obsessive-compulsive disorder. *Journal of Affective Disorders* 24, 1–10.

Bejerot S, Bodlund O (1998). Response to high doses of citalopram in treatment-resistant obsessive compulsive disorder. *Acta Psychopharmacologica Scandinavia* 98, 423–424.

Bergeron R, Ravindran AV, Chaput Y et al. (2001). Sertraline and fluoxetine treatment of obsessive compulsive disorder: results of a double-blind, 6-month treatment study. *Journal of Clinical Psychopharmacology* 22, 148–154.

Berlin HA, Koran LM, Jenike MA et al. (2010). Double-blind, placebo-controlled trial of topiramate augmentation in treatment-resistant obsessive-compulsive disorder. *Journal of Clinical Psychiatry.* Aug 10. [Epub ahead of print]

Bisserbe JC, Lane RM, Flament MF (1997). A double-blind comparison of sertraline and clomipramine in outpatients with obsessive-compulsive disorder. *European Psychiatry* 12, 82–93.

Blier P, Bergeron R (1996). Sequential administration of augmentation strategies in treatment resistant obsessive compulsive disorder: preliminary findings. *International Clinical Psychopharmacology* 11, 37–44.

Bloch MH, McGuire J, Landeros-Weisenberger A, Leckman JF, Pittenger C (2010). Meta-analysis of the dose-response relationship of SSRI in obsessive-compulsive disorder. *Molecular Psychiatry* 15(8), 850–855. Epub 2009 May 26.

Bloch MH, Craiglow BG, Landeros-Weisenberger A et al. (2009). Predictors of early adult outcomes in pediatric-onset obsessive-compulsive disorder. *Pediatrics* 124(4), 1085–1093. Epub 2009 Sep 28.

Bobes J, González MP, Bascarán MT et al. (2001). Quality of life and disability in patients with obsessive–compulsive disorder. *European Psychiatry Jun* 16(4): 239–245.

Bogetto F, Albert U, Maina G (2002). Sertraline treatment of obsessive-compulsive disorder: efficacy and tolerability of a rapid titration regimen. *European Neuropsychopharmacology* 12, 181–186.

Bridge JA, Iyengar S, Salary CB et al. (2007). Clinical response and risk for reported suicidal ideation and suicide attempts in pediatric antidepressant treatment: a meta-analysis of randomized controlled trials. *Journal of the American Medical Association* 297(15), 1683–1696.

Byerly MJ, Goodman WK, Christenen R (1996). High doses of sertraline for treatment-resistant obsessive compulsive disorder. *American Journal of Psychiatry* 153, 1232–1233.

Bystritsky A, Ackerman DL, Rosen RM et al. (2004). Augmentation of serotonin reuptake inhibitors in refractory obsessive-compulsive disorder using adjunctive olanzapine: a placebo-controlled trial. *Journal of Clinical Psychiatry* 65, 565–568.

Carey PD, Vythilingum B, Seedat S et al. (2005). Quetiapine augmentation of SRIs in treatment refractory obsessive-compulsive disorder: a double-blind, randomised, placebo-controlled study. *BMC Psychiatry* 5, 5.

Chouinard G, Goodman W, Greist J, et al. (1990). Results of a double-blind placebo-controlled trial of a new serotonin reuptake inhibitor, sertraline, in the treatment of obsessive-compulsive disorder. *Psychopharmacology Bulletin* 26, 279–284.

Cleveland WL, DeLaPaz RL, Fawwaz RA, Challop RS (2009). High-dose glycine treatment of refractory obsessive-compulsive disorder and body dysmorphic disorder in a 5-year period. *Neural Plasticity* 2009, 768398. Epub 2010 Feb 18.

Clomipramine Collaborative Study Group (1991). Clomipramine in the treatment of patients with obsessive compulsive disorder. *Archives of General Psychiatry* 48, 730–738.

Coric C, Sarper T, Pittenger C et al. (2005). Riluzole augmentation in treatment-resistant obsessive-compulsive disorder: an open label trial. *Biological Psychiatry.* Sep 1; 58(5), 424–428.

Cottraux J, Mollard E, Bouvard M, et al. (1990). A controlled study of fluvoxamine and exposure in obsessive-compulsive disorder. *International Clinical Psychopharmacology* 5, 17–30.

Culpepper L (2002). Escitalopram: a new SSRI for the treatment of depression in primary care. *Primary Care Companion Journal of Clinical Psychiatry* 4, 209–214.

D'Amico G, Cedro C, Muscatello MR et al. (2003). Olanzapine augmentation of paroxetine-refractory obsessive-compulsive disorder. *Progress in Neuropsychopharmacology and Biological Psychiatry* 27, 619–623.

Dannon PN, Sasson Y, Hirschmann S et al. (2000). Pindolol augmentation in treatment resistant obsessive compulsive disorder. A double-blind placebo-controlled trial. *European Neuropsychopharmacology* 10, 165–169.

Denys D, De Geus F, Van Megen HJ, Westenberg HG (2004). A double-blind, randomized, placebo-controlled trial of quetiapine addition in patients with obsessive-compulsive disorder refractory to serotonin reuptake inhibitors. *Journal of Clinical Psychiatry* 65, 1040–1048.

Denys D, Fineberg N, Carey PD, Stein DJ (2007). Quetiapine addition in obsessive-compulsive disorder: is treatment outcome affected by type and dose of serotonin reuptake inhibitors? *Biological Psychiatry* 61, 412–414.

Denys D, van der Wee N, van Megen HJ, Westenberg HG (2003). A double blind comparison of venlafaxine and paroxetine in obsessive-compulsive disorder. *Journal of Clinical Psychopharmacology* 23, 568–575.

De Veaugh-Geiss J, Landau P, Katz R (1989). Treatment of obsessive compulsive disorder with clomipramine. *Psychiatric Annals* **19**, 97–101.

De Veaugh-Geiss J, Moroz G, Biederman J *et al.* (1992). Clomipramine hydrochloride in childhood and adolescent obsessive compulsive disorder: a multicenter trial. *Journal of the American Academy of Child and Adolescent Psychiatry* **31**, 45–49.

Diniz JB, Shavitt RG, Pereira CA *et al.* (2010). Quetiapine versus clomipramine in the augmentation of selective serotonin reuptake inhibitors for the treatment of obsessive-compulsive disorder: a randomized, open-label trial. *Journal of Psychopharmacology* **24**, 297–307. Epub 2009 Jan 22.

Drummond LM (1993). The treatment of severe, chronic, resistant obsessive-compulsive disorder. An evaluation of an in-patient programme using behavioural psychotherapy in combination with other treatments. *British Journal of Psychiatry* **163**, 223–229.

Dunbar G, Steiner M, Bushnell WD, Gergel I, Wheadon DE (1995). Long-term treatment and prevention of relapse of obsessive compulsive disorder with paroxetine. *European Neuropsychopharmacology* **5**, 372 (P-D-11).

Eddy KT, Dutra L, Bradley R, Weston D (2004). A multi-dimensional meta-analysis of psychotherapy and pharmacotherapy for obsessive-compulsive disorder. *Clinical Psychology Review* **24**, 1011–1030.

Eisen JL, Mancebo MA, Pinto A *et al.* (2006). Impact of obsessive-compulsive disorder on quality of life. *Comprehensive Psychiatry* **47**(4), 270–275.

Englisch S, Esslinger C, Inta D *et al.* (2009). Clozapine-induced obsessive-compulsive syndromes improve in combination with aripiprazole. *Clinical Neuropharmacology* **32**(4), 227–229.

Eser D, Baghai TC, Möller HJ (2010). Agomelatine: the evidence for its place in the treatment of depression. *Core Evidence* **4**, 171–179.

Fallon BA, Liebowitz MR, Campeas R *et al.* (1998). Intravenous clomipramine for obsessive-compulsive disorder refractory to oral clomipramine: a placebo-controlled study. *Archives of General Psychiatry* **55**, 918–924.

Farre JM, Fora F, Lasheras MG (2004). Specific aspects of erectile dysfunction in psychiatry. *International Journal of Impotence Research* **16** (Suppl. 2), S46–S49.

Fernandez CE, Lopez-Ibor JJ (1967). Monochlorimipramine in the treatment of psychiatric patients resistant to other therapies. *Actas Luso-Españ olas de Neurología Psíquiatría y Ciencias Afines* **26**, 119–147.

Feusner JD, Kerwin L, Saxena S, Bystritsky A (2009). Differential efficacy of memantine for obsessive-compulsive disorder vs. generalized anxiety disorder: an open-label trial. *Psychopharmacology Bulletin* **42**, 81–93.

Fineberg N, Pampaloni I, Pallanti S, Ipser J, Stein D (2007*a*). Sustained response versus relapse: the pharmacotherapeutic goal for obsessive compulsive disorder. *International Clinical Psychopharmacology* **22**(6), 313–322.

Fineberg NA, Gale TM (2005). Evidence-based pharmacotherapy of obsessive-compulsive disorder. *International Journal of Neuropsychopharmacology* **8**, 107–129.

Fineberg NA, Hawley C, Gale T (2006*b*). Are placebo-controlled trials still important for obsessive compulsive disorder? *Progress in Neuropsychopharmacology and Biological Psychiatry* **30**, 413–422.

Fineberg NA, Robbins TW, Bullmore E *et al.* (2010). Probing compulsive and impulsive behaviors, from animal models to endophenotypes: a narrative review. *Neuropsychopharmacology* **35**, 591–604. Epub 2009 Nov 25.

Fineberg NA, Sivakumaran T, Roberts A, Gale T (2005). Adding quetiapine to SRI in treatment-resistant obsessive-compulsive disorder: a randomized controlled treatment study. *International Clinical Psychopharmacology* **20**(4), 223–226.

Fineberg NA, Stein DJ, Prekumar P *et al.* (2006*a*) Adjunctive quetiapine for serotonin reuptake inhibitor-resistant obsessive-compulsive disorder: a meta-analysis of randomized controlled treatment trials. *International Clinical Psychopharmacology* **21**(6), 337–343.

Fineberg NA, Tonnoir B, Lemming O, Stein DJ (2007*b*). Escitalopram prevents relapse of obsessive-compulsive disorder. *European Neuropsychopharmacology* 17(6–7), 430–439.

Flament MF, Rapoport JL, Berg CJ *et al.* (1985). Clomipramine treatment of childhood obsessive-compulsive disorder. A double-blind controlled study. *Archives of General Psychiatry* 42, 977–983.

Foa EB, Steketee G, Kozak MJ, Dugger D (1987). Imipramine and placebo in the treatment of obsessive-compulsives: their effect on depression and obsessional symptoms. *Psychopharmacology Bulletin* 23, 8–11.

Fux M, Benjamin J, Belmaker RH (1999). Inositol versus placebo augmentation of serotonin reuptake inhibitors in the treatment of obsessive-compulsive disorder: a double-blind cross-over study. *International Journal of Neuropsychopharmacology* 2, 193–195.

Garcia AM, Sapyta JJ, Moore PS, *et al.* (2010). Predictors and moderators of treatment outcome in the Pediatric Obsessive Compulsive Treatment Study (POTS I). *Journal of the American Academy of Child and Adolescent Psychiatry* 49, 1024–33; quiz 1086. Epub 2010 Sep 6.

Geller DA, Biederman J, Stewart SE *et al.* (2003*a*). Which SSRI? A meta-analysis of pharmacotherapy trials in paediatric obsessive-compulsive disorder. *American Journal of Psychiatry* 160, 1919–1928.

Geller DA, Biederman J, Stewart SE *et al.* (2003*b*). Impact of comorbidity on treatment response to paroxetine in paediatric obsessive compulsive disorder: is the use of exclusion criteria empirically supported in randomised controlled trials? *Journal of Child and Adolescent Psychopharmacology* 13 (Suppl.), S19–S29.

Geller DA, Hoog SL, Heiligenstein JH *et al.* (2001). Fluoxetine treatment for obsessive-compulsive disorder in children and adolescents: a placebo-controlled clinical trial. *Journal of the American Academy of Child and Adolescent Psychiatry* 40, 773–779.

Goodman WK, Kozak MJ, Liebowitz M, White KL (1996). Treatment of obsessive-compulsive disorder with fluvoxamine: a multicentre, double-blind, placebo-controlled trial. *International Clinical Psychopharmacology* 11, 21–29.

Goodman WK, Price LH, Delgado PL *et al.* (1990). Specificity of serotonin reuptake inhibitors in the treatment of obsessive-compulsive disorder: comparison of fluvoxamine and desipramine. *Archives of General Psychiatry* 47, 577–585.

Goodman WK, Price LH, Rasmussen SA, *et al.* (1989*c*). Efficacy of fluvoxamine in obsessive-compulsive disorder. A double-blind comparison with placebo. *Archives of General Psychiatry* 46, 36–44.

Goodman WK, Price LH, Rasmussen SA *et al.* (1989*a*). The Yale–Brown obsessive compulsive scale, I: development, use and reliability. *Archives of General Psychiatry* 46(11), 1006–1011.

Goodman WK, Price LH, Rasmussen SA *et al.* (1989*b*). The Yale Brown Obsessive Compulsive Scale, II: validity. *Archives of General Psychiatry* 46(11), 1012–1016.

Grady TA, Pigott TA, L'Heureux F *et al.* (1993). Double-blind study of adjuvant buspirone for fluoxetine-treated patients with obsessive-compulsive disorder. *American Journal of Psychiatry* 150, 819–821.

Grant P, Lougee L, Hirschtritt M, Swedo SE (2007). An open-label trial of riluzole, a glutamate antagonist, in children with treatment-resistant obsessive-compulsive disorder. *Journal of Child and Adolescent Psychopharmacology* 17, 761–767.

Grant P, Song JY, Swedo SE (2010). Review of the use of the glutamate antagonist riluzole in psychiatric disorders and a description of recent use in childhood obsessive-compulsive disorder. *Journal of Child and Adolescent Psychopharmacology* 20, 309–315.

Greenberg WM, Benedict MM, Doerfer J *et al.* (2009). Adjunctive glycine in the treatment of obsessive-compulsive disorder in adults. *Journal of Psychiatric Research* 43, 664–670. Epub 2008 Nov 30.

Greenblatt DJ, von Moltke LL, Harmatz JS, Shader RI (1998). Drug interactions with newer antidepressants: role of human cytochromes P450. *Journal of Clinical Psychiatry*. 59 (Suppl 15):19–27.

Greist J, Chouinard G, DuBoff E et al. (1995b).
Double-blind parallel comparison of three
dosages of sertraline and placebo in
outpatients with obsessive-compulsive
disorder. Archives of General Psychiatry 52,
289–295.

Greist JH, Bandelow B, Hollander E et al.
(2003). Long-term treatment of
obsessive-compulsive disorder in adults. CNS
Spectrums 8, 7–16.

Greist JH, Jefferson JW, Kobak KA et al.
(1995a). A one year double-blind
placebo-controlled fixed dose study of
sertraline in the treatment of obsessive-
compulsive disorder. International Clinical
Psychopharmacology 10, 57–65.

Greist JH, Jefferson JW, Kobak KA, Katzelnick
DJ, Serlin RC (1995c). Efficacy and
tolerability of serotonin transport inhibitors
in obsessive-compulsive disorder: a
meta-analysis. Archives of General Psychiatry
52, 53–60.

Greist JH, Jefferson JW, Rosenfeld R et al.
(1990). Clomipramine and obsessive
compulsive disorder: a placebo-controlled
double-blind study of 32 patients. Journal of
Clinical Psychiatry 51, 292–297.

Guy, W. (1976) ECDEU Assessment Manual for
Psychopharmacology (Revised). Bethesda,
MD: US Department of Health, Education
and Welfare.

Hamilton M (1960). A rating scale for
depression. Journal of Neurology,
Neurosurgery and Psychiatry 23, 56–
62.

Harris E, Eng HY, Kowatch R, Delgado SV,
Saldaña SN (2010). Disinhibition as a side
effect of treatment with fluvoxamine in
pediatric patients with obsessive-
compulsive disorder. Journal of Child and
Adolescent Psychopharmacology 20, 347–
353.

Hewlett WA, Vinogradov S, Agras WS (1992).
Clomipramine, clonazepam, and clonidine
treatment of obsessive-compulsive disorder.
Journal of Clinical Psychopharmacology 12,
420–430.

Heyman I, Fombonne E, Meltzer H, Goodman
R (2001). Prevalence of obsessive-compulsive
disorder in the British nationwide survey of
child mental health. British Journal of
Psychiatry 179, 324–329.

Hodgson RJ, Rachman S (1977). Obsessional-
compulsive complaints. Behavior Research
and Therapy 15, 389–395.

Hoehn-Saric R, Ninan P, Black DW et al.
(2000). Multicentre double-blind
comparison of sertraline and desipramine for
concurrent obsessive-compulsive and major
depressive disorders. Archives of General
Psychiatry 57, 76–82.

Hohagen F, Winkelmann G, Rasche-Ruchle H
et al. (1998). Combination of behaviour
therapy with fluvoxamine in comparison
with behaviour therapy and placebo: results
of a multicentre study. British Journal of
Psychiatry 173, 71–78.

Hollander E, Allen A, Steiner M et al. (2003b).
Acute and long-term treatment and
prevention of relapse of obsessive-
compulsive disorder with paroxetine.
Journal of Clinical Psychiatry 64, 1113–
1121.

Hollander E, Greenwald S, Neville D (1998).
Uncomplicated and comorbid
obsessive-compulsive disorder in an
epidemiological sample. CNS Spectrums 3,
10–18.

Hollander E, Kaplan A, Stahl SM (2003c). A
double-blind placebo-controlled trial of
clonazepam in obsessive-compulsive
disorder. World Journal of Biological
Psychiatry 4, 30–34.

Hollander E, Koran LM, Goodman WK et al.
(2003a). A double-blind placebo-controlled
study of the efficacy and safety of controlled
release fluvoxamine in patients with
obsessive-compulsive disorder. Journal of
Clinical Psychiatry 64, 640–647.

Hollander E, Rossi NB, Sood E, Pallanti S
(2003d). Risperidone augmentation in
treatment-resistant obsessive compulsive
disorder: a double-blind, placebo controlled
study. International Journal of
Neuropsychopharmacology 6,
397–401.

Hollander E, Stein D, Fineberg NA, Legault M
(2010). Quality of life outcomes in patients
with obsessive-compulsive disorder:
relationship to treatment response and
symptom relapse. Journal of Clinical
Psychiatry 71(6), 784–792.

Hollander E, Wong C (1998). Psychosocial
function and economic costs of obsessive

compulsive disorder. *CNS Spectrums*
3 (5, Suppl. 1), 48–58.
Insel TR, Murphy DL, Cohen RM *et al.* (1983).
Obsessive-compulsive disorder – a
double-blind trial of clomipramine and
clorgyline. *Archives of General Psychiatry* **40**,
605–612.
Jenike MA, Baer L, Greist JH (1990c).
Clomipramine versus fluoxetine in
obsessive-compulsive disorder: a
retrospective comparison of side effects and
efficacy. *Journal of Clinical
Psychopharmacology* **10**, 122–124.
Jenike MA, Baer L, Minichiello WE, Raunch SL,
Buttolph ML (1997). Placebo-controlled trial
of fluoxetine and phenelzine for
obsessive-compulsive disorder. *American
Journal of Psychiatry* **154**, 1261–1264.
Jenike MA, Baer L, Summergrad P *et al.* (1989).
Obsessive-compulsive disorder: a
double-blind, placebo-controlled trial of
clomipramine in 27 patients. *American
Journal of Psychiatry* **146**, 1328–1330.
Jenike MA, Baer L, Summergrad P *et al.* (1990b).
Sertraline in obsessive-compulsive disorder:
a double-blind comparison with placebo.
American Journal of Psychiatry **147**, 923–928.
Jenike MA, Hyman S, Baer L *et al.* (1990a). A
controlled trial of fluvoxamine in
obsessive-compulsive disorder: implications
for a serotonergic theory. *American Journal
Psychiatry* **147**, 1209–1215.
Katz RJ, DeVeaugh-Geiss J, Landau P (1990).
Clomipramine in obsessive-compulsive
disorder. *Biological Psychiatry* **28**, 401–
404.
Kim SW, Shin IS, Kim JM *et al.* (2009). The
5-HT2 receptor profiles of antipsychotics in
the pathogenesis of obsessive-compulsive
symptoms in schizophrenia. *Clinical
Neuropharmacology* **32**(4), 224–226.
Kobak KA, Greist JH, Jefferson JW, Katzelnick
DJ, Henk HJ (1998). Behavioural versus
pharmacological treatments of obsessive
compulsive disorder: a meta-analysis.
Psychopharmacology **136**, 205–216.
Koran LM, Gamel NN, Choung HW, Smith EH,
Aboujaoude EN (2005). Mirtazapine for
obsessive-compulsive disorder: an open trial
followed by double-blind discontinuation.
Journal of Clinical Psychiatry **66**,
515–520.

Koran LM, Hackett E, Rubin A, Wolkow R,
Robinson D (2002). Efficacy of sertraline in
the long-term treatment of obsessive-
compulsive disorder. *American Journal of
Psychiatry* **159**, 89–95.
Koran LM, Hanna GL, Hollander E, Nestadt G,
Simpson HB (2007). *Practice guideline for the
treatment of patients with obsessive-
compulsive disorder.* Arlington, VA:
American Psychiatric Association. Available
at http//www.psych.org/psych_pract/treatg/
pg/prac_ guide.cfm
Koran LM, Pallanti S, Querciolil L (2001).
Sumatriptan, 5-HT(1D) receptors and
obsessive compulsive disorder. *European
Neuropsychopharmacology* **11**, 169–172.
Koran LM, Sallee FR, Pallanti S (1997). Rapid
benefit of intravenous pulse-loading of
clomipramine in obsessive compulsive
disorder. *American Journal of Psychiatry* **154**,
396–401.
Koran LM, Thienemann ML, Davenport R
(1996). Quality of life for patients with
obsessive–compulsive disorder. *American
Journal of Psychiatry* **153**, 783–788.
Kordon A, Wahl K, Koch N *et al.* (2008).
Quetiapine addition to serotonin reuptake
inhibitors in patients with severe obsessive-
compulsive disorder: a double-blind,
randomized, placebo-controlled study.
Journal of Clinical Psychopharmacology **28**,
550–554.
Kronig MH, Apter J, Asnis G *et al.* (1999).
Placebo-controlled, multicenter study of
sertraline treatment for obsessive-
compulsive disorder. *Journal of Clinical
Psychopharmacology* **19**, 172–176.
Kruger S, Cooke RG, Hasey GM, Jorna T,
Persad E (1995). Comorbidity of obsessive
compulsive disorder in bipolar disorder.
Journal of Affective Disorders **34**, 117–120.
Kumar S, Ng B, Howie W (2003). The
improvement of obsessive-compulsive
symptoms in a patient with schizophrenia
treated with clozapine. *Psychiatry and
Clinical Neurosciences* **57**, 235–236.
Kushner MG, Kim SW, Donahue C *et al.* (2007).
D-cycloserine augmented exposure therapy
for obsessive-compulsive disorder. *Biological
Psychiatry* **62**, 835–838. Epub 2007 Jun 22.
Kwon JS, Joo YH, Nam HJ *et al.* (2009).
Association of the glutamate transporter

gene SLC1A1 with atypical antipsychotics-induced obsessive-compulsive symptoms. *Archives of General Psychiatry* **66**, 1233–1241.

Landeros-Weisenberger A, Bloch MH, Kelmendi B *et al.* (2010). Dimensional predictors of response to SRI pharmacotherapy in obsessive-compulsive disorder. *Journal of Affective Disorders* **121**(1–2), 175–179. Epub 2009 Jul 3.

Leckman JF, Grice DE, Barr LC *et al.* (1994). Tic-related vs. non-tic-related obsessive compulsive disorder. *Anxiety* **1**, 208–215.

Lee KU, Lee YM, Nam JM *et al.* (2010). Antidepressant-induced sexual dysfunction among newer antidepressants in a naturalistic setting. *Psychiatry Investigation* **7**, 55–59. Epub 2010 Feb 8.

Leibowitz MR, Turner SM, Piacentini J *et al.* (2002). Fluoxetine in children and adolescents with OCD: a placebo-controlled trial. *Journal of the American Academy of Child and Adolescent Psychiatry* **41**, 1431–1438.

Leonard HL, Swedo SE, Lenane MC *et al.* (1991). A double-blind desipramine substitution during long-term clomipramine treatment in children and adolescents with obsessive-compulsive disorder. *Archives of General Psychiatry* **48**, 922–927.

Leonard HL, Swedo S, Rapoport JL, Coffey M, Cheslow D (1988). Treatment of childhood obsessive compulsive disorder with clomipramine and desmethylimipramine: a double-blind crossover comparison. *Psychopharmacology Bulletin* **24**, 93–95.

Li X, May RS, Tolbert LC *et al.* (2005). Risperidone and haloperidol augmentation of serotonin reuptake inhibitors in refractory obsessive-compulsive disorder: a crossover study. *Journal of Clinical Psychiatry* **66**, 736–743.

Lopez-Ibor Jr J, Saiz J, Cottraux J *et al.* (1996). Double-blind comparison of fluoxetine versus clomipramine in the treatment of obsessive compulsive disorder. *European Neuropsychopharmacology* **6**, 111–118.

Maina G, Albert U, Ziero S, Bogetto F (2003*b*). Antipsychotic augmentation for treatment-resistant obsessive compulsive disorder: what if antipsychotic is

discontinued? *International Clinical Psychopharmacology* **18**, 23–28.

Maina G, Pessina E, Albert U, Bogetto F (2008). 8-week, single-blind, randomized trial comparing risperidone versus olanzapine augmentation of serotonin reuptake inhibitors in treatment-resistant obsessive-compulsive disorder. *European Neuropsychopharmacology* **18**(5), 364–372. Epub 2008 Feb 15.

Maina G, Salvi V, Bogettoa (2003*a*). Weight-gain during long-term drug treatment of obsessive compulsive disorder. *European Neuropsychopharmacology* **13** (Suppl.), S357.

Marazziti D, Pfanner C, Dell'Osso B *et al.* (2005). Augmentation strategy with olanzapine in resistant obsessive compulsive disorder: an Italian long term open-label study. *Journal of Psychopharmacology* **19**, 392–394.

March JS (2004). Cognitive-behavior therapy, sertraline, and their combination for children and adolescents with obsessive-compulsive disorder: the Pediatric OCD Treatment Study (POTS) randomized controlled trial. *Journal of the American Medical Association* **16**, 1969–1976.

March JS, Biederman J, Wolkow R *et al.* (1998). Sertraline in children and adolescents with obsessive compulsive disorder: a multicenter randomised controlled trial. *Journal of the American Medical Association* **28**, 1752–1756.

March JS, Frances A, Kahn DA, Carpenter D (1997). The Expert Consensus Guideline series. Treatment of obsessive-compulsive disorder. *Journal of Clinical Psychiatry* **58** (Suppl.), 1–72.

March JS, Klee BJ, Kremer CM (2006). Treatment benefit and the risk of suicidality in multicenter, randomized, controlled trials of sertraline in children and adolescents. *Journal of Child and Adolescent Psychopharmacology* **16**(1–2), 91–102.

Marks IM, Lelliott P, Basoglu M *et al.* (1988). Clomipramine, self-exposure and therapist-aided exposure for obsessive-compulsive rituals. *British Journal of Psychiatry* **152**, 522–534.

Marks IM, Stern RS, Mawson D, Cobb J, McDonald R (1980). Clomipramine and exposure for obsessive-compulsive rituals. *British Journal of Psychiatry* **136**, 1–25.

Mataix-Cols D, Rauch SL, Manzo PA, Jenike MA, Baer L (1999). Use of factor-analysed symptom dimensions to predict outcome with serotonin reuptake inhibitors and placebo in the treatment of obsessive-compulsive disorder. *American Journal of Psychiatry* **156**, 1409–1416.

Matsunaga H, Nagata T, Hayashida K *et al.* (2009). A long-term trial of the effectiveness and safety of atypical antipsychotic agents in augmenting SSRI-refractory obsessive-compulsive disorder. *Journal of Clinical Psychiatry* **70**, 863–868. Epub 2009 May 5.

Mavissakalian M, Turner SM, Michelson L, Jacob R (1985). Tricyclic antidepressants in obsessive-compulsive disorder: antiobsessional or antidepressant agents? II. *American Journal of Psychiatry* **142**, 572–576.

McDougle CJ, Barr LC, Goodman WK *et al.* (1995). Lack of efficacy of clozapine monotherapy in refractory obsessive-compulsive disorder. *American Journal of Psychiatry* **152**, 1812–1814.

McDougle CJ, Epperson CN, Pelton GH, Wasylink S, Price LH (2000). A double-blind, placebo-controlled study of risperidone addition in serotonin reuptake inhibitor refractory obsessive-compulsive disorder. *Archives of General Psychiatry* **57**, 794–801.

McDougle CJ, Goodman WK, Leckman JF *et al.* (1993). Limited therapeutic effect of addition of buspirone in fluvoxamine-refractory obsessive compulsive disorder. *American Journal of Psychiatry* **150**, 647–649.

McDougle CJ, Goodman WK, Leckman JF, et al. (1994). Haloperidol addition in fluvoxamine-refractory obsessive-compulsive disorder: a double-blind placebo-controlled study in patients with and without tics. *Archives of General Psychiatry* **51**, 302–308.

McDougle CJ, Goodman WK, Price LH *et al.* (1990). Neuroleptic addition in fluvoxamine-refractory obsessive compulsive disorder. *American Journal of Psychiatry* **147**, 652–654.

McDougle CJ, Price LH, Goodman WK, Charney DS, Heninger GR (1991). A controlled trial of lithium augmentation in fluvoxamine-refractory obsessive compulsive disorder: lack of efficacy. *Journal of Clinical Psychopharmacology* **11**, 175–184.

McDougle CJ, Walsh KH (2001). Treatment of refractory OCD. In Fineberg NA, Marazitti D, Stein D (Eds.), *Obsessive Compulsive Disorder: A Practical Guide* (pp. 135–152). London: Martin Dunitz.

Micali N, Heyman I, Perez M *et al.* (2010). Long-term outcomes of obsessive-compulsive disorder: follow-up of 142 children and adolescents. *British Journal of Psychiatry* **197**, 128–134.

Miguel EC, Diniz JB, Joaquim M *et al.* (2009). Clomipramine and quetiapine augmentation for obsessive compulsive disorder compared with sustained fluoxetine treatment. (Poster Presentation) Annual Meeting of American College of Neuropsychopharmacology 5–9 December Florida.

Monteiro WO, Noshirvani HF, Marks IM, Lelliott PT (1987). Anorgasmia from clomipramine in obsessive-compulsive disorder: a controlled trial. *British Journal of Psychiatry* **151**, 107–112.

Montgomery SA (1980). Clomipramine in obsessional neurosis: a placebo-controlled trial. *Pharmacological Medicine* **1**, 189–192.

Montgomery SA, Fineberg N, Montgomery DB (1990). The efficacy of serotonergic drugs in OCD: power calculations compared with placebo. In Montgomery SA, Goodman WK, Goeting N (Eds.), *Current Approaches in Obsessive Compulsive Disorder* (pp. 54–63). Southampton, UK: Ashford Colour Press for Duphar Medical Relations.

Montgomery SA, Fineberg NA, Montgomery DB, Bullock T (1992). L-tryptophan in obsessive compulsive disorder: a placebo-controlled study. *European Neuropsychopharmacology* **2** (Suppl. 2), 384.

Montgomery SA, Kasper S, Stein DJ, Bang Hedegaard K, Lemming OM (2001). Citalopram 20 mg, 40 mg, and 60 mg are all effective and well tolerated compared with placebo in obsessive-compulsive disorder. *International Clinical Psychopharmacology* **16**, 75–86.

Montgomery SA, McIntyre A, Osterheider M *et al.* (1993). A double-blind placebo-controlled study of fluoxetine in patients with DSM–IIIR obsessive compulsive disorder. *European Neuropsychopharmacology* **3**, 143–152.

Moritz S, Ruferb M, Fricke S *et al.* (2005). Quality of life in obsessive–compulsive disorder before and after treatment. *Comprehensive Psychiatry* **46**, 453– 459.

Mundo E, Bareggi SR, Pirola R, Bellodi L (1999). Effect of acute intravenous clomipramine and antiobsessional response to proserotonergic drugs: is gender a predictive variable? *Biological Psychiatry* **45**, 290–294.

Mundo E, Bareggi SR, Pirola R, Bellodi L, Smeraldi E (1997*b*). Long-term pharmacotherapy of obsessive-compulsive disorder; a double-blind controlled study. *Journal of Clinical Psychopharmacology* **17**, 4–10.

Mundo E, Bianchi L, Bellodi L (1997*a*). Efficacy of fluvoxamine, paroxetine, and citalopram in the treatment of obsessive-compulsive disorder; a single-blind study. *Journal of Clinical Psychopharmacology* **17**, 267–271.

Mundo E, Guglielmo E, Bellodi L (1998). Effect of adjuvant pindolol on the antiobsessional response to fluvoxamine; a double-blind, placebo-controlled study. *International Clinical Psychopharmacology* **13**, 219–224.

Mundo E, Rouillon F, Figuera ML, Stigler M (2001). Fluvoxamine in obsessive-compulsive disorder: similar efficacy but superior tolerability in comparison with clomipramine. *Human Psychopharmacology* **16**, 461–468.

Muscatello MR, Bruno A, Pandolfo G *et al.* (2011). Effect of aripiprazole augmentation of serotonin reuptake inhibitors or clomipramine in treatment-resistant obsessive-compulsive disorder: a double-blind, placebo-controlled study. *Journal of Clinical Psychopharmacology* **31**(2), 174–179.

National Institute for Health and Clinical Excellence (NICE) (2006). *Obsessive-Compulsive Disorder: Core Interventions in the Treatment of Obsessive-Compulsive Disorder and Body Dysmorphic Disorder.* www.NICE.org.uk

Ninan PT, Koran LM, Kiev A *et al.* (2006). High-dose sertraline strategy for nonresponders to acute treatment for obsessive-compulsive disorder: a multicenter double-blind trial. *Journal of Clinical Psychiatry* **67**, 15–22.

Pallanti S, Bernardi S, Antonini S, Singh N, Hollander E (2009). Ondansetron augmentation in treatment-resistant obsessive-compulsive disorder: a preliminary, single-blind, prospective study. *CNS Drugs* **23**, 1047–1055.

Pallanti S, Hollander E, Bienstock C *et al.* (2002*a*). Treatment-non-response in OCD: methodological issues and operational definitions. *International Journal of Neuropsychopharmacology* **5**, 181–191.

Pallanti S, Quercioli L, Bruscoli M (2004). Response acceleration with mirtazapine augmentation of citalopram in obsessive-compulsive disorder patients without comorbid depression: a pilot study. *Journal of Clinical Psychiatry* **65**, 1394–1399.

Pallanti S, Quercioli L, Koran LM (2002*b*). Citalopram infusions in resistant obsessive compulsive disorder: an open trial. *Journal of Clinical Psychiatry* **63**, 796–801.

Pallanti S, Quercioli L, Paiva RS, Koran LM (1999). Citalopram for treatment-resistant obsessive-compulsive disorder. *European Psychiatry* **14**, 101–106.

Pampaloni I, Sivakumaran T, Hawley CJ, *et al.* (2009). High-dose selective serotonin reuptake inhibitors in OCD: a systematic retrospective case notes survey. *Journal of Psychopharmacology* **24**, 1439–1445. Epub 2009 Apr 7.

Pasquini M, Biondi M (2006). Memantine augmentation for refractory obsessive–compulsive disorder. *Progress in Neuro-Psychopharmacology & Biological Psychiatry* **30**(6), 1173–1175. Epub 2006 May 30.

Pasquini M, Garavini A, Biondi M (2005). Nicotine augmentation for refractory obsessive-compulsive disorder. A case report. *Progress in Neuro-Psychopharmacology & Biological Psychiatry* **29**(1), 157–159.

Pato MT, Zohar-Kadouch R, Zohar J (1988). Return of symptoms after discontinuation of clomipramine in patients with obsessive compulsive disorder. *American Journal of Psychiatry* **145**, 211–214.

Perse T, Greist JH, Jefferson JW, Rosenfeld R, Dar R (1987). Fluvoxamine treatment of obsessive compulsive disorder. *American Journal of Psychiatry* **144**, 1543–1548.

Pessina E, Albert U, Bogetto F, Maina G (2009). Aripiprazole augmentation of serotonin reuptake inhibitors in treatment-resistant obsessive-compulsive disorder: a 12-week open-label preliminary study. *International Clinical Psychopharmacology* **24**(5), 265–269.

Piacentini J, Langley AK (2004). Cognitive-behavioral therapy for children who have obsessive-compulsive disorder. *Journal of Clinical Psychology* **60**(11), 1181–1194.

Piccinelli M, Pini S, Bellantuono C, Wilkinson G (1995). Efficacy of drug treatment in obsessive compulsive disorder. *British Journal of Psychiatry* **166**, 424–443.

Pigott TA, L'Heureux F, Dubbert B, *et al.* (1994). Obsessive compulsive disorder: comorbid conditions. *Journal of Clinical Psychiatry* **55** (Suppl.), 15–32.

Pigott TA, L'Heureux F, Hill JL *et al.* (1992*a*). A double-blind study of adjuvant buspirone hydrochloride in clomipramine-treated patients with obsessive compulsive disorder. *Journal of Clinical Psychopharmacology* **12**, 11–18.

Pigott TA, L'Heureux F, Rubinstein CF, Hill JL, Murphy DL (1992*b*). A controlled trial of clonazepam augmentation in OCD patients treated with clomipramine or fluoxetine. New Research Abstracts NR 144 presented at the 145th Annual Meeting of the American Psychiatric Association, Washington, DC, USA.

Pigott TA, Pato MT, L'Heureux F *et al.* (1991). A controlled comparison of adjuvant lithium carbonate or thyroid hormone in clomipramine-treated patients with obsessive compulsive disorder. *Journal of Clinical Psychopharmacology* **11**, 242–248.

Pigott TA, Seay SM (1999). A review of the efficacy of selective serotonin reuptake inhibitors in obsessive compulsive disorder. *Journal of Clinical Psychiatry* **60**, 101–106.

Pittenger C, Coric V, Banasr M, *et al.* (2008*a*). Riluzole in the treatment of mood and anxiety disorders. *CNS Drugs.* **22**(9): 761–786.

Pittenger C, Kelmendi B, Wasylink S, Bloch MH, Coric V (2008*b*). Riluzole augmentation in treatment-refractory obsessive-compulsive disorder: a series of 13 cases, with long-term follow-up. *Journal of Clinical Psychopharmacology* **28**, 363–367.

Rasmussen S, Hackett E, Duboff E *et al.* (1997). A 2-year study of sertraline in the treatment of obsessive-compulsive disorder. *International Clinical Psychopharmacology* **12**, 309–316.

Rasmussen SA, Eisen JL (1990). Epidemiology of obsessive compulsive disorder. *Journal of Clinical Psychiatry* **51**, 10–13.

Ravizza L, Albert U, Ceregato A (2001). *Venlafaxine in OCD.* Presented at the International Obsessive Compulsive Disorder Conference, Sardinia, Italy.

Ravizza L, Maina G, Bogetto F *et al.* (1998). Long term treatment of obsessive compulsive disorder. *CNS Drugs* **10**, 247–255.

Reddy YC, Alur AM, Manjunath S, Kandavel T, Math SB (2010). Long-term follow-up study of patients with serotonin reuptake inhibitor-nonresponsive obsessive-compulsive disorder. *Journal of Clinical Psychopharmacology* **30**(3), 267–272.

Reynghe de Voxrie GV (1968). Anafranil (G34586) in obsessive neurosis. *Acta Neurologia Belgica* **68**, 787–792.

Riddle MA, Reeve EA, Yaryura-Tobias J *et al.* (2001). Fluvoxamine for children and adolescents with obsessive compulsive disorder; a randomised, controlled multicentre trial. *Journal of the American Academy of Child and Adolescent Psychiatry* **40**, 222–229.

Riddle MA, Scahill L, King RA, *et al.* (1992). Double-blind crossover trial of fluoxetine and placebo in children and adolescents with obsessive compulsive disorder. *Journal of the American Academy of Child and Adolescent Psychiatry* **31**, 1062–1069.

Robins LN, Helzer JE, Weissman MM *et al.* (1984). Lifetime prevalence of specific psychiatric disorders in three sites. *Archives of General Psychiatry* **41**, 949–958.

Rodriguez-Salgado B, Dolengevich-Segal H, Arrojo-Romero M *et al.* (2006). Perceived quality of life in obsessive-compulsive disorder: related factors. *BMC Psychiatry* **6**, 20. doi:10.1186/1471–244X-6–20.

Romano S, Goodman WK, Tamura R *et al.* (2001). Long-term treatment of obsessive-compulsive disorder after an acute response: a comparison of fluoxetine versus placebo. *Journal of Clinical Psychopharmacology* **21**, 46–52.

Rosenbaum JF, Fava M, Hoog S, Ascroft RC, Krebs WB (1998). Selective serotonin reuptake inhibitor discontinuation syndrome; a randomised clinical trial. *Biological Psychiatry* **44**, 77–87.

Rouillon F (1998). A double-blind comparison of fluvoxamine and clomipramine in OCD. *European Neuropsychopharmacology* **8** (Suppl.), 260–261.

Sa AR, Hounie AG, Sampaio AS, *et al.* (2009). Obsessive-compulsive symptoms and disorder in patients with schizophrenia treated with clozapine or haloperidol. *Comprehensive Psychiatry* **50**(5), 437–442. Epub 2009 Jan 15.

Savas H, Yumru M, Özen ME (2008). Quetiapine and ziprasidone as adjuncts in treatment-resistant obsessive-compulsive disorder. *Clinical Drug Investigation* **28**(7), 439–442.

Scahill L, Riddle MA, McSwiggin-Hardin M *et al.* (1997). Children's Yale-Brown Obsessive Compulsive Scale: reliability and validity. *Journal of the American Academy of Child and Adolescent Psychiatry* **36**, 844–852.

Shapira NA, Ward HE, Mandoki M *et al.* (2004). A double-blind, placebo-controlled trial of olanzapine addition in fluoxetine-refractory obsessive-compulsive disorder. *Biological Psychiatry* **55**, 553–555.

Sheehan DV, Harnett-Sheehan K, Raj BA (1996). The measurement of disability. *International Clinical Psychopharmacology* **11** (Suppl.), 89–95.

Simpson HB, Foa EB, Liebowitz MR *et al.* (2008). A randomized, controlled trial of cognitive-behavioral therapy for augmenting pharmacotherapy in obsessive-compulsive disorder. *American Journal of Psychiatry* **165**, 621–630.

Skapinakis P, Papatheodorou T, Mavreas V (2007). Antipsychotic augmentation of serotonergic antidepressants in treatment-resistant obsessive-compulsive disorder: a meta-analysis of the randomized controlled trials. *European Neuropsychopharmacology* **17**, 79–93. Epub 2006 Aug 10.

Soltani F, Sayyah M, Feizy F *et al.* (2010). A double-blind, placebo-controlled pilot study of ondansetron for patients with obsessive-compulsive disorder. *Human Psychopharmacology* **25**, 509–513.

Soomro GM, Altman D, Rajagopal S, Oakley-Browne M (2008). Selective serotonin re-uptake inhibitors (SSRIs) versus placebo for obsessive-compulsive disorder (OCD). *Cochrane Database of Systematic Reviews* **23** (1).

Stahl S (2008). Antidepressants. In *Stahl's Essential Psychopharmacology – Neuroscientific Basis and Practical Applications* (pp. 511–666) Cambridge: Cambridge University Press.

Stein D, Montgomery SA, Kasper S, Tanghoj P (2001). Predictors of response to pharmacotherapy with citalopram in obsessive compulsive disorder. *International Clinical Psychopharmacology* **16**, 357–361.

Stein D, Tonnoir B, Andersen EW, Fineberg NA (2007). Escitalopram in OCD: a randomised, placebo-controlled, fixed-dose, paroxetine referenced, 24-week study. *Current Medical Research and Opinion* **23**(4), 701–711.

Stein DJ, Carey PD, Lochner C *et al.* (2008). Escitalopram in obsessive-compulsive disorder: response of symptom dimensions to pharmacotherapy. *CNS Spectrums* **13** 492–498.

Stein DJ, Spadaccini E, Hollander E (1995). Meta-analysis of pharmacotherapy trials of obsessive compulsive disorder. *International Clinical Psychopharmacology* **10**, 11–18.

Stewart SE, Jenike AE, Hezel DM *et al.* (2010). A single-blind case-control study of memantine in severe obsessive-compulsive disorder. *Journal of Clinical Psychopharmacology* **30**, 34–39.

Storch EA, Lewin AB, De Nadai AS, Murphy TK (2010*b*). Defining treatment response and remission in obsessive-compulsive disorder: a signal detection analysis of the Children's Yale-Brown Obsessive Compulsive Scale. *Journal of the American Academy of Child and Adolescent Psychiatry* **49**, 708–717. Epub 2010 Jun 2.

Storch EA, Merlo LJ, Bengtson M *et al.* (2008*a*). D-cycloserine does not enhance exposure-response prevention therapy in obsessive-compulsive disorder. *International Clinical Psychopharmacology* **22**(4), 230–237.

Storch EA, Merlo LJ, Larson MJ *et al.* (2008*b*). Impact of comorbidity on cognitive-behavioral therapy response in pediatric obsessive-compulsive disorder. *Journal of the American Academy of Child and Adolescent Psychiatry* **47**, 583–592.

Storch EA, Murphy TK, Goodman WK et al. (2010a). A preliminary study of d-cycloserine augmentation of cognitive-behavioral therapy in pediatric obsessive-compulsive disorder. *Biological Psychiatry* Sept 1 [Epub ahead of print].

Szegedi A, Wetzel H, Leal M, Hartter S, Hiemke C (1996). Combination treatment with clomipramine and fluvoxamine: drug monitoring, safety and tolerability data. *Journal of Clinical Psychiatry* **57**, 257–264.

Tenney NH, Denys DA, Van Megen HJGM, Glas G, Westenberg HGM (2003). Effect of a pharmacological intervention on quality of life in patients with obsessive-compulsive disorder. *International Clinical Psychopharmacology* **18**, 29–33.

Thoren P, Asberg M, Cronholm B, Jornestedt L, Traskman L (1980). Clomipramine treatment and obsessive compulsive disorder. *Archives of General Psychiatry* **37**, 1281–1285.

Tollefson G, Rampey A, Potvin J et al. (1994). A multicenter investigation of fixed-dose fluoxetine in the treatment of obsessive-compulsive disorder. *Archives of General Psychiatry* **51**, 559–567.

Ushijima S, Kamijima K, Asai M, et al. (1997). Clinical evaluation of sertraline hydrochloride, a selective serotonin reuptake inhibitor, in the treatment of obsessive-compulsive disorder: a double blind placebo-controlled trial. *Japanese Journal of Neuropsychopharmacology* **19**, 603–623.

Uzun O (2010). Lamotrigine as an augmentation agent in treatment-resistant obsessive-compulsive disorder: a case report. *Journal of Psychopharmacology* **24**(3), 425–427. Epub 2008 Nov 14.

Van Ameringen M, Mancini C, Patterson B, Bennet M (2006). Topiramate augmentation in treatment-resistant obsessive-compulsive disorder: a retrospective, open label case series. *Depression and Anxiety* **23**, 1–5.

Vïsänen E, Ranta P, Nummikko-Pelkonen A, Tienari P (1977). Mianserin Hydrochloride

(Org GB 94) in the treatment of obsessional traits. *Journal of International Medical Research* **5**(4), 289–291.

Volavka J, Neziroglu F, Yaryura-Tobias JA (1985). Clomipramine and imipramine in obsessive compulsive disorder. *Psychiatry Research* **14**, 85–93.

Vulink NC, Denys D, Fluitman SB, Meinardi JC, Westenberg HG (2009). Quetiapine augments the effect of citalopram in non-refractory obsessive-compulsive disorder: a randomized, double-blind, placebo-controlled study of 76 patients. *Journal of Clinical Psychiatry* **70**, 1001–1008. Epub 2009 Jun 2.

Wagner KD, March J, Landau P (1999). Safety and efficacy of sertraline in long-term paediatric OCD treatment: a multicentre study. Presented at the 39th Annual Meeting of the New Clinical Drug Evaluation Unit, FL, USA.

Watson HJ, Rees CS (2008). Meta-analysis of randomized, controlled treatment trials for pediatric obsessive-compulsive disorder. *Journal of Child Psychology and Psychiatry* **49**(5), 489–498.

Weissman MM, Bland RC, Canino GJ et al. (1994). The cross national epidemiology of obsessive compulsive disorder. *Journal of Clinical Psychiatry* **55** (Suppl.), 5–10.

Wheadon D, Bushnell W, Steiner M (1993). A fixed dose comparison of 20, 40 or 60 mg paroxetine to placebo in the treatment of obsessive compulsive disorder. Poster presented at Annual Meeting of the American College of Neuropsycho-pharmacology, Honolulu, Hawaii, USA.

Wilens TE, Biederman J, March J et al. (1999). Absence of cardiovascular and adverse effects of sertraline in children and adolescents. *Journal of American Academy of Child and Adolescent Psychiatry* **38**, 573–577.

Wilhelm S, Buhlmann U, Tolin DF et al. (2008). Augmentation of behavior therapy with D-cycloserine for obsessive-compulsive disorder. *American Journal of Psychiatry* **165**, 335–341; quiz 409. Epub 2008 Feb 1.

Wittchen HU, Jacobi F. (2005). Size and burden of mental disorders in Europe – a critical review. *European Neuropsychopharmacology* **15**, 357–376.

Wood A, Tollefson GD, Burkitt M (1993).
Pharmacotherapy of obsessive compulsive
disorder: experience with fluoxetine.
International Clinical Psychopharmacology 8,
301–306.

World Health Organization (1999). *The "Newly
Defined" Burden of Mental Problems*. Fact
Sheets no 217. Geneva: WHO.

Yaryura-Tobias JA, Neziroglu FA (1996).
Venlafaxine in obsessive compulsive
disorder. *Archives of General Psychiatry* 53,
653–654.

Zohar J, Judge R (1996). Paroxetine versus
clomipramine in the treatment of obsessive
compulsive disorder. *British Journal of
Psychiatry* 169, 468–474.

Evidence-based pharmacotherapy of post-traumatic stress disorder

9

Jonathan C. Ipser and Dan J. Stein

Introduction

It is estimated that as many as 80% to 100% of all people are exposed to traumatic events during their lifetimes (Breslau *et al.*, 1998; Frans *et al.*, 2005). Depending on the nature of the trauma, approximately 5–9% of the general population go on to develop post-traumatic stress disorder (PTSD), a condition characterized by the experience of persistent flashbacks of the event (re-experiencing/intrusion symptoms), a state of high arousal when exposed to reminders of the trauma (hyperarousal symptoms), and concomitant avoidance/emotional numbing in response to these reminders (avoidance/emotional numbing symptoms) (Breslau *et al.*, 1998; Frans *et al.*, 2005; Kessler *et al.*, 2005). This constellation of symptoms satisfy the criteria for PTSD when they extend beyond a month after exposure to the trauma and cause clinically significant functional disability, as conceptualized in current psychiatry diagnostic systems such as the *Diagnostic and Statistical Manual of Mental Disorders, 4th edition* (DSM–IV) (American Psychiatric Association, 1994).

PTSD is frequently chronic and associated with significant morbidity, poor quality of life, and high personal, social, and economic costs. It additionally represents a risk factor for developing other mood and anxiety disorders, as well as substance-use disorders. It has been estimated that the US economy alone loses in the region of 3 billion dollars annually due to PTSD-related loss in productivity (Brunello *et al.*, 2001).

PTSD is characterized by a range of neurobiological disruptions, including changes in the hypothalamus–pituitary–adrenal axis, as well as alterations in the serotonergic and noradrenergic neurotransmitter systems. Chemical modulation of these systems by means of medication therefore holds promise as a treatment for this disorder. Conversely, reports of the efficacy of the selective serotonin reuptake inhibitors, or SSRIs, in treating PTSD implicates involvement of the serotonin system in its etiology. Indeed, on the basis of both open-label and controlled trials of these agents the majority of clinical practice guidelines have recommended the SSRIs as first-line agents in treating PTSD. The SSRIs paroxetine and sertraline are currently the only medications approved by the Federal Drug Agency in the USA for the treatment of PTSD.

Despite the general acceptance of SSRIs as first-line medication interventions for treating PTSD, a recent analysis of clinical practice treatment guidelines revealed considerable variability in conclusions regarding their efficacy (Stein *et al.*, 2009). This is reflected in a review conducted by the Institute of Medicine, in which it was concluded that there is insufficient evidence that any of the SSRIs reduce PTSD symptom severity (Institute of Medicine (IOM),

2009). In addition, there is recognition that not all patients with PTSD respond to the SSRIs, leading to the need for augmentation or combination treatment strategies, and to interest in agents such as tiagabine that employ novel mechanisms of action. A comprehensive review of the efficacy of medication in treating PTSD is therefore warranted.

Accordingly, a narrative review was conducted of the effectiveness of medication in reducing PTSD symptoms, as reported by randomized controlled trials (RCTs) of pharmacotherapy for PTSD. The quantitative summary of these findings in published meta-analyses was also reviewed. A more current estimate of efficacy was obtained through updating a prior meta-analysis of PTSD pharmacotherapy, using the guidelines established by the Cochrane Collaboration (Higgins & Altman, 2008). Finally, a review of pharmacotherapy RCTs for treatment-resistant patients was also conducted.

This review addresses the following questions:

(1) Is medication effective in treating PTSD?
(2) Are some agents more effective than others?
(3) How long should medications be administered?
(4) Are augmentation strategies effective in treating resistant PTSD?

RCTs of pharmacotherapy for PTSD in adults who are not receiving concurrent psychotropics were identified in February 2010 by systematically searching the following databases: MEDLINE, the Cochrane Central Register of Controlled Trials, the Cochrane Collaboration Depression, Anxiety and Neurosis Controlled Trials Register and the National PTSD Center Pilots database (contact author for queries used). Unpublished studies were located using the metaRegister module [mRCT] of the Controlled Trials database (http://www.controlled-trials.com), by searching the bibliographies of published articles, and contacting experts in the field. Study characteristics and outcomes are provided in Table 9.1.

Monoamine oxidase inhibitors

MOA-A is a deaminater of both norepinephrine and serotonin, neurotransmitters that have been implicated in PTSD (Baker et al., 1995). Nevertheless, two RCTs of phenelzine, a monoamine oxidase inhibitor (MAOI), provide mixed evidence for its efficacy in treating this patient population. No differences were detected in a 5-week cross-over RCT (Shestatzky et al., 1988), with over half of the participants (7/13) withdrawing during the course of the study while receiving phenelzine. A placebo-controlled comparison of phenelzine and the tricyclic antidepressant imipramine in 60 male combat veterans reported a significant decrease after 3 weeks of treatment with phenelzine in the score on the primary PTSD symptom severity scale, the self-rated Impact of Event Scale (IES) (Kosten et al., 1991).

Reversible inhibitors of monoamine oxidase A (RIMAs)

The clinical utility of the MAOIs is limited by the potential for serious drug-related adverse events, such as hypertensive crises, and stringent dietary restrictions that reduce the likelihood of compliance. These shortcomings have been largely overcome in the case of the reversible inhibitors of monoamine oxidase A (RIMAs), with their more selective inhibition of monoamine oxidase A reuptake.

Table 9.1. Placebo-controlled randomized studies included in the review.

Medication agents	P.I.	Year	Duration (weeks)	Sample size	% Males	Dose (mg/day)	Response rates (%) Drug	Response rates (%) Control	Response criteria[a]	Efficacy[b]	Tx-related dropouts (%)
MAOIs											
Phenelzine	Shestatzky	1988	5	13	–	30–75	–	–	CGI-I < 4	↔	44
Phenelzine	Kosten	1991	8	37	100	15–75	68	28		↔	17
RIMAs											
Brofaromine	Katz	1995	14	60	76	50–150	55	26	no PTSD diagnosis	↔	5
Brofaromine	Baker	1995	12	114	81	150 (max)	–	–		↔	18
SSRIs											
Citalopram	Tucker	2003	10	35	29	20–50	–	–		↔	–
Fluoxetine	v.d. Kolk	1994	5	64	66	20–60	–	–		↑	–
Fluoxetine	Connor	1999	12	54	9	10–60	85	62	DGRP-I < 3	↔	0
Fluoxetine	Hertzberg	2000	12	12	100	10–60	17	33	DGRP-I < 3	↔	17
Fluoxetine	Martenyi[c]	2002	12/24	301	81	20–80	60	44	CGI < 3, TOP-8 <= 50%	↑	3
Fluoxetine	Davidson[c]	2005	24/24	62	50		–	–		↔	3
Fluoxetine	Martenyi	2007	12	411	29	20, 20–40	41, 39	38	CGI < 3, TOP-8 <= 50%, no PTSD diag.	↔	4 & 13
Fluoxetine	v.d. Kolk	2007	8	59	14	10–60	81	65	CGH < 3	↔	–
Paroxetine	Marshall	2001	12	376	32	20, 20–40	62, 54	37	CGH < 3	↑	11 & 15
Paroxetine	Tucker	2001	12	323	34	20–50	59	38	CGI < 3	↑	11
Paroxetine	SKB627		12	322	46	20–50	–	–	–	–	–
Paroxetine	SKB650		36	176	34	–	–	–	–	–	–
Paroxetine	Marshall[c]	2007	10/12	52	33	20–60	67	27	CGH < 3,	↔	0
Sertraline	Brady[‡]	2000	12/24/28	187	27	25–200	53	32	CGH < 3, CAPS < 20	↑	5
Sertraline	Davidson[c]	2001	12/24/28	208	22	25–200	60	38	CGI < 3	↑	9
Sertraline	Zohar	2002	10	42	88	50–200	53	20	CGI < 3	↔	13
Sertraline	Tucker	2003	10	35	29	50–200	–	–		–	–
Sertraline	Pfizer		11	193	25	156 (mean)	–	–		–	–
Sertraline	Brady	2005	12	94	54	150	–	–		↔	0
Sertraline	Davidson	2006	12	352	–	25–200	–	–		↔	13
Sertraline	Friedman	2007	10	169	80	25–200	37	42	CGI-I < 3	↔	13

(cont.)

Table 9.1. (cont.)

Medication agents	P.I.	Year	Duration (weeks)	Sample size	% Males	Dose (mg/day)	Response rates (%) Drug	Response rates (%) Control	Response criteria	Efficacy	Tx-related dropouts (%)
TCAs											
Desipramine	Reist	1989	4	18	100	50–200	–	–		↔	7
Amitriptyline	Davidson	1990	8	46	100	50–300	50	17	CGI-I < 3	↔	12
Imipramine	Kosten	1991	8	41	100	50–300	65	28	CGI-I < 4	↔	17
ANTICONVULSANTS											
Divalproex	Davis	2008	8	85	98	500–3000	–	–		↔	7
Lamotrigine	Hertzberg	1999	12	15	64	25–500	50	25	DGRP-I < 3	–	18
Tiagabine	Connor[c]	2006	12/12	18	–	2 (BID) – 16	–	–		↔	0
Tiagabine	Davidson	2007	12	232	34	4–16	49	54	CGI < 3	↔	8
Topiramate	Tucker	2007	12	40	21	25–400	42	21	CAPS < 20	↔	20
ANTIPSYCHOTICS											
Olanzapine	Butterfield	2001	10	15	7	5–20	60	60	CGI < 3	↔	20
Risperidone	Reich	2004	8	21	0	0.5–8	–	–		←	8
Risperidone	Padala	2006	10	20	0	0.5–6	–	–		←	9
OTHER											
Alprazolam	Braun	1990	5	16	–	1.5–6	–	–		↔	0
Inositol	Kaplan	1996	4	13	62	12000	–	–		↔	–
Mirtazapine	Davidson	2003	8	26	–	15–45	65	22	SPRINT-I < 3	↔	18
Nefazodone	Davis	2004	12	42	98	200–600	47	42	CAPS >= 30% improvement	←	19
Venlafaxine	Davidson	2006	12	358	–	37.5–300	–	–		←	10
Venlafaxine	Davidson	2006	24	329	46	37.5–300	78	64	CAPS-SX >= 30% improvement at 12 weeks	←	9

[a] CGI-I: Clinical Global Impressions Scale – Improvement item, DGRP-I: Duke Global Rating of PTSD – Improvement item, SPRINT-I: Short PTSD Rating Interview – Improvement item, CAPS: Clinician Administered PTSD Scale, –, no data provided.

[b] Significant differences in PTSD symptom severity in favor of medication are indicated by an upward pointing arrow (↑) and non-significant differences by a double-headed horizontal arrow (↔). Symptom severity data were collected for the CAPS, or from other primary efficacy measures where the CAPS was not employed.

[c] Sample included in maintenance trial.

Nevertheless, results from the two placebo-controlled trials of the RIMA brofaromine conducted to date have been disappointing. In the first, Katz *et al.* (1994) observed no evidence of reductions in the total score of the gold-standard observer-rated measure of symptom severity, the Clinician Administered PTSD scale (CAPS) (Blake *et al.*, 1995), following 14 weeks of treatment. However, a significant treatment effect emerged when restricting the sample of 60 patients to those diagnosed for at least 1 year. A larger 12-week study of 118 patients failed to detect difference on the CAPS following a similar dosing regimen (Baker *et al.*, 1995).

Selective serotonin reuptake inhibitors

The SSRIs represent the medication class that has been most frequently investigated in placebo-controlled trials, with a total of 18 RCTs conducted to date. It is primarily on the basis of these studies that these agents are regarded as first-line treatments for PTSD.

Paroxetine

Paroxetine is registered by the FDA for the short-term treatment of PTSD. All three published randomized placebo-controlled trials of this medication have reported favorable results. In the first two trials, improvements in symptom severity on the CAPS were detected after 4 weeks of paroxetine, with medication effective for all three symptom clusters (Marshall *et al.*, 2001; Tucker *et al.*, 2001). In Tucker *et al.* (2001) almost a third of patients (29.4%) went into remission after 12 weeks of paroxetine. A large placebo-controlled comparison of fixed doses of paroxetine (20 mg/day versus 40 mg/day) failed to detect a difference in treatment response as a function of dosage or comorbid depression (Marshall *et al.*, 2001). Marshall *et al.* (2007) reported significant differences in treatment response on the improvement item of the Clinical Global Impressions scale (CGI-I) after 10 weeks of treatment with paroxetine, with a third (14/21) of patients in a sample of 52 mostly Hispanic adults responding to treatment (Guy, 1976).

Fluoxetine

Six RCTs of fluoxetine have been conducted to date. This includes the first published placebo-controlled trial of an SSRI for the treatment of PTSD, a small 5-week trial in which significant reductions in PTSD symptom severity were observed on the CAPS (van der Kolk *et al.*, 1994). This effect was not observed in this trial in a subsample from a VA site, however.

In a second trial in civilian subjects ($n = 54$) differences in treatment response only reached significance for subjects classified as very much improved (Connor *et al.*, 1999). Using a composite measure, almost half of the subjects on fluoxetine (41%) were regarded as displaying minimal levels of symptoms and non-disability by study end-point. No differences were observed on any of the self- or clinician-rated symptom severity measures after 12 weeks of fluoxetine treatment in a small sample ($n = 12$) of combat veterans with high levels of comorbid depression (Hertzberg *et al.*, 2000). In a larger sample of predominantly male participants a significant effect of medication (average dose: 57 mg/day) emerged after 6 weeks on the observer-rated TOP-8 symptom severity scale (Connor & Davidson, 1999; Martenyi *et al.*, 2002*b*).

A subsequent placebo-controlled trial comparing treatment with 20 or 40 mg/day of fluoxetine in a sample composed primarily of women did not detect superiority of medication after 12 weeks between any of the comparison groups ($n = 411$) (Martenyi *et al.*, 2007). Similar results were reported for a study comparing 8 weeks of treatment with fluoxetine or eye movement desensitization and reprocessing (EMDR) (van der Kolk *et al.*, 2007). No patients on fluoxetine in this study were asymptomatic (CAPS score < 20) at 6-month follow-up.

Sertraline

Sertraline is licensed by the FDA for the short- and long-term treatment of PTSD. There have been seven published placebo-controlled RCTs of sertraline conducted to date. Evidence for the efficacy of sertraline has been mixed, with negative results reported for under-powered studies, or typically treatment-resistance populations (veterans). Significant differences in symptom severity were observed in two 12-week placebo-controlled trials employing similar designs. Brady and colleagues (2000) detected differences on the CAPS after only 2 weeks of sertraline in 187 outpatients, with 70% of the reductions on the CAPS and the IES apparent after 4 weeks. Davidson *et al.* (2001*a*) reported significant differences on all primary severity measures by trial end in the intent-to-treat sample of 202 outpatients.

Two small 10-week placebo-controlled trials of sertraline, one in a sample of Israeli military veterans and the other in predominantly female outpatients, both failed to detect an effect of medication on the efficacy scales employed (Tucker *et al.*, 2003; Zohar *et al.*, 2002). No differences on intent-to-treat analyses were observed for either drinking or PTSD severity outcomes in a 12-week fixed-dose study of 150 mg/day sertraline in 94 subjects with comorbid PTSD and alcohol abuse/dependence (Brady *et al.*, 2005). Additionally, a 12-week placebo-controlled comparison of sertraline and the serotonin norepinephrine reuptake inhibitor (SNRI) venlafaxine in 538 mixed-trauma subjects did not detect differences between sertraline and placebo on the CAPS-SX (Davidson *et al.*, 2006*b*).

In the final RCT of sertraline for PTSD, a total of 169 combat veterans were randomized to 25 to 200 mg/day of sertraline for 12 weeks (Friedman *et al.*, 2007). However, Tucker and colleagues (2003) also observed negative effects in the citalopram arm of their study, suggesting the study had insufficient power to detect treatment effects. An equivalent number of treatment responders were observed in the sertraline (36.9%) and placebo (41.5%) groups, as assessed on the CGI-I. The majority of patients treated with sertraline experienced treatment-emergent adverse events (86%), with diarrhea and headaches being most common. Combat trauma was associated with a significantly smaller placebo response than non-combat traumas.

Citalopram

A single published RCT of citalopram (described above), failed to demonstrate an effect on PTSD symptom severity after 10 weeks compared with either sertraline or placebo (Tucker *et al.*, 2003).

Tricyclic antidepressants (TCAs)

The tricyclic antidepressants (TCAs) represent one of the most established classes of antidepressants, although only three relatively small controlled trials of TCAs for PTSD have been published. In the first study, 18 male US war veterans with high levels of comorbid psychopathology, including affective disorder and substance abuse, completed 4 weeks of treatment with desipramine (25–200 mg/day) or placebo, administered in a randomized cross-over design (Reist et al., 1989). No difference was observed between groups in the reduction of PTSD symptom severity.

In a placebo-controlled study of amitriptyline (50–300 mg/day) in 46 veterans, medication demonstrated superiority after 8 weeks on self-rated PTSD severity scales only (Davidson et al., 1990). An 8-week comparison of the TCA imipramine and phenelzine detected a significant reduction on the self-rated IES after 5 weeks of imipramine (50–300 mg/day) (Kosten et al., 1991). However, a relatively large proportion of patients on imipramine dropped out due to treatment-related side-effects (17.4%, 4/23).

Anticonvulsants

The possibility that limbic hypersensitization or kindling might underlie increased arousal to traumatic stimuli in PTSD suggests that anticonvulsants might be effective in treating this disorder (Post et al., 2003). A placebo-controlled trial of 10 weeks of lamotrigine (mean: 380 mg/day) was conducted in war veterans to test this hypothesis (Hertzberg et al., 1999). Although a larger proportion of participants responded to treatment in the medication than placebo group (2/5 vs. 1/4, respectively), the small sample (n = 15) precluded the estimation of a treatment-effect size.

More recently, 232 patients from 38 centers in the USA were treated for 12 weeks with the selective GABA reuptake inhibitor tiagabine (Davidson et al., 2007). No differences were observed in any of the efficacy outcomes assessed. A similar pattern was observed in a 12-week trial of topiramate (25–400 mg/day) in 40 outpatients (Tucker et al., 2007), with the exception that a reduction in overall PTSD symptom severity on the TOPS-8 was reported following medication treatment. No effect of treatment was detected on any outcome measure after 8 weeks of placebo-controlled treatment with the selective GABA inhibitor divalproex in 85 US military veterans with PTSD (Davis et al., 2008).

Antipsychotics

Three small randomized controlled trials have evaluated the effectiveness of antipsychotic medication as monotherapy in treating PTSD. An initial trial of the atypical antipsychotic olanzapine (5–20 mg/day) was unable to detect a treatment response in 15 mostly female patients with non-combat PTSD over 10 weeks (Butterfield et al., 2001). Patients treated with olanzapine gained significantly more weight than those given placebo by study end (11.5 lb vs. 0.9 lb, respectively).

Two small studies provide preliminary evidence that risperidone may be effective in treating PTSD in female patients, however. In a trial of 21 women with PTSD from childhood physical, sexual, verbal, and emotional abuse, 8 weeks of risperidone (average dose: 1.4 mg/day) resulted in a significant reduction of symptom severity on the CAPS-2 (Reich et al., 2004). Almost half of the subjects were receiving concurrent antidepressants or benzodiazepines. A similar superiority of risperidone over placebo was detected on the CAPS after 10 weeks of treatment in 20 women exposed to domestic violence and sexual assault (Padala et al., 2006).

Benzodiazepines

In a small controlled trial, 16 outpatients were administered 1.5 to 6 mg/day of alprazolam or placebo for two 5-week periods in a cross-over fashion, separated by a 2-week placebo-substitution washout period (Braun et al., 1990). Analysis of data from the 10 patients who completed the study revealed a significant reduction in depression symptoms only.

Table 9.2. Meta-analyses of pharmacotherapy for post-traumatic stress disorder.

Study	Year	Intervention	Databases*	Date range	Trials[†]	PTSD Outcomes[‡]	ES[§]	Limitations
Penava	1996	All controlled trials of medication	psycINFO, MEDLINE	1974–July 1996	6	PTSD effect, or the "best overall measure of specific PTSD symptomatology".	$0.41(-)^a$	Small number of studies; no explicit criteria for "best" measure of PTSD; variability of effect sizes not reported; combination of data from self- and observer-rated scales; multiple data points for different studies
Van Etten	1998	All medication and psychological studies	MEDLINE, PILOTS, Psychological Abstracts, Current Contents library	1984–1996	16(19)	(1) observer-rated PTSD scales (2) self-rated PTSD scales	(1) 1.05^a, (2) 0.69^a	Meta-analysis included open-label trials without controls; combination of wait-list, supportive psychotherapy and pill placebo as primary control group; likelihood of false positive findings increased through setting statistical threshold to 0.1; analyses limited to data from trial completers
Stein	2006	All medication RCTs	MEDLINE, psycINFO, PILOTS, CCDAN-TR, Controlled Trials metaregister	Up till December, 2004	35(17)	CAPS-2	-5.76^b $(-8.16, -3.36)$	Possible publication bias in the funnel plot for the CAPS
Stewart	2009	All medication and psychotherapy trials for combat-related PTSD (except case studies)	psycINFO	1988–2006	13(10)	Clinician- and self-rated PTSD scales	1^a	Included open-label studies that did not control for placebo effect; pre-/post-treatment within group analyses; two of the studies employed the medication as adjunctive agents to existing pharmacotherapy; multiple studies reporting on the same sample included

* AMED, Allied and Complementary Medicine Database; CCDAN-TR, Cochrane Collaboration Depression, Anxiety and Neurosis Trial Registry; CINAHL, Cumulative Index to Nursing and Allied Health Literature; PILOTS, Published International Literature on Traumatic Stress; SIGLE, System for Information on Grey Literature in Europe.
[†] Total number of pharmacotherapy trials included in study, with the specific number of trials included in meta-analysis in parentheses.
[‡] CAPS: Clinician Administered PTSD Scale, IES: Impact of Events Scale, DTS: Davidson Trauma Scale.
[§] Effect size estimates and 95% confidence intervals reported using standardized (a) or non-standardized (b) mean difference metrics.

Other medications

A total of six placebo-controlled RCTs of medications with novel mechanisms of action have been conducted. In the first trial inositol (12 g) or placebo were administered over 4 weeks in a cross-over fashion to 17 outpatients with mixed trauma, with no discernable effect of medication on the IES amongst the 13 subjects who completed the trial (Kaplan *et al.*, 1996).

The second trial compared the effectiveness of 8 weeks of treatment with mirtazapine or placebo in 26 subjects with PTSD, the majority of whom had comorbid depression (David-son *et al.*, 2003). A greater number of treatment responders were observed in the medication group, with mirtazapine also demonstrating an antidepressant effect. Davis *et al.* (2004) detected superiority of 12 weeks of nefazodone (mean dose: 435 mg/day) to placebo in 42 combat veterans on the continuous total CAPS score. The high dropout rate amongst those treated with medication (46%) raises questions regarding the tolerability of this agent, however.

A 6-month study of the SNRI venlafaxine assessed its effectiveness in patients sampled from 56 outpatient centers outside of the USA (Davidson *et al.*, 2006a). An improvement was observed on the CAPS-SX on a mean dose of 181.7 mg/day, as well as on measures of quality of life, functional disability, resilience to stress, and comorbid depression. A subsequent trial by the same group detected significant reductions in symptom severity following venlafaxine treatment in 538 outpatients on the CAPS-SX total score. Differences were observed as early as 2 weeks following the initiation of treatment (Davidson *et al.*, 2006b).

Review of meta-analyses of pharmacotherapy for PTSD

This brief review highlights the inconsistency of the evidence for the efficacy of medication in treating PTSD. Of the 37 short-term studies included in this review that conducted between-group comparisons, only 12 detected a significant reduction in PTSD symptom severity on the CAPS or an alternative primary outcome measure (see Table 9.1). This divergence in findings was detected even amongst first-line agents, with 9 of the 15 SSRI trials employing the CAPS unable to distinguish statistically between the effects of medication and placebo.

Poor sensitivity to treatment effects may be partially due to variation in study methodology and the clinical characteristics of patient groups, as well as insufficient power to detect a treatment effect in small studies. The quantitative synthesis or meta-analysis of treatment outcome data allows one to maximize power in detecting an effect. Overall treatment effects are typically summarized in the form of a mean difference (MD) or effect-size estimate that can be standardized to accommodate the use of different outcome scales (Cohen, 1988).

A brief description of PTSD pharmacotherapy meta-analyses will follow (Table 9.2).[1] Although several meta-analyses have focused on individual agents, including valproate (Adamou *et al.*, 2007) and sertraline (Mooney *et al.*, 2004), we will limit our scope to those which compare the efficacy of a range of medication classes in treating PTSD. The findings of these studies will be supplemented with results from a meta-analysis conducted by the authors.

---

[1] Interested readers should consult Stein *et al.* (2009) for a summary of the evidence synthesized in relevant clinical practice guidelines.

The first meta-analysis to assess the effectiveness of medication for treating PTSD was published in 1996. Penava *et al.* (1996) combined data from "the best overall measure of specific PTSD symptomatology" for six RCTs, yielding an overall effect-size estimate of 0.41. Fluoxetine demonstrated the largest treatment effect (0.77), with the smallest effect observed for the benzodiazepine alprazolam (0.25). The authors observed that larger effects were observed for those agents that possess greater specificity for serotonin.

Van Etten and colleagues published a meta-analysis in 1998 comparing the effectiveness of all open-label and controlled psychological and medication studies of PTSD (Van Etten & Taylor, 1998). Data from 61 treatment arms in 39 trials of chronic PTSD were included in the meta-analysis. Drug therapies ($n = 19$) were found to be significantly more effective than controls for both self and observer-rated PTSD symptoms, with effect sizes of 0.69 and 1.05, respectively. Drug therapies possessed a greater attrition rate (31.9%) than either psychological therapies (14%) or control groups (16.6%). The authors concluded that there was little evidence for the effectiveness of benzodiazepines.

Efficacy data from a total of 35 randomized controlled trials ($n = 4597$) of pharmacotherapy for PTSD were synthesized by Stein *et al.* in an update of a Cochrane review (Stein *et al.*, 2006). They found an average reduction of symptom severity on the CAPS following medication treatment (relative to the placebo control) across 17 trials (2507 participants) of close to 6 points (MD $= -5.76$, 95% CI $= -8.16, -3.36$). Over half of patients in the medication groups (59.1%, $n = 644$) and 38.5% ($n = 628$) in the control groups responded on the CGI-I (number needed to treat (NNT) $=$ five patients). The majority of the evidence of efficacy was for the SSRIs, with paroxetine reducing symptom severity to a greater extent than sertraline. A greater effect of treatment was observed on the CAPS for multi-center studies, with a reduced impact of medication in trials including combat veterans.

Finally, Stewart & Wrobel (2009) included 13 pharmacotherapy and 12 psychotherapy trials in a review of pharmacotherapy and psychotherapy for combat-related PTSD. A significantly larger effect was observed for medication than placebo on PTSD symptom severity ($t = -2.74$, $p = 0.01$). The mean difference was approximately twice as large for drug than for psychotherapy treatments (-1 *vs.* -0.52 standardized units, respectively), though average baseline PTSD symptoms were less severe in the psychotherapy trials.

Meta-analysis of pharmacotherapy for PTSD

A number of limitations reduce the strength of the conclusions that can be drawn from previous meta-analyses (see Table 9.2). Accordingly, we conducted a meta-analysis of placebo-controlled RCTs of PTSD in adults that was restricted to between-group comparisons of outcome data from validated scales.

Primary outcomes included the reduction in total symptom severity on the Clinician Administered PTSD Scale and the number of subjects rated as "much improved" or "very much improved" on the improvement item of the Clinical Global Impressions scale (CGI-I) (or closely related measure). Secondary outcomes included the efficacy of medication in alleviating the severity of PTSD symptom clusters, as assessed by the respective subscales of the observer-rated CAPS and the self-rated DTS. The total proportion of participants who withdrew from the RCTs due to treatment-emergent adverse events was used as a proxy for medication acceptability.

The assessment of RCTs for inclusion and study data extraction was conducted independently by two raters. Where information was missing, the reviewers contacted investigators by email in an attempt to obtain this information.

Weighted mean differences (WMD) for continuous measures and relative risks for categorical outcomes were obtained from a random-effects model and were expressed in terms of the average and 95% CI of the effect size for each subgroup. Treatment response on the CGI-I was converted into a number needed to treat (NNT) for each medication agent (see footnotes in Table 9.2 for the exact procedure). Efficacy analyses (detailed below) were conducted using the metafor package in the R statistical software, and employing the DerSimonian–Laird estimator of heterogeneity (DerSimonian & Laird, 1986; Viechtbauer, 2010). Differences in the efficacy of classes of medication were assessed by means of Deeks' stratified test of heterogeneity (Deeks $et al.$, 2001).

A total of 37 short-term RCTs (4–24 weeks), containing data for 5008 patients treated with medication for an average of 10 weeks, were included in the review. The greatest number of trials assessed the effectiveness of the SSRIs ($n = 20$).

Medication treatment resulted in a significant reduction in PTSD symptom severity, with a reduction of about 6 points on the CAPS total score relative to placebo ($n = 23$, MD = -6.10, 95% CI = $-7.98, -4.23, n = 4112$). A moderate degree of variation was evident in the results of the SSRI ($I^2 = 35\%$) and brofaromine trials ($I^2 = 31\%$). Of the four SSRI agents for which there were data (citalopram, fluoxetine, paroxetine, and sertraline), evidence of efficacy was only available for paroxetine ($n = 4$, MD = -10.65, 95% CI = $-14.16, -7.14$, $n = 1100$) and sertraline ($n = 8$, MD = -4.35, 95% CI = $-6.76, -1.93, n = 1260$). Paroxetine was significantly more effective than sertraline and fluoxetine in reducing symptom severity using a fixed-effects model (chi-squared = 10.37, $p = 0.001$ and chi-squared = 3.08, $p = 0.08$, respectively).

Medication was more likely to result in a global clinical response on the CGI-I than placebo ($n = 16$, RR = 1.4, 95% CI = 1.17, 1.66, $n = 1821$). A larger proportion of patients were responders on this scale in the medication (57.2%) than placebo (40.2%) groups. The corresponding NNT indicates that, relative to patients in the placebo groups, approximately 7–10 patients have to be treated for an average of 11 weeks with medication in order for an additional patient to respond to treatment (see Table 9.3 for details).

Significant treatment effects were observed for the intrusion/re-experiencing, avoidance/numbing, and hyperarousal symptoms on the CAPS. Comorbid depression but not anxiety were reduced following medication treatment (HAM-D: $n = 10$, MD = -2.31, 95% CI = $-3.6, -1.02, n = 930$). Significant improvements were also observed in functional disability following medication treatment ($n = 10$, MD = -1.87, 95% CI = $-2.72, -1.02, n = 1852$). Finally, a larger number of patients on medication withdrew from treatment due to adverse events than on placebo ($n = 29$, relative risk = 1.38, 95% CI = 1.10, 1.72, $n = 4045$), though the absolute proportion that withdrew was relatively small (9.5%).

Length of treatment

The available pharmacotherapy evidence base suggests that treatment effects may emerge as early as 2–4 weeks for the SSRIs and the SNRI venlafaxine. Less is known about how long patients should be treated to achieve a maximal response, and when it is safe to discontinue pharmacotherapy without risking relapse.

Table 9.3. Summary measures of effect size and statistical heterogeneity across medication agents.

Medication	Studies	Sample	CAPS Effect & 95% CI[a]	Heterogeneity[b]	NNT[c]
SSRIs	13	2642	−6.64 (−9.11, −4.16)	Moderate	6–9
Sertraline	7	1072	−4.84 (−7.37, −2.31)	Minimal	7–11
Paroxetine	3	888	−12.17 (−15.68, −8.65)	Minimal	4–7
Fluoxetine	2	356	−4.76 (−10.79, 1.27)	Minimal	8–12
Citalopram	1	33	−13.41 (−34.73, 7.91)	na	–
Brofaromine	2	178	−5.06 (−15.93, 5.81)	Moderate	16–25
Venlafaxine	2	687	−8.11 (−12.30, −3.92)	Minimal	–
Divalproex	1	82	−0.70 (−11.69, 10.29)	na	–
Nefazodone	1	41	−5.60 (−21.26, 10.06)	na	–
Risperidone	1	21	−11.00 (−30.55, 8.55)	na	–
Tiagabine	1	202	−0.50 (−7.60, 6.60)	na	25–40
Topirimate	1	38	−14.00 (−36.33, 8.33)	na	–

[a] Effect sizes reported as (non-standardized) mean differences.
[b] Heterogeneity classified as minimal, moderate and large, based on an I^2 statistic of less than 30%, between 30% and 50%, and over 50%, respectively.
[c] The number needed to treat (NNT) was calculated from the risk ratio estimates of treatment response, defined as "much improved" or "very much improved" on the Clinical Global Impressions Improvement item (or related scale). The NNT is based on a high and low estimate of response in the control group of 0.25 and 0.4, respectively, calculated by rounding the limits of the interquartile range for the placebo group response rate in the included studies to the nearest 5 percentage points. Baseline risk was calculated using the metannt command of the Metan package in Stata 11.

Davidson and colleagues administered 28 weeks of placebo or sertraline to patients who completed a 12-week placebo-controlled trial of sertraline, and who responded to a subsequent 24 weeks of open-label treatment with this agent (50–200 mg/day) (Davidson et al., 2001a). Response to acute-treatment with sertraline was maintained in the majority of patients during open-label continuation, with more than half of the non-responders to sertraline (54%) during the acute phase responding during the continuation phase (Londborg et al., 2001). Relapse, defined as a composite measure consisting of reductions in clinical improvement scores, increasing PTSD symptom severity and investigators' opinion of clinical deterioration, was 6.4 times as frequent in responders to continuation treatment who were subsequently randomized to placebo (26%) than sertraline (5%).

Responders to medication in a 12-week double-blind placebo-controlled trial of fluoxetine for PTSD were randomized to another 24 weeks of treatment with fluoxetine or placebo (Martenyi et al., 2002a). Relapse was defined as an increase from baseline at week 12 of acute treatment by 40% on the TOP-8 score and an increase ≥ 2 on the CGI-S. Time to relapse was significantly longer in the medication than the placebo group, with a lower proportion of the 131 responders to acute-phase fluoxetine treatment relapsing (5.8%) after continuation with medication than placebo (16.1%). Patients who were randomized to fluoxetine continued to improve significantly on the clinical and PTSD severity scores, as well as in anxiety and depression symptoms.

Davidson et al. (2005) randomized 62 subjects to 6-months continuation treatment with fluoxetine or placebo after the same period of open-label treatment (max. 60 mg/day) with fluoxetine. Relapse was defined as either an untoward clinical event (e.g. psychiatric hospitalization) during the randomization phase, or an increase of at least 2 points on the CGI-I since randomization, or as no improvement or worsening of symptoms on the CGI-I relative to open-label baseline. Although a relatively strong effect of medication was observed in preventing relapse during the maintenance phase of the study, relapse rates were high for both the participants who continued receiving a stable dose of fluoxetine (22%) as well as for those whose medication was discontinued (50%).

The efficacy of maintenance treatment with the selective GABA reuptake inhibitor tiagabine was tested by randomizing 18 completers of 12 weeks of open-label treatment with tiagabine (max. dose: 16 mg/day) to ongoing medication treatment or placebo for an additional 12 weeks (Connor et al., 2006). No differences in clinical response were detected.

The limited evidence reviewed above suggests that treatment with SSRIs may be beneficial over the long term. These agents also appear to be well tolerated amongst those patients who have achieved stable doses, with no drug-related adverse events reported for more than 20% of subjects in any of the relapse prevention studies reviewed.

Treatment-refractory cases

A large proportion of patients with PTSD fail to respond to treatment. This is evident from the controlled trials included in this review, where approximately half of the patients in the 23 RCTs that provided this information responded to treatment (mean: 55.8%, SD: 14.8) (Table 9.1). In a recent review, Ipser et al. (2006) identified only three RCTs that assessed augmentation strategies for treating PTSD in populations that could be defined as treatment resistant using strict criteria (Bartzokis et al., 2005; Raskind et al., 2003; Stein et al., 2002) (Table 9.4). These trials are briefly described below, as well as a small study of the antipsychotic risperidone that was subsequently published (Rothbaum et al., 2008).

Dysregulation of the sympathetic system and the centrality of hyperarousal symptoms in PTSD suggest that antagonists of adrenergic receptors might be effective in treating refractory patients. A small 20-week double-blinded cross-over study of the efficacy of the alpha-1 adrenergic antagonist prazosin in treating sleep disturbances in patients with chronic PTSD reported clinically significant improvement following medication treatment in PTSD and sleep symptoms (Raskind et al., 2003).

The presence of psychotic symptoms in complicated cases of PTSD, and possible dysregulation of the dopaminergic system in PTSD, suggests that antipsychotic agents might be effective in augmenting treatment with serotonergic agents. The first antipsychotic tested in an RCT for PTSD was olanzapine (Stein et al., 2002). This agent was administered for the treatment of chronic PTSD in war veterans who did not respond to a minimum of 12 weeks of prior treatment with a psychotropic medication (Stein et al., 2002). Olanzapine significantly reduced symptom severity on the CAPS and sleep disturbance after 8 weeks of double-blind treatment, despite the absence of psychosis in any of the patients.

The effectiveness of risperidone has been assessed in two RCTs. Sixty-five veterans with non-psychotic PTSD who participated in a 5-week psychotherapy residential program were randomized to a placebo-controlled trial of risperidone (maximum dose = 3 mg at bedtime) (Bartzokis et al., 2005). Superiority of medication was observed after 16 weeks in reducing PTSD symptoms as well as anxiety and negative and positive psychotic symptoms. In one of the few trials to assess pharmacotherapy for treatment-resistant PTSD in a non-veteran population, Rothbaum et al. (2008) administered 0.5–3 mg/day of add-on risperidone for

Table 9.4. Randomized placebo-controlled augmentation studies.

Medication agents	P.I.	Year	Duration (weeks)	Sample size	% Males	% War trauma	% other meds	Min. Severity	Outcome scales
Alpha-adrenergic agonists									
Prazosin	Raskind	2003	10	10	100	100	70	CAPS distressing dreams item => 6	CAPS, CGI-I
Antipsychotics									
Olanzapine	Stein	2002	8	21	100	100	100	–	CAPS, CGI-I, CES-D PSQI
Risperidone	Bartzokis	2005	16	65	100	100	92	CAPS => 65	CAPS, HAM-D, HAM-A, PANSS-P
	Rothbaum	2008	8	20	20	0	100	CAPS => 50	CAPS, DTS, PANSS, BDI, CGI-I

CAPS, Clinician Administered PTSD Scale; BDI, Becks Depression Inventory; CES-D, Center for Epidemiologic Studies Depression Scale; CGI-I, Clinical Global Impression scale – Improvement item; DTS, Davidson Trauma Scale; HAM-A, Hamilton Anxiety scale; HAM-D, Hamilton Depression scale; PANSS, Positive and Negative Syndrome Scale; PANSS-P, Positive and Negative Syndrome Scale-Positive; PSQI, Pittsburgh Sleep Quality Index.

8 weeks to patients who failed to achieve a 75% reduction in total score on the CAPS after 8 weeks of open-label treatment with sertraline (25–200 mg/day). Virtually identical differences were observed on the CAPS at end-point in the placebo and medication groups. Approximately a third of the patients treated with risperidone (4/11) dropped out due to possibly treatment-related adverse events.

The majority of controlled trials of pharmacotherapy in combating anxiety disorders add a course of antipsychotics to ongoing treatment with SSRIs (Ipser *et al.*, 2006). In general, findings from trials of PTSD appear to support the efficacy of this strategy, at least with respect to combat-related traumas. There is less evidence regarding the management of PTSD in civilian populations. There is evidence that prazosin may be particularly effective in treating sleep disturbances associated with PTSD, a finding that has been replicated in at least one other RCT (Taylor *et al.*, 2008).

Conclusion

Medication appears to be effective in treating PTSD over the short term, with the largest body of evidence of efficacy for the SSRIs and venlafaxine. The agents appear relatively fast-acting, with response reported as early as the first 2–4 weeks of treatment. Nevertheless, maximizing response to medication might require treatment for substantially longer, with RCTs of paroxetine and fluoxetine observing substantial improvements in clinical response beyond 12 weeks of treatment (Martenyi *et al.*, 2002a). No evidence of efficacy was available for the benzodiazepines, despite their continued popularity in clinical practice (Cloos & Ferreira, 2009).

The current evidence-base supports the efficacy and tolerability of treatment with the SSRIs over the longer term. The finding that over a quarter of patients relapsed after discontinuation of fluoxetine treatment after up to 26 weeks of treatment (Davidson et al., 2001a) provides some support to the consensus that treatment of chronic PTSD with medication should be continued for at least 1 year. Of the two FDA-approved agents for the treatment of PTSD, stronger support is available for the efficacy of paroxetine than sertraline. This calls into question the usefulness of including sertraline as the gold-standard comparator in trials comparing the efficacy of different medications (Chung et al., 2004; McRae et al., 2004; Saygin et al., 2002; Smajkic et al., 2001).

War trauma is commonly perceived as being prognostic of a poorer response to treatment, with nine of the 11 trials that included a majority of trauma veterans failing to demonstrate efficacy for pharmacotherapy. The finding in a 12-week trial of fluoxetine of increased response in patients recently exposed to combat suggests that the salient characteristic with regards to medication response might be duration of PTSD, rather than combat trauma or gender, per se (Martenyi et al., 2002b).

Neither of the dose-comparison studies of fluoxetine or paroxetine were able to detect significant differences in efficacy between higher and lower doses (Marshall et al., 2001; Martenyi et al., 2007). This is consistent with the general observation of a flat response curve for the SSRIs, and suggests that it might be prudent to initiate medication treatment at the low end of the recommended dose range, with the aim of minimizing potential treatment-related adverse events. Future research should address the comparative efficacy of doses of venlafaxine, as there is evidence in studies of depression that the efficacy of venlafaxine is dose-dependent (Stahl et al., 2005). It is notable that the maximum dose of venlafaxine in both of the RCTs of this agent in PTSD conducted to date were higher than the FDA guidelines for the licensed prescription of this medication for depression (Davidson et al., 2006a, 2006b).

There has recently been interest shown in the treatment of PTSD with medications that employ extra-serotonergic mechanisms of action, including the anticonvulsants, atypical antipsychotics, and venlafaxine. With the exception of risperidone and venlafaxine, the results of these trials have been disappointing. Positive results from small under-powered studies of risperidone need to be followed up with larger placebo-controlled trials. Similarly, although medications such as prazosin and the atypical antipsychotics appear to hold promise as augmenting agents, much additional work is needed to determine how best to manage PTSD symptoms in treatment-refractory patients.

Acknowledgments

The authors would like to thank Carli Sager for assisting with trial selection and data extraction. We are also grateful to the PIs who responded to requests for information required to determine the eligibility of trials for inclusion in the review. Drs Mark Hamner, Mark Pollack, Gina Manguno-Mire, and Jonathan Davidson were particularly helpful in this regard. Finally, Dr. Michael Hertzberg kindly responded to queries concerning trial methodology.

Statement of interest

Jonathan Ipser declares no conflicts of interest.

Dan Stein has received research grants and/or consultancy honoraria from AstraZeneca, Eli-Lilly, GlaxoSmithKline, Lundbeck, Orion, Pfizer, Pharmacia, Roche, Servier, Solvay, Sumitomo, and Wyeth.

References

Adamou M, Puchalska S, Plummer W, Hale AS (2007). Valproate in the treatment of PTSD: systematic review and meta analysis. *Current Medical Research and Opinion* 23(6), 1285–1291.

American Psychiatric Association (APA) (1994). *Diagnostic and Statistical Manual of Mental Disorders (3rd edn – revised)*. Washington, DC: American Psychiatric Association.

Baker DG, Diamond BI, Gillette G et al. (1995). A double-blind, randomized, placebo-controlled, multi-center study of brofaromine in the treatment of post-traumatic stress disorder. *Psychopharmacology (Berlin)* 122(4), 386–389.

Bartzokis G, Lu PH, Turner J et al. (2005). Adjunctive risperidone in the treatment of chronic combat-related posttraumatic stress disorder. *Biological Psychiatry* 57, 474–479.

Blake DD, Weathers FW, Nagy LM et al. (1995). The development of a clinician-administered PTSD scale. *Journal of Traumatic Stress* 8, 75–90.

Brady K, Pearlstein T, Asnis GM et al. (2000). Efficacy and safety of sertraline treatment of posttraumatic stress disorder: a randomized controlled trial. *Journal of the American Medical Association* 283(14), 1837–1844.

Brady KT, Sonne S, Anton RF et al. (2005). Sertraline in the treatment of co-occurring alcohol dependence and posttraumatic stress disorder. *Alcoholism: Clinical and Experimental Research* 29, 395–401.

Braun P, Greenberg D, Dasberg H, Lerer B (1990). Core symptoms of posttraumatic stress disorder unimproved by alprazolam treatment. *Journal of Clinical Psychiatry* 51(6), 236–238.

Breslau N, Kessler RC, Chilcoat HD et al. (1998). Trauma and posttraumatic stress disorder in the community: the 1996 Detroit Area Survey of Trauma. *Archives of General Psychiatry* 55, 626–632.

Brunello N, Davidson JR, Deahl M et al. (2001). Posttraumatic stress disorder: diagnosis and epidemiology, comorbidity and social consequences, biology and treatment. *Neuropsychobiology* 43(3), 150–162.

Butterfield MI, Becker ME, Connor KM et al. (2001). Olanzapine in the treatment of post-traumatic stress disorder: a pilot study. *International Clinical Psychopharmacology* 16(4), 197–203.

Chung MY, Min KH, Jun YJ et al. (2004). Efficacy and tolerability of mirtazapine and sertraline in Korean veterans with posttraumatic stress disorder: a randomized open label trial. *Human Psychopharmacology* 19(7), 489–494.

Cloos JM, Ferreira V (2009). Current use of benzodiazepines in anxiety disorders. *Current Opinion in Psychiatry* 22(1), 90–95.

Cohen J (1988). *Statistical Power Analysis for the Behavioral Sciences (2nd edition)*. New York, NY: Academic Press.

Connor KM, Davidson JR (1999). Further psychometric assessment of the TOP-8: a brief interview-based measure of PTSD. *Depression and Anxiety* 9(3), 135–137.

Connor KM, Davidson JR, Weisler RH et al. (2006). Tiagabine for posttraumatic stress disorder: effects of open-label and double-blind discontinuation treatment. *Psychopharmacology* 184, 21–25.

Connor KM, Sutherland SM, Tupler LA et al. (1999). Fluoxetine in post-traumatic stress disorder. Randomised, double-blind study. *British Journal of Psychiatry* 175, 17–22.

Davidson J, Baldwin D, Stein DJ et al. (2006a). Treatment of posttraumatic stress disorder with venlafaxine extended release: a 6-month randomized controlled trial. *Archives of General Psychiatry* 63, 1158–1165.

Davidson J, Kudler H, Smith R et al. (1990). Treatment of posttraumatic stress disorder with amitriptyline and placebo. *Archives of General Psychiatry* 47, 259–266.

Davidson J, Pearlstein T, Londborg P et al. (2001a). Efficacy of sertraline in preventing relapse of posttraumatic stress disorder: results of a 28-week double-blind, placebo-controlled study. *American Journal of Psychiatry* 158, 1974–1981.

Davidson J, Rothbaum BO, Tucker P *et al.* (2006*b*). Venlafaxine extended release in posttraumatic stress disorder: a sertraline- and placebo-controlled study. *Journal of Clinical Psychopharmacology* **26**, 259–267.

Davidson JR, Brady K, Mellman TA, Stein MB, *et al.* (2007). The efficacy and tolerability of tiagabine in adult patients with post-traumatic stress disorder. *Journal of Clinical Psychopharmacology*, **27**(1): 85–88.

Davidson JR, Connor KM, Hertzberg MA *et al.* (2005). Maintenance therapy with fluoxetine in posttraumatic stress disorder: a placebo-controlled discontinuation study. *Journal of Clinical Psychopharmacology* **25**, 166–169.

Davidson JR, Rothbaum BO, van der Kolk BA *et al.* (2001*b*). Multicenter, double-blind comparison of sertraline and placebo in the treatment of posttraumatic stress disorder. *Archives of General Psychiatry* **58**, 485–492.

Davidson JR, Weisler RH, Butterfield MI *et al.* (2003). Mirtazapine vs. placebo in posttraumatic stress disorder: a pilot trial. *Biological Psychiatry* **53**, 188–191.

Davis LL, Davidson JR, Ward LC *et al.* (2008). Divalproex in the treatment of posttraumatic stress disorder: a randomized, double-blind, placebo-controlled trial in a veteran population. *Journal of Clinical Psychopharmacology* **28**, 84–88.

Davis LL, Jewell ME, Ambrose S *et al.* (2004). A placebo-controlled study of nefazodone for the treatment of chronic posttraumatic stress disorder: a preliminary study. *Journal of Clinical Psychopharmacology* **24**, 291–297.

Deeks J, Altman D, Bradburn M (2001). Statistical methods for examining heterogeneity and combining results from several studies in meta-analysis. In Egger, M, Davey, SG, Altman, DG (Eds.), *Systematic Reviews in Health Care: Meta-Analysis in Context (2nd edition).* London: BMJ Publication Group.

DerSimonian R, Laird N (1986). Meta-analysis in clinical trials. *Controlled Clinical Trials* **7**(3), 177–188.

Frans O, Rimmö PA, Aberg L, Fredrikson M (2005). Trauma exposure and post-traumatic stress disorder in the general population. *Acta Psychiatrica Scandinavica* **111**(4), 291–299.

Friedman MJ, Marmar CR, Baker DG *et al.* (2007). Randomized, double-blind comparison of sertraline and placebo for posttraumatic stress disorder in a Department of Veterans Affairs setting. *Journal of Clinical Psychiatry* **68**, 711–720.

Guy W (1976). *ECDEU Assessment Manual for Psychopharmacology.* Washington, DC: National Institute of Health.

Hertzberg MA, Butterfield MI, Feldman ME *et al.* (1999). A preliminary study of lamotrigine for the treatment of posttraumatic stress disorder. *Biological Psychiatry* **45**, 1226–1229.

Hertzberg MA, Feldman ME, Beckham JC *et al.* (2000). Lack of efficacy for fluoxetine in PTSD: a placebo controlled trial in combat veterans. *Annals of Clinical Psychiatry* **12**, 101–105.

Higgins JPT, Altman DG (2008). *Cochrane Handbook for Systematic Reviews of Interventions Version 5.0.0* (updated February 2008). The Cochrane Collaboration.

Institute of Medicine (IOM) (2009). *Treatment of Posttraumatic Stress Disorder: An Assessment of the Evidence.* Washington, DC: Institute of Medicine.

Ipser JC, Carey P, Dhansay Y *et al.* (2006). Pharmacotherapy augmentation strategies in treatment-resistant anxiety disorders. *Cochrane Database of Systematic Reviews* **4**, 1. CD005473.

Kaplan Z, Amir M, Swartz M, Levine J (1996). Inositol treatment of post-traumatic stress disorder. *Anxiety* **2**, 51–52.

Katz RJ, Lott MH, Arbus P *et al.* (1994). Pharmacotherapy of post-traumatic stress disorder with a novel psychotropic. *Anxiety* **1**, 169–174.

Kessler RC, Berglund P, Demler O *et al.* (2005). Lifetime prevalence and age-of-onset distributions of DSM–IV disorders in the National Comorbidity Survey Replication. *Archives of General Psychiatry* **62**, 593–602.

Kosten TR, Frank JB, Dan E *et al.* (1991). Pharmacotherapy for posttraumatic stress disorder using phenelzine or imipramine. *Journal of Nervous Mental Disorders* **179**(6), 366–370.

Londborg PD, Hegel MT, Goldstein S *et al.* (2001). Sertraline treatment of posttraumatic stress disorder: results of 24 weeks of open-label continuation treatment. *Journal of Clinical Psychiatry* **62**, 325–331.

Marshall RD, Beebe KL, Oldham M, Zaninelli R (2001). Efficacy and safety of paroxetine treatment for chronic PTSD: a fixed-dose, placebo-controlled study. *American Journal of Psychiatry* **158**, 1982–1988.

Marshall RD, Lewis-Fernandez R, Blanco C, Simpson HB *et al.* (2007). A controlled trial of paroxetine for chronic PTSD, dissociation, and interpersonal problems in mostly minority adults. *Depression and Anxiety* **24**(2), 77–84.

Martenyi F, Brown EB, Caldwell CD (2007). Failed efficacy of fluoxetine in the treatment of posttraumatic stress disorder: results of a fixed-dose, placebo-controlled study. *Journal of Clinical Psychopharmacology* **27**, 166–170.

Martenyi F, Brown EB, Zhang H *et al.* (2002a). Fluoxetine v. placebo in prevention of relapse in post-traumatic stress disorder. *British Journal of Psychiatry* **181**, 315–320.

Martenyi F, Brown EB, Zhang H *et al.* (2002b). Fluoxetine versus placebo in posttraumatic stress disorder. *Journal of Clinical Psychiatry* **63**, 199–206.

McRae AL, Brady KT, Mellman TA *et al.* (2004). Comparison of nefazodone and sertraline for the treatment of posttraumatic stress disorder. *Depression and Anxiety* **19**(3), 190–196.

Mooney P, Oakley J, Ferriter M, Travers R (2004). Sertraline as a treatment for PTSD: a systematic review and meta-analysis. *Irish Journal of Psychological Medicine* **21**, 100–103.

Padala PR, Madison J, Monnahan M *et al.* (2006). Risperidone monotherapy for post-traumatic stress disorder related to sexual assault and domestic abuse in women. *International Clinical Psychopharmacology* **21**(5), 275–280.

Penava SJ, Otto MW, Pollack MH, Rosenbaum JF (1996). Current status of pharmacotherapy for PTSD: an effect size analysis of controlled studies. *Depression and Anxiety* **4**(5), 240–242.

Post RM, Chalecka-Franaszek E, Hough CJ (2003). Mechanisms of action of anticonvulsants and new mood stabilizers. In Soares JC, Gershon S (Eds.), *Handbook of Medical Psychiatry* (pp. 767–791). New York, NY: Marcel Dekker.

Raskind MA, Peskind ER, Kanter ED *et al.* (2003). Reduction of nightmares and other PTSD symptoms in combat veterans by prazosin: a placebo-controlled study. *American Journal of Psychiatry* **160**, 371–373.

Reich DB, Winternitz S, Hennen J *et al.* (2004). A preliminary study of risperidone in the treatment of posttraumatic stress disorder related to childhood abuse in women. *Journal of Clinical Psychiatry* **65**, 1601–1606.

Reist C, Kauffmann CD, Haier RJ *et al.* (1989). A controlled trial of desipramine in 18 men with posttraumatic stress disorder. *American Journal of Psychiatry* **146**, 513–516.

Rothbaum BO, Killeen TK, Davidson JR *et al.* (2008). Placebo-controlled trial of risperidone augmentation for selective serotonin reuptake inhibitor-resistant civilian posttraumatic stress disorder. *Journal of Clinical Psychiatry* **69**, 520–525.

Saygin MZ, Sungur MZ, Sabol EU, Cetinkaya P (2002). Nefazodone versus sertraline in the treatment of posttraumatic stress disorder. *Bulletin of Clinical Psychopharmacology* **12**(1), 1–5.

Shestatzky M, Greenberg D, Lerer B (1988). A controlled trial of phenelzine in posttraumatic stress disorder. *Psychiatry Research* **24**, 149–155.

Smajkic A, Weine S, Djuric-Bijedic Z *et al.* (2001). Sertraline, paroxetine, and venlafaxine in refugee posttraumatic stress disorder with depression symptoms. *Journal of Traumatic Stress* **14**, 445–452.

Stahl SM, Grady MM, Moret C, Briley M (2005). SNRIs: the pharmacology, clinical efficacy, and tolerability in comparison with other classes of antidepressants. *CNS Spectrums* **10**, 732–747.

Stein DJ, Ipser J, McAnda N (2009). Pharmacotherapy of posttraumatic stress disorder: a review of meta-analyses and treatment guidelines. *CNS Spectrums* **14**(1 Suppl. 1), 25–31.

Stein DJ, Ipser JC, Seedat S (2006). Pharmacotherapy for post traumatic stress disorder (PTSD). *Cochrane Database of Systematic Reviews* **1**, CD002795.

Stein MB, Kline NA, Matloff JL (2002). Adjunctive olanzapine for SSRI-resistant combat-related PTSD: a double-blind, placebo-controlled study. *American Journal of Psychiatry* **159**, 1777–1779.

Stewart C, Wrobel T (2009). Evaluation of the efficacy of pharmacotherapy and psychotherapy in treatment of combat-related post-traumatic stress disorder: a meta-analytic review of outcome studies. *Military Medicine* **174**, 460–469.

Taylor FB, Martin P, Thompson C et al. (2008). Prazosin effects on objective sleep measures and clinical symptoms in civilian trauma posttraumatic stress disorder: a placebo-controlled study. *Biological Psychiatry* **63**, 629–632.

Tucker P, Potter-Kimball R, Wyatt DB et al. (2003). Can physiologic assessment and side effects tease out differences in PTSD trials? A double-blind comparison of citalopram, sertraline, and placebo. *Psychopharmacology Bulletin* **37**(3), 135–149.

Tucker P, Trautman RP, Wyatt DB et al. (2007). Efficacy and safety of topiramate monotherapy in civilian posttraumatic stress disorder: a randomized, double-blind, placebo-controlled study. *Journal of Clinical Psychiatry* **68**(2), 201–206.

Tucker P, Zaninelli R, Yehuda R et al. (2001). Paroxetine in the treatment of chronic posttraumatic stress disorder: results of a placebo-controlled, flexible-dosage trial. *Journal of Clinical Psychiatry* **62**, 860–868.

van der Kolk BA, Dreyfuss D, Michaels M et al. (1994). Fluoxetine in posttraumatic stress disorder. *Journal of Clinical Psychiatry* **55**(12), 517–522.

van der Kolk BA, Spinazzola J, Blaustein ME et al. (2007). A randomized clinical trial of eye movement desensitization and reprocessing (EMDR), fluoxetine, and pill placebo in the treatment of posttraumatic stress disorder: treatment effects and long-term maintenance. *Journal of Clinical Psychiatry* **68**(1), 37–46.

Van Etten ML, Taylor S (1998). Comparative efficacy of treatments for post-traumatic stress disorder: a meta-analysis. *Clinical Psychology and Psychotherapy* **5**, 126–144.

Viechtbauer W (2010). Conducting meta-analyses in R with the metafor package. *Journal of Statistical Software* **36**(3), 1–48.

Zohar J, Amital D, Miodownik C et al. (2002). Double-blind placebo-controlled pilot study of sertraline in military veterans with posttraumatic stress disorder. *Journal of Clinical Psychopharmacology* **22**(2), 190–195.

Evidence-based pharmacotherapy of eating disorders

Martine F. Flament, Hany Bissada, and Wendy Spettigue

Introduction

Eating disorders (EDs) are widespread, disabling, and often chronic psychiatric disorders. Anorexia nervosa (AN) and bulimia nervosa (BN) share a morbid preoccupation with weight and shape. AN is characterized by an ego-syntonic restriction of food intake resulting in a body weight lower than 85% of normal, and can be of restricting type (dieting and excessive exercise) or binge eating/purging type (associated binge/purge behaviors) (American Psychiatric Association, 1994). The eating pattern in BN consists of recurring disinhibition of restraint, resulting in cycles of binge eating and compensatory behaviors to prevent weight gain, including self-induced vomiting and abuse of laxatives/diuretics in the purging type, or extreme exercise and fasting in the non-purging type. Most individuals with BN maintain an average body weight (Fairburn & Harrison, 2003). Binge-eating disorder (BED) is characterized by recurrent binge-eating episodes accompanied by a sense of distress, loss of control, and feelings of disgust, depression, or guilt (Spitzer *et al.*, 1991). Most persons with BED are obese, and often seek treatment for weight loss rather than for disturbed eating behaviors. Night eating syndrome (NES) is a form of BED characterized by consumption of at least 25% of food intake after the evening meal, conscious nocturnal eating at least twice a week for 3 months, or both (Allison *et al.*, 2010). The American Psychiatric Association is recommending modifications to some of the diagnostic criteria for EDs in the forthcoming revision of the DSM (DSM–V). Suggested changes include: "markedly low body weight" to replace 'body weight less than 85% of that expected," and removal of the amenorrhea criterion for AN; listing of BED as a stand-alone diagnosis, and NES as a form of BED; restricting the diagnosis of BN to the purging form, with the non-purging form classified as BED; and a frequency criterion of at least once a week (rather than twice a week) for binge eating and/or inappropriate compensatory behaviors in the diagnosis of BN or BED (www.DSM5.org).

In young women, lifetime prevalence rates have been estimated at 0.3–0.9% for AN, 1–2% for BN, 3.5% for BED, and up to 10% for eating disorders not otherwise specified (EDNOS); among males, lifetime prevalence estimates are 0.3% for AN, 0.5% for BN, and 2.0% for BED (Grucza *et al.*, 2007; Hoek, 2006; Hoek & Van Hoeken, 2003; Hudson *et al.*, 2007; Machado *et al.*, 2007). In children and adolescents, EDs profoundly affect physical, emotional, and psychosocial development. In both youth and adults, psychiatric

Essential Evidence-Based Psychopharmacology, Second Edition, ed. Dan J. Stein, Bernard Lerer, and Stephen M. Stahl. Published by Cambridge University Press. © Cambridge University Press.

complications include social isolation, major depression, severe anxiety, substance abuse, and suicide (Hudson *et al.*, 2007), and medical complications encompass cardiac problems, osteopenia, and infertility (Mitchell & Crow, 2006). The mortality among women with an ED is as high as 20% (Nielsen, 2001), and the impact of EDs on the healthcare system is enormous (Simon *et al.*, 2005).

The objective of this paper is to review currently available evidence for efficacy and safety of pharmacotherapy in adults and children with EDs. We conducted a computer search of MEDLINE and PsycINFO databases for pharmacotherapy of AN, BN, and BED from 1960 to May 2010. The search included: randomized controlled trials (RCTs); if none were available (e.g. for pediatric EDs), open trials or case reports suggesting benefits, systematic reviews, meta-analyses, and guidelines. Pharmacotherapy for AN, BN, BED, and NES are presented consecutively. Findings from clinically relevant RCTs are summarized in Tables 10.1–10.9. Other studies and meta-analyses are described in the text. For AN and BN, studies conducted in pediatric populations are reported separately (whenever available). Based on the evidence reviewed, we address three questions: (1) What is the first-line pharmacotherapy of choice for EDs? (2) What is the evidence for maintenance treatment? (3) What is the best approach to treatment resistance?

Pharmacotherapy of AN

Antipsychotics (Table 10.1)

It was initially argued that patients with AN should be treated with antipsychotics because their obsessions regarding weight and body shape could be viewed as delusional. Early RCTs have tested chlorpromazine (Dally & Sargant, 1966), pimozide (Vandereycken & Pierloot, 1982), and sulpiride (Vandereycken, 1984), with trends for higher weight gain, but no advantage on eating attitudes and behaviors. Given their potential for short- and long-term side-effects, and the fact that weight gain in anorexic patients tends not to persist if not accompanied by changes in attitudes towards eating and body shape, the treatment of AN with traditional antipsychotics is no longer recommended.

The atypical antipsychotics have a side-effect profile that often includes weight gain and an increased serotonin to dopamine blockade ratio, which make them potential candidates for pharmacotherapy of AN (see Table 10.1). In a small randomized trial, olanzapine was superior to chlorpromazine for reduction of anorexic ruminations (Mondraty *et al.*, 2005). Brambilla *et al.* (2007) compared individual cognitive–behavioral treatment (CBT) with and without olanzapine. There was a greater improvement in depression, anxiety, obsessive-compulsiveness, and aggressiveness in the olanzapine group. The increase in body mass index (BMI) was larger for participants with AN binge/purge type receiving olanzapine. Bissada *et al.* (2008) compared olanzapine with placebo, and concluded that olanzapine may be safely used in AN to achieve more rapid weight gain and reduce obsessive symptoms, as measured on the Yale–Brown Obsessive–Compulsive Rating Scale (YBOCS); there were no serious side-effects, and no evidence of impaired glucose tolerance. Quetiapine (50–800 mg/day) has been investigated in two small open studies, with significant changes in BMI and the Eating Disorder Examination (EDE) restraint subscale in one study (Bosanac *et al.*, 2007), and decreases in measures of anxiety, depression, and the Positive and Negative Syndrome Scale (PANSS) score, but no significant change in BMI in another (Powers *et al.*, 2007). Trunko

Table 10.1. Controlled pharmacological trials with atypical antipsychotics in anorexia nervosa (AN).

Authors, country	N (drug/ placebo):[a] ITT, Completers Inclusion criteria	Study design and duration	Medication (daily dose)	Results	Follow-up data
Mondraty et al. (2005) Australia	8/7 In-patients with AN (DSM-IV)	Parallel olanzapine (mean 46 days) vs. chlorpromazine (mean 53 days)	Olanzapine (maximum 20 mg) chlorpromazine (maximum 200 mg)	Olanzapine > chlorpromazine for reduction of anorexic ruminations Olanzapine = chlorpromazine for weight gain	n.a.
Brambilla et al. (2007) Italy	15/15 Outpatients with AN (DSM-IV)	Parallel CBT + olanzapine vs. CBT + placebo 12 weeks	Olanzapine (maximum 5 mg)	CBT + olanzapine > CBT + placebo for weight gain (binge/purge type only), and improvement of depression, anxiety, obsessive symptoms and aggressiveness	n.a.
Bissada et al. (2008) Canada	16/18 14/14 Day hospital patients with AN (DSM-IV)	Parallel Olanzapine vs. placebo 13 weeks	Olanzapine (maximum 10 mg)	Olanzapine > placebo for weight gain and improvement of obsessive symptoms	n.a.

CBT, Cognitive behavioral treatment; n.a., not available.
[a] When available, sample sizes are indicated with both intent-to-treat (ITT) (normal text) and completers (*italics*) numbers, in this and the following tables.

et al. (2010) reported on eight patients (five with AN, three with BN) treated with aripiprazole, in addition to an antidepressant, for 4 months to 3 years. They described a significant reduction in eating-specific anxiety as well as obsessional thoughts about food, weight, and body image, and full or partial weight restoration in all AN patients; the drug was well tolerated.

Antipsychotics in children and adolescents

Small case series using olanzapine in children and adolescents suggested: decrease in body-image concerns, agitation, and anxiety regarding eating (Mehler *et al.*, 2001); decreased agitation and anxiety, and improved weight gain (Boachie *et al.*, 2003); and decreased eating anxiety and ruminations (Dennis *et al.*, 2006). Barbarich *et al.* (2004a) conducted a 6-week open trial of olanzapine in 17 adolescent or adult patients with AN. Olanzapine significantly reduced depression, anxiety, and ED symptoms, and significantly increased weight; there were no dropouts from the study, and no abnormal biological findings. In a retrospective chart review, Norris *et al.* (2011) compared 43 adolescents with AN treated with olanzapine (2.5–7.5 mg/day) to controls. Those on olanzapine had greater illness severity and higher rates of comorbidity. Side-effects (albeit mild) were reported in 56%, including abnormal lipid profiles in 29%. Two single case reports indicated possible benefits of risperidone for treating pediatric AN (Fisman *et al.*, 1996; Newman-Toker, 2000), and Mehler-Wex *et al.* (2008) reported three cases treated successfully with adjunctive quetiapine.

Tricyclic antidepressants (TCAs)

Due to clinical and biological similarities between AN and depression (Halmi *et al.*, 1991), the tricyclic antidepressants (TCAs) were seen, 30 years ago, as the most promising drug treatment for AN. Unfortunately, findings from a few RCTs using amitriptyline (Biederman *et al.*, 1985; Halmi *et al.*, 1986) or clomipramine (Crisp *et al.*, 1987; Lacey & Crisp, 1980) have not been encouraging. Given, on the one hand, the limited evidence for any clinical benefit and, on the other, the lethal risk with overdose and the potential for fatal arrhythmia at low body weight, particularly in youth, this type of medication is not recommended today for AN.

Selective serotonin reuptake inhibitors (SSRIs) (Table 10.2)

In the last decades, selective serotonin reuptake inhibitors (SSRIs) have been increasingly used to treat AN, but only two have been tested in RCTs, with mostly negative results. Fluoxetine conveyed no advantage over placebo for underweight AN inpatients (Attia *et al.*, 1998), nor for AN outpatients treated with fluoxetine plus serotonin precursors (Barbarich *et al.*, 2004b). Kaye *et al.* (2001) randomly assigned restricting AN patients to fluoxetine or placebo after inpatient weight gain. In the following year, women receiving fluoxetine had a significantly lower rate of relapse than those treated with placebo. However, limitations of this study include its small size (only 13 completers), and the lack of standardized psychological treatment during the medication trial. In a larger RCT including 93 weight-restored outpatients randomized to CBT plus fluoxetine or placebo, Walsh *et al.* (2006) found no difference in relapse rate after 1 year. Fassino *et al.* (2002) conducted a RCT comparing citalopram with a waitlist condition in restricting AN patients. Weight gain was similar in both groups, but citalopram appeared to improve depression, obsessive–compulsive symptoms, impulsiveness, and trait-anger.

SSRIs in children and adolescents

Holtkamp *et al.* (2005) retrospectively compared 19 partially weight-restored adolescents with AN treated with fluoxetine (mean 35 mg/day), fluvoxamine (35 mg/day), or sertraline (100 mg/day) with 13 unmedicated adolescent patients. They found no group differences in BMI, ED, depression or obsessive–compulsive scores, and concluded that there was no effect of SSRIs on the course of illness. Given the limited evidence to support their use, SSRIs should be reserved for treating comorbid depression or anxiety in pediatric patients with AN who have been weight-restored. Due to concerns about possibly increased suicidal ideation in young people on SSRIs, medication should be monitored closely. Currently, fluoxetine has the most evidence favoring its use for treating depression and anxiety in children and adolescents.

Other antidepressants

Mirtazapine is a non-SSRI sedative antidepressant which increases appetite and induces weight gain. One open trial by Schüle *et al.* (2006) reported weight gain on mirtazapine in five AN inpatients.

Table 10.2. Controlled pharmacological trials with selective serotonin reuptake inhibitors (SSRIs) in anorexia nervosa (AN).

Authors, country	N (drug/ placebo): ITT, *Completers* Inclusion criteria	Study design and duration	Medication (daily dose)	Results	Follow-up data
Attia *et al.* (1998) USA	15/16 *11/12* Underweight inpatients with AN (DSM–IV)	Parallel fluoxetine vs. placebo 7 weeks	Fluoxetine (mean 56 mg)	Fluoxetine = placebo for weight gain and changes in ED or associated symptoms	n.a.
Barbarich *et al.* (2004b) USA	15/11 *7/2* Underweight inpatients with AN (DSM–IV)	Parallel fluoxetine + nutritional supplements vs. fluoxetine + placebo 6 months	Fluoxetine (20–60 mg)	Nutritional supplements are ineffective in increasing the efficacy of fluoxetine	n.a.
Kaye *et al.* (2001) USA	16/19 *10/3* Weight-restored outpatients with restricting and binge/purge type AN (DSM–IV)	Relapse prevention study, parallel fluoxetine vs. placebo 52 weeks	Fluoxetine (20–60 mg)	Fluoxetine > placebo for completion rate (63% vs. 16%) Fluoxetine > placebo for weight gain, reduction of ED and associated symptoms, and decreased relapse rate Study did not control for drug dose or other treatments received during study period	
Fassino *et al.* (2002) Italy	26/26 *19/20* Outpatients with restricting type AN (DSM–IV)	Parallel citalopram vs. waitlist 12 weeks	Citalopram (10–20 mg)	Citalopram > placebo for improvement of depression, obsessive symptoms, impulsiveness, trait anger Citalopram = placebo for weight gain	n.a.
Walsh *et al.* (2006) USA	49/44 *24/16* Weight-restored outpatients with restricting and binge/purge type AN (DSM–IV)	Relapse prevention study parallel fluoxetine vs. placebo 52 weeks	Fluoxetine (mean 63.5 mg)	Fluoxetine = placebo for completion rate, outcome status and time-to-relapse	

ED, Eating disorder; ITT, intent-to-treat; n.a., not available.

Mood stabilizers and anticonvulsants

Lithium is known to induce weight gain and has been used for AN patients in a small RCT, with greater average weight gain on lithium than placebo (Gross *et al.* 1981). However, the use of lithium is not recommended in AN, because sodium and fluid depletion may lead to reduced lithium clearance, resulting in increased potential toxicity. Only a few case reports were found for the use of anti-epileptic medications with mood-stabilizing properties. Available data are mixed, preventing definitive conclusions (McElroy *et al.*, 2009).

Medications that improve gastric emptying (prokinetic agents)

Anorexic patients commonly complain of feelings of fullness, early satiety and bloating. Biological measures of gastric motility may be abnormal (Stacher et al., 1986). Prokinetic agents such as metoclopramide, bethanecol, cisapride, and domperidone, have been suggested as adjuvants to reduce post-prandial abdominal bloating in anorexic patients. Cisapride has been removed from the market because of concerns about potentially fatal cardiac effects.

Opiate antagonists

The opioid peptide system helps modulate appetite and feeding behaviors in animals, and disturbance in the opioid function has been shown in patients with AN (Baranowska et al., 1984).

A RCT by Marrazzi et al. (1995) assessed the efficacy of 200 mg/day of naltrexone in six patients with AN or BN. Although the amount of weight gain was not analyzed, the binge/purge frequency was reduced on naltrexone. However, at the dose used (four times the recommended dose), there is a high risk for significant elevation in hepatic transaminases, reflected in the "black box" warning that "naltrexone can cause hepato-cellular injury at excessive doses."

Appetite enhancers

Cyproheptadine, a serotonin and histamine antagonist noted to produce weight gain in children with asthma, has been tested in controlled trials in anorexic patients, with disappointing results (Goldberg et al., 1979). Halmi et al. (1986) compared amitriptyline (160 mg/day), cyproheptadine (32 mg/day), and placebo in 72 females aged 13–36 years. An unexpected finding was that cyproheptadine decreased the length of time to achieve a healthy weight for the restricting anorexic patients, but significantly impaired treatment efficiency for the binge/purge anorectic patients, compared with amitriptyline and placebo. Tetrahydrocannabinol (THC) has an appetite-stimulating effect and has been tested in a small RCT vs. diazepam in 11 anorexic adults; no significant effect of THC was found on weight gain, while side-effects included sleep disturbance, paranoia, and dysphoria (Gross et al., 1983). It should be emphasized that AN patients are not without appetite (Garfinkel & Garner, 1982), but are frightened about losing control over their hunger; thus, increasing appetite could potentially increase anxiety.

Other medications

AN patients often lose bone mass – 92% develop early osteopenia and 40% progress to osteoporosis – at a time (adolescence and young adulthood) when they should be optimizing bone growth (Grinspoon et al., 2000). Given the effectiveness of bisphosphonates and hormone therapy in the treatment of osteopenic post-menopausal women, their use in AN was evaluated. In a RCT using bisphosphonates, the increase in bone mass density did not differ between active treatment and control groups (Golden et al., 2005). Mehler & MacKenzie (2009) reviewed three RCTs using estrogens in AN. None demonstrated any significant improvement in bone mass density over the control group.

Table 10.3. Controlled pharmacological trials with other medications in anorexia nervosa (AN).

Authors, country	N (drug/placebo): ITT, Completers Inclusion criteria	Study design Duration	Medication (daily dose)	Results	Follow-up data
Katz et al. (1987) USA	7/7 6/7 Adolescents with AN (DSM-III)	Parallel zinc sulfate vs. placebo 6 months	Zinc sulfate (50 mg)	Zinc sulfate = placebo for weight gain Zinc sulfate > placebo for improvement of depression and anxiety	n.a.
Lask et al. (1993) USA	Total N: 26 9- to 14-yr-olds with AN (DSM-III-R)	Cross-over zinc sulfate vs. placebo 6 weeks	Zinc sulfate (50 mg)	Zinc sulfate = placebo for weight gain Zinc levels correlated with degree of malnutrition and returned to normal with refeeding	n.a.
Birmingham et al. (1994) Canada	6/28 16/19 ≥ 15-year-old in-patients with AN (DSM-III-R)	Parallel zinc gluconate vs. placebo. As needed to achieve 10% BMI increase	Zinc gluconate (100 mg)	Rate of BMI increase in zinc supplemented group = twice that in placebo group	n.a.

BMI, Body mass index; ITT, intent-to-treat; n.a., not available.

Other medications in children and adolescents (Table 10.3)

Individuals with zinc deficiency seem to exhibit symptoms similar to AN, i.e. weight loss, depression, appetite and taste changes, and amenorrhea (Zhu & Walsh, 2002). Given the nutritional deprivation in anorexic patients, zinc supplementation has been suggested. Three RCTs conducted in children and adolescents (Birmingham et al., 1994; Katz et al., 1987; Lask et al., 1993) have produced mixed results, and the role of zinc supplementation in AN remains controversial.

Pharmacotherapy of BN

TCAs

Seven RCTs have been published using TCAs for treatment of BN in adults (two with imipramine, four with desipramine, and one with amitriptyline). In all but one, the active drug (imipramine or desipramine) led to a mean reduction in frequency of binge eating (47–91%) significantly superior to that on placebo. However, because TCAs often cause unpleasant side-effects and have the potential to be fatal in overdose, this class of medication is not considered as a first-line pharmacological treatment for BN in adults, and should not be used to treat BN in children or adolescents.

Monoamine oxidase inhibitors (MAOIs)

Four RCTs have used monoamine oxidase inhibitors (MAOIs) (two phenelzine, one isocarboxazid, one brofaromine) in patients with BN. In the Walsh et al. (1988) study, phenelzine

(60–90 mg/day) was superior to placebo for both reduction of binge frequency (64% vs. 5%) and the total number of participants achieving remission after 10 weeks (35% vs. 4%). However, follow-up data indicated that all initial responders had relapsed at 6 months, and by 4 years, 3/15 had experienced severe hypertensive episodes, including one with a fatal outcome (Fallon et al., 1991). In a RCT by Kennedy et al. (1988), 18 women with BN were assigned to either isocarboxazid (60 mg/day) or placebo for 13 weeks; on isocarboxazid, there was a significant reduction in binge eating and vomiting, and no serious adverse effects. A later RCT using phenelzine (75 mg/day) in 18 depressed bulimic patients resulted in significant reduction of both bulimic and depressive symptoms (Rothschild et al., 1994). Brofaromine is a reversible MAOI reported as somewhat effective in individuals with BN (Kennedy et al., 1993), but is not commercially available in the USA. Overall, due to the risk of adverse reactions or drug interactions associated with the use of MAOIs, and the potential for the ingestion of tyramine-containing food during a binge episode causing a hypertensive crisis, MAOIs are not a first-line treatment for BN.

SSRIs (Table 10.4)

Fluoxetine has been the most studied of the SSRIs. A large multicenter trial (Fluoxetine Bulimia Nervosa Collaborative Study Group, 1992) compared two dosages of fluoxetine to placebo. At 60 mg/day, fluoxetine was superior to placebo for reduction of binging (median reduction: 67% vs. 33% on placebo) and vomiting frequency (56% vs. 5%). At 20 mg/day, fluoxetine had an intermediate effect (median reduction: 45% for bingeing, and 29% for purging frequency). Fluoxetine at 60 mg also improved depression, carbohydrate binges, and eating attitudes, as demonstrated by reduced scores on most subscales of the Eating Attitudes Test (EAT) and the Eating Disorder Inventory (EDI). On the higher dosage of fluoxetine, side-effects were most frequent, and there was a mean weight loss of 1.7 kg. In another large RCT, subjects receiving 60 mg/day fluoxetine showed superior improvement in binge and purge behaviors, as well as significant decreases on the EDI total score and the drive for thinness (but not the other) subscale (Goldstein et al., 1995). Treatment of BN with fluvoxamine has yielded mixed results. In one study including 103 outpatients, fluvoxamine did not prove to be efficacious relative to placebo in reducing the frequency or intensity of any aspect of bulimic symptomatology (Flament et al., 1994). In 54 female patients discharged from intensive inpatient treatment, fluvoxamine had several significant effects in preventing relapse or deterioration of eating behaviors, as measured by patients and clinician ratings; however, it had no effect on body image or eating attitudes, and nine subjects in the fluvoxamine group discontinued treatment because of side-effects (Fichter et al., 1996). Milano et al. (2004) compared sertraline to placebo in 20 patients with BN, and found sertraline effective in decreasing binging and purging symptoms.

SSRIs for BN in children and adolescents

One open trial included 10 adolescents treated with fluoxetine (60 mg/day) for 8 weeks (Kotler et al., 2003). At treatment end, binging and purging symptoms had decreased significantly, with 70% rated as improved or much improved, and another 30% slightly improved. There were no dropouts due to adverse effects. Given the strength of evidence for fluoxetine in treating adults with BN, along with its widespread use in treating pediatric depression, most clinicians would recommend fluoxetine as part of a treatment program for adolescents with BN.

Table 10.4. Controlled pharmacological trials with selective serotonin reuptake inhibitors (SSRIs) in bulimia nervosa (BN).

Authors, country	N (drug/placebo): ITT, Completers Inclusion criteria	Study design Duration	Medication (daily dose)	Results	Follow-up data
Fluoxetine Bulimia Nervosa Collaborative Study Group (1992) USA	129 (FLX 20 mg)/129 (FLX 60 mg)/129 (Pla) 89 (FLX 20 mg)/98 (FLX 60 mg)/79 (Pla) BN (DSM–III–R)	Parallel Fluoxetine (FLX) 20 mg vs. fluoxetine (FLX) 60 mg vs. placebo (Pla) 8 weeks	Fluoxetine (20 mg or 60 mg)	Fluoxetine (FLX) 60 mg > placebo for reduction in binge/purge frequency, and improvement of depression, carbohydrate craving, and eating attitudes. Intermediate effect of FLX 20 mg for reduction in binge/purge frequency and improvement on some other measures. Binge remission: 27% on FLX 60 mg and 14% on FLX 20 mg. Side-effects (insomnia, nausea, fatigue, tremors) most frequent on FLX 60 mg, but no group difference for dropout rate	n.a.
Flament et al. (1994) France, Belgium, Netherlands	53/50 38/39 BN (DSM–III–R)	Phase 1. Parallel Fluvoxamine vs. placebo 8 weeks Phase 2. Drug-free period 4 weeks	Fluvoxamine (mean 233 mg)	Fluvoxamine = placebo for reduction of binge/purge frequency and changes on ED and associated measures. No change in weight in either group. Responder rate: 27% on FLV and placebo. 40% treatment discontinuations for adverse reactions. Plasma concentrations of fluvoxamine satisfactory	Relapse during Phase 2: 5/7 in fluoxetine vs. 2/10 in placebo group
Goldstein et al. (1995) USA	296/102 229/62 BN (DSM–III–R)	Parallel Fluoxetine vs. placebo 16 weeks	Fluoxetine (60 mg)	Fluoxetine > placebo for decrease in binge (50% vs. 18%) and purge frequency (50% vs. 21%). Binge remission: 19% vs. 12%	n.a.
Fichter et al. (1996) Germany, Belgium	37/35 23/30 BN (DSM–III–R)	Parallel Fluvoxamine vs. placebo 15 weeks (3 weeks in-patient + 12 weeks outpatient)	Fluvoxamine (mean 188 mg)	Fluvoxamine > placebo for reduction of binge/purge frequency, and improvement of eating attitudes and behaviors. Dropout rate: 38% on fluvoxamine vs. 14% on placebo	At 1-month follow-up, no effect of drug discontinuation (no rebound or withdrawal symptom)
Milano et al. (2004) Italy	10/10 10/10 BN (DSM–IV)	Parallel Sertraline vs. placebo 12 weeks	Sertraline (100 mg)	Sertraline > placebo for reduction of binge/purge frequency	n.a.

ED, Eating disorder; ITT, intent to treat; n.a., not available.

Table 10.5. Controlled pharmacological trials with mood stabilizers and anticonvulsants in bulimia nervosa (BN).

Authors, country	N (drug/placebo): ITT, *Completers* Inclusion criteria	Study design Duration	Medication (daily dose)	Results	Follow-up data
Hsu et al. (1991) USA	47/44 *38/30* BN (DSM–III)	Parallel Lithium vs. placebo 8 weeks	Lithium (300 mg)	Compared with placebo, lithium was effective only in depressed BN patients	n.a.
Hoopes et al. (2003) USA	31/33 BN (DSM–IV)	Parallel Topiramate vs. placebo 10 weeks	Topiramate (25–400 mg)	Topiramate > placebo for reduction of binge/purge frequency and weight loss	n.a.
Nickel et al. (2005) Germany	30/30 *25/24* BN (DSM–IV)	Parallel Topiramate vs. placebo 10 weeks	Topiramate (25–250 mg)	Topiramate > placebo for reduction of binge/purge frequency and weight loss	n.a.

ITT, Intent-to-treat; n.a., not available.

Mood stabilizers and anticonvulsants (Table 10.5)

In a RCT, lithium resulted in significant improvement, compared with placebo, only in depressed bulimic patients; however, plasma concentrations of lithium were relatively low (Hsu *et al.*, 1991). Phenytoin and carbamazepine have been anecdotally tried in BN, with no significant effects (Kaplan *et al.*, 1983; Wermuth *et al.*, 1977). Topiramate has been found to induce weight loss in patients with seizure disorder (Langtry *et al.*, 2003), and has been studied for BN in two RCTs (Hoopes *et al.*, 2003; Nickel *et al.*, 2005). In both, it was well tolerated and associated with improvement in binge and purge behaviors, and also weight loss.

Opiate antagonists

Despite preliminary work indicating that i.v. opiate antagonists decreased the duration and quantity of food eaten during a binge meal (Mitchell *et al.*, 1986), naltrexone appeared ineffective for BN in two small RCTs (Igoin-Apfelbaum & Apfelbaum, 1987; Mitchell *et al.*, 1989). In another, Jonas & Gold (1988) noted modest improvement in 16 bulimic patients who received high doses (200–300 mg/day) of naltrexone. As noted above, naltrexone should not be used at such a high dose because it can cause significant elevations in hepatic transaminases.

Other medications (Table 10.6)

In one RCT, the norepinephrine dopamine reuptake inhibitor (NDRI) bupropion was found superior to placebo, but was associated with unexplained occurrence of seizures in four (5.8%) participants (Horne *et al.*, 1988). Therefore, bupropion is contraindicated in BN.

Table 10.6. Controlled pharmacological trials with other medications in bulimia nervosa (BN).

Authors, country	N (drug/ placebo): ITT, Completers Inclusion criteria	Study design Duration	Medication (daily dose)	Results	Follow-up data
Home et al. (1988) USA	55/26 37/12 BN (DSM–III)	Parallel Bupropion vs. placebo 8 weeks	Bupropion (maximum 450 mg)	Bupropion > placebo for reduction of binge/purge frequency Unexplained seizures in 4 participants on bupropion	n.a.
Hudson et al. (1989) USA	20/22 20/22 BN (DSM–III–R)	Parallel Trazodone vs. placebo 6 weeks	Trazodone (200–100 mg at bedtime)	Trazodone > placebo for reduction of binge/purge frequency 10% patients abstinent and 30% improved on trazodone vs. 0% improved on placebo	9–19 month follow-up of 36/42 subjects on trazodone ± other antide- pressant: 72 % improved, 50% remitted
Faris et al. (2000) USA	14/12 13/12 Severe BN (7 binges/week) (DSM–IV)	Parallel Odansetron vs. placebo 4 weeks	Odansetron (24 mg)	Odansetron > placebo for reduction of binge/ purge frequency	n.a.

ITT, Intent-to-treat; n.a., not available.

Trazodone, an antidepressant with sedative properties, was superior to placebo for reducing binge-eating frequency; only drowsiness and dizziness were reported as side-effects (Hudson et al., 1989). Ondansetron, a 5-HT$_3$ antagonist marketed for the treatment of nausea and vomiting induced by chemotherapeutic agents and radiation treatment, was administered to 26 severely bulimic women, with reduction of binge/purge frequency compared with no change on placebo (Faris et al., 2000).

Pharmacotherapy of BED

TCAs
Despite some evidence of efficacy, TCAs are not considered a first-line pharmacological treatment for BED, because of their side-effect profile, which includes lethality in overdose.

SSRIs (Table 10.7)
RCTs against placebo have been conducted in BED patients using fluvoxamine (Hudson et al., 1998), sertraline (McElroy et al., 2000), fluoxetine (Arnold et al., 2002), citalopram (McElroy et al., 2003a), and escitalopram (Guerdjikova et al., 2008). All have been associated with significant reduction in the frequency of binge-eating episodes (except escitalopram), decrease in BMI, and overall clinical improvement. Ricca et al. (2001) randomized BED patients to fluoxetine, fluvoxamine, CBT, CBT + fluoxetine, or CBT + fluvoxamine. At treatment end,

Table 10.7. Controlled pharmacological trials with selective serotonin reuptake inhibitors (SSRIs) and norepinephrine reuptake inhibitors (NRIs) in binge-eating disorder (BED) and night eating syndrome (NES).

Authors, country	N (drug/ placebo): ITT, Completers Inclusion criteria	Study design Duration	Medication (daily dose)	Results	Follow-up data
Hudson et al. (1998) USA	42/43 29/38 BED (DSM–IV)	Parallel fluvoxamine vs. placebo 9 weeks	Fluvoxamine (50–300 mg)	Fluvoxamine > placebo for reduction of binge frequency and BMI. Remission rate: 45% on fluvoxamine vs. 24% on placebo. More patients on fluvoxamine dropped out for adverse events	n.a.
McElroy et al. (2000) USA	18/16 13/13 BED (DSM–IV)	Parallel sertraline vs. placebo 6 weeks	Sertraline (50–200 mg)	Sertraline > placebo for reduction of binge frequency, BMI and severity of illness	n.a.
Ricca et al. (2001) Italy	Total N: 108 21 (FLX)/22 (FLV)/20 (CBT)/22(CBT + FLX)/23(CBT + FLV) BED (DSM–IV)	Parallel FLX vs. FLV vs. CBT vs. CBT + FLX vs. CBT + FLV 24 weeks	Fluoxetine (FLX) (60 mg) Fluvoxamine (FLV) (300 mg)	CBT, CBT + FLX, CBT + FLV > FLX and FLV for reduction of BMI and improvement of eating behaviors Addition of FLV but not FLX enhanced effects of CBT on eating behaviors	Improvement of eating behaviors maintained at 1 year, although weight loss was partially regained
Arnold et al. (2002) USA	30/30 23/13 BED (DSM–IV)	Parallel fluoxetine vs. placebo 6 weeks	Fluoxetine (20–80 mg)	Fluoxetine > placebo for reduction of binge-eating frequency, weight and severity of illness	n.a.
McElroy et al. (2003a) USA	19/19 16/15 BED (DSM–IV)	Parallel citalopram vs. placebo 6 weeks	Citalopram (20–60 mg)	Citalopram > placebo for reduction of binge frequency, BMI, and severity of illness	n.a.
O'Reardon et al. (2006) USA	17/17 NES	Parallel sertraline vs. placebo 8 weeks	Sertraline (50–200 mg)	Sertraline > placebo for frequency of nocturnal awakenings and ingestions, nocturnal caloric intake, weight, quality of life, severity of illness 71% improved in sertraline vs. 18% in placebo group Mean weight loss: 2.9 kg on sertraline	n.a.
McElroy et al. (2007a) USA	20/20 14/11 BED (DSM–IV)	Parallel atomoxetine vs. placebo 10 weeks	Atomoxetine (mean 106 mg)	Atomoxetine > placebo for reduction of binge eating frequency, BMI, hunger, and severity of illness	n.a.
Guerdjikova et al. (2008) USA	20/23 15/19 BED (DSM–IV)	Parallel escitalopram vs. placebo 12 weeks	Escitalopram (10–30 mg)	Escitalopram > placebo for reduction of weight and severity of illness. No conclusion regarding binge frequency due to low statistical power	n.a.

BMI, Body mass index; CBT, cognitive–behavioral treatment; ITT, intent-to-treat; n.a., not available.

both BMI and total score on the EDE were reduced in the three groups treated by CBT, with or without medication, and the group receiving fluvoxamine was superior to the other two for reduction of the EDE score. At 1-year follow-up, the BMI was significantly higher than at treatment end-point, but still significantly lower than at baseline in the three groups which had received CBT, while the EDE score remained unchanged in all groups. Thus, the addition of fluvoxamine seemed to have enhanced the effects of CBT on eating behaviors, and the treatment effects were partially maintained post-treatment.

Norepinephrine uptake inhibitors and serotonin norepinephrine reuptake inhibitors

There has been one RCT indicating that the norepinephrine reuptake inhibitor (NRI) atomoxetine (40–120 mg/day) was superior to placebo and fairly well tolerated in BED patients (McElroy *et al.*, 2007*a*) (see Table 10.7). In one retrospective review including 35 outpatients with BED and obesity, the serotonin norepinephrine reuptake inhibitor (SNRI) venlafaxine was associated with significant reduction in binge-eating frequency (Malhotra *et al.*, 2002).

Mood stabilizers and anticonvulsants (Table 10.8)

Phenytoin was the first anticonvulsant used to treat BED. However, early promising results have not been replicated, and weight gain was a common side-effect. Because they also increase appetite, valproate and carbamazepine are of little value for BED (Carter *et al.*, 2003). Topiramate induces appetite suppression and weight loss. In a flexible dose study comparing topiramate with placebo in obese outpatients with BED, topiramate was associated with a higher reduction of weekly and daily binge frequency, and with greater weight loss; no serious adverse events were reported (McElroy *et al.*, 2003*b*). A larger RCT showed that topiramate significantly reduced frequency of binge-eating days and binge-eating episodes, weight, and BMI (McElroy *et al.*, 2007*b*). Claudino *et al.* (2007) compared CBT + topiramate to CBT + placebo. In the topiramate group, patients lost more weight, and were more likely to achieve binge remission. Zonisamide, which is approved for the treatment of epilepsy in the USA, has been associated with anorexia and weight loss (Gadde *et al.*, 2003). In obese outpatients with BED, zonisamide was superior to placebo for reduction in binge frequency and weight (McElroy *et al.*, 2006). In many countries, lamotrigine is approved for maintenance treatment of bipolar disorder (Goodwin *et al.*, 2004). Guerdjikova *et al.* (2009) evaluated its efficacy and safety in BED associated with obesity. Due to an exceptionally high placebo response, the study was incapable of detecting drug–placebo differences. However, lamotrigine was associated with a numerically greater amount of weight loss.

Antiobesity medications (Table 10.9)

In obese patients, Stunkard *et al.* (1996) showed that D-fenfluramine was superior to placebo for reducing binge frequency. Shortly after, D-fenfluramine was withdrawn from the market. The SNRI sibutramine is FDA-approved for inducement and maintenance of weight loss, and its efficacy for treatment of obesity has been well established (Arterburn *et al.*, 2004). Appolinario *et al.* (2003) reported significant weight loss and reduction of binge frequency in BED patients receiving sibutramine, compared with placebo. In a larger RCT, sibutramine

Table 10.8. Controlled pharmacological trials with mood stabilizers and anticonvulsants in binge-eating disorder (BED).

Authors, country	N (drug/placebo): ITT, Completers Inclusion criteria	Study design Duration	Medication (daily dose)	Results	Follow-up data
McElroy et al. (2003b) USA	30/31 24/28 Obese BED (DSM–IV)	Parallel Topiramate vs. placebo 14 weeks	Topiramate (mean 212 mg)	Topiramate > placebo for reduction of binge frequency and weight (mean weight loss: 5.9 kg vs. 1.2 kg)	n.a.
McElroy et al. (2007b) USA	195/199 BED (DSM–IV)	Parallel Topiramate vs. placebo 16 weeks	Topiramate (25–300 mg)	Topiramate > placebo for reduction of binge frequency, weight and BMI	n.a.
McElroy et al. (2006) USA	30/30 22/26 Obese BED (DSM-IV)	Parallel zonisamide vs. placebo 16 weeks	Zonisamide (100–600 mg)	Zonisamide > placebo for reduction of binge frequency and weight	n.a.
Claudino et al. (2007) Brazil	37/36 30/26 Obese BED (DSM–IV)	Parallel CBT + topiramate vs. CBT + placebo 21 weeks	Topiramate (mean 206 mg)	CBT + topiramate > CBT + placebo for weight loss (6.8 kg vs. 0.9 kg) and frequency of binge remission	n.a.
Guerdjikova et al. (2009) USA	26/25 BED (DSM–IV)	Parallel lamotrigine vs. placebo 16 weeks	Lamotrigine (236 mg)	Lack of group differences due to very high placebo response Lamotrigine associated with weight loss (1.17 kg) and decrease in serum concentration of glucose, insulin, triglycerides	n.a.

BMI, Body mass index; CBT, cognitive–behavioral treatment; ITT, intent-to-treat; n.a., not available.

was superior to placebo for reduction in BMI, binge frequency and binge days, and was associated with greater global clinical improvement (Wilfley et al., 2008). However, in October 2010, Abbott Laboratories announced the voluntary withdrawal of sibutramine from the US market because of an increased risk of heart attack and stroke. Orlistat, a pancreatic lipase inhibitor available over-the-counter in the USA, has modest efficacy for treatment of obesity (Padwal et al., 2003). Golay et al. (2005) randomized patients with BED to placebo or orlistat, in conjunction with dietary modification, and reported greater weight loss and a significant decrease in ED symptoms for those taking orlistat. Although antiobesity medications have been studied for the treatment of obesity in adolescents, trials are lacking for adolescent BED.

Pharmacotherapy of NES

The pharmacotherapy literature for NES only includes one RCT (see Table 10.7), in which the SSRI sertraline demonstrated significant improvement, compared with placebo, for night eating symptoms, general illness severity, and quality of life (O'Reardon et al., 2006). Case reports have suggested beneficial effects of fluoxetine (Howell & Schenck, 2009).

Table 10.9. Controlled pharmacological trials with antiobesity medication in binge-eating disorder (BED).

Authors, country	N (drug/placebo): ITT, Completers Inclusion criteria	Study design Duration	Medication (daily dose)	Results	Follow-up data
Appolinario et al. (2003) Brazil	30/30 23/25 Obese BED (DSM–IV)	Parallel sibutramine vs. placebo 12 weeks	Sibutramine (15 mg)	Sibutramine > placebo for weight loss and reduction in binge frequency	n.a.
Golay et al. (2005) Switzerland	44/45 39/34 BED (DSM–IV) with BMI ≥ 30	Parallel orlistat vs. placebo 24 weeks	Orlistat (360 mg)	Orlistat > placebo for weight loss, reduction of fat intake, and improvement of binge eating behavior	n.a.
Wilfley et al. (2008) USA	152/152 100/86 BED (DSM–IV)	Parallel sibutramine vs. placebo 24 weeks	Sibutramine (15 mg)	Sibutramine > placebo for reduction in binge frequency, weight loss, and improvement of illness severity	n.a.

ITT, Intent-to-treat; n.a., not available.

First-line pharmacotherapy for EDs

Meta-analyses

AN

A Cochrane review of antidepressants for AN (Claudino et al., 2006) has included seven RCTs. Major methodological limitations such as small sample sizes and large confidence intervals were found to decrease the power of the studies to detect differences between treatments, and meta-analysis of data was not possible for the majority of outcomes. Four RCTs did not find evidence that antidepressants improved weight gain, ED or associated psychopathology. Isolated findings favoring amineptine (not available in the USA) and nortriptyline emerged from antidepressant vs. antidepressant comparisons, but could not be conceived as evidence of efficacy of a specific drug or class of antidepressant in light of the negative findings from the placebo comparisons.

BN

Several meta-analyses of medication trials for BN concluded to a significant, albeit moderate efficacy of treatment. In the Whittal et al. (1999) meta-analysis including nine medication trials, the pooled effect sizes (ESs) were 0.66 for binge frequency, 0.39 for purge frequency, 0.73 for depression, and 0.71 for eating attitudes (self-reported restraint, weight/shape concerns). The Nakash-Eisikovits et al. (2002) meta-analysis (16 studies) noted that ~50% of potential participants were excluded from research trials because of psychiatric or medical comorbidity, but that only 10% of those included dropped out due to side-effects. The average ES of medication also was moderate (Cohen's $d = 0.6$) on both binge and purge frequency. Overall remission rate of bingeing episodes among completers was higher after treatment with MAOIs (35%) than with SSRIs (19%) or atypical antidepressants such as trazodone or bupropion (20%). Improvement rate was higher in studies using TCAs than in those using SSRIs, MAOIs, or atypical antidepressants. In intent-to-treat analysis of all classes of medications together, the recovery rate was 25% for remission of both binge and purge episodes, 17% for remission of bingeing episodes only, and 23% for remission of purging episodes only. A Cochrane review of antidepressants for BN (Bacaltchuk & Hay, 2003) has included 19 RCTs. Efficacy results were similar for all classes of drugs. The pooled risk ratio (RR) for remission of binge episodes was 0.87 (95% CI 0.81–0.93, $p < 0.001$) favoring medication. The number needed to treat (NNT) for a mean duration of 8 weeks was 9 (95% CI 6–16). For clinical improvement (50% reduction in binge episodes), the RR was 0.63 (95% CI 0.55–0.74), and the NNT was 4 (95% CI 3–6). Patients treated with antidepressants were more likely to interrupt treatment prematurely due to adverse events, except for fluoxetine.

BED

A meta-analysis of pharmacotherapy for BED included 14 RCTs with a total of 1279 patients (Reas & Grilo, 2008). There were no significant differences between medication and placebo for attrition. Pharmacological treatments had a moderate though clinically significant advantage over placebo for short-term remission from binge eating (48.7% vs. 28.5%), and the average weight loss on medication was −3.42 kg (95% CI −4.25 to −2.58).

Treatment guidelines

American Psychiatric Association's guidelines

In the acute treatment of AN, weight gain is critical and often requires a combined approach including psychological support, nutritional rehabilitation, CBT and, for children and adolescents, family interventions. The APA guidelines (APA, 2006) support with substantial clinical confidence (level I) that SRRIs do not confer advantage regarding weight gain in patients receiving treatment in an organized ED program. The guidelines also state with moderate clinical confidence (level II) that adding fluoxetine after weight restoration does not confer additional benefits with respect to preventing relapse. On the basis of individual circumstances (level III), it is suggested that second-generation antipsychotics, particularly olanzapine, risperidone, and quetiapine, may be useful in patients with severe, unremitting resistance to gaining weight, severe obsessional thinking, or denial that assumes delusional proportions. Based on level II evidence, pro-motility agents such as metoclopramide may be used for bloating and abdominal pains that occur during refeeding in some AN patients.

For BN, the APA guidelines convey level I evidence that antidepressants are effective as one component of the initial treatment for most BN patients. To date, fluoxetine is the best-studied SSRI and is FDA-approved for BN; sertraline is the only other SSRI that has been shown effective. Dosages of SSRIs higher than those used for depression (e.g. fluoxetine 60 mg/day) are recommended in the treatment of bulimic symptoms. TCAs and MAOIs are not recommended as initial treatment.

Regarding BED, there is level I evidence that antidepressant medications, particularly SSRIs at the high end of the recommended dose, are associated with at least short-term reduction in binge-eating behavior but, in most cases, not with substantial weight loss. The guidelines convey level II evidence that: the anticonvulsant topiramate is effective in binge reduction and weight loss, although adverse effects may limit its clinical utility in some individuals; and that adding antidepressant medication to behavioral weight control and/or CBT may confer additional benefits in weight reduction.

National Institute for Clinical Excellence (NICE) guidelines

According to the 2004 NICE guidelines (www. nice.org.uk/CG009NICEguidelines), the key priorities for treating EDs include psychological treatments (CBT for BN), and family interventions for children and adolescents. Based on expert opinion/clinical experience (Grade C evidence), it is recommended that medication not be used as the sole or primary treatment for AN. A range of drugs may be used in the treatment of comorbid conditions, but caution should be exercised given the physical vulnerability of many people with AN, and because comorbid conditions such as depressive or obsessive–compulsive features may resolve with weight gain alone. For adults with BN, a trial of an antidepressant drug is proposed as an alternative or additional first step to using an evidence-based self-help program, based on Grade B evidence (well-conducted clinical studies). Grade C evidence suggests that SSRIs (specifically fluoxetine) are the drugs of choice in terms of acceptability, tolerability, and reduction of symptoms. No drugs, other than antidepressants, are recommended for the treatment of BN. For patients with BED, there is Grade B evidence that a trial of a SSRI may be offered as an alternative or additional first step to using an evidence-based self-help program.

EDNOS

The category of EDNOS represent patients with subsyndromal AN or BN who meet most but not all DSM–IV criteria. Although evidence is still lacking, both the APA and NICE guidelines recommend that patients with EDNOS receive treatment similar to that for the corresponding diagnosis which their illness most resembles.

Evidence for maintenance treatment

Scientific evidence is scarce, but clinical experience suggests that treatment interventions shown to date to have value in the acute management of the EDs do not guarantee long-term recovery. As discussed above, the utility of maintenance treatment with the SSRI fluoxetine in AN after weight restoration is still uncertain. For persons with BN, the Cochrane review of antidepressants *vs.* placebo trials (Bacaltchuk & Hay, 2003) demonstrated that the mean clinical improvement significantly favored medication in the pooled shorter clinical trials (6–8 weeks: RR 0.63, 95% CI 0.51–0.77) but not in the longer trials (>8 weeks: RR 0.53, 95% CI 0.23–1.20). As shown in Tables 10.4–10.7, only a few of the acute medication trials for BN or BED have followed participants past treatment end. In a 4-month maintenance study (Pyle *et al.*, 1990), 47% of bulimic patients who had responded to imipramine were randomized to imipramine alone, intensive group psychotherapy plus placebo, or combined treatment. Relapse rate was high (30%), but those patients receiving group psychotherapy alone or combined with imipramine, were the least likely to relapse. Romano *et al.* (2002) conducted a single-blind placebo-controlled study comparing fluoxetine (60 mg/day) and placebo in preventing relapse of BN during a 52-week period following successful fluoxetine therapy. In acute treatment responders, continued treatment with fluoxetine improved outcome and decreased the likelihood of relapse. However, attrition rate was high. No data exist on long-term effects of pharmacotherapy for BED. Carter *et al.* (2003) recommend that once a successful response is achieved, medication should be continued for at least 6–12 months.

Best approaches for treatment resistance

AN is a disease characterized by denial of illness, frequent treatment refusal, and non-compliance with pharmacological treatment due to fear of gaining weight (McKnight & Park, 2010). The ego-syntonic nature of the illness leads to fear of and resistance to treatment that is a core feature of the disorder. It is often aggravated by cognitive impairment resulting from a state of starvation that deprives the brain of nutrients required to synthesize adequate amounts of neurotransmitters, a factor that also contributes to the poor medication response (Crow et al., 2009). Typically, anorexic patients will initially decline nutritional rehabilitation and pharmacotherapy out of fear of weight gain and loss of control. Motivational interviewing strategies may help move them from the pre-contemplative stage to a contemplative stage where they become less resistant to treatment. Addressing the patient's malnutrition status will also improve cognition and reduce the patient's psychological resistance. For patients who have a life-threatening AN, an argument can be made for coercive treatment including involuntary hospitalization and enteral feeding if the patient adamantly refuses oral feeding. For pediatric AN, treatment is generally more aggressive, and involves family-based therapy to empower parents to compassionately renourish their child.

To date, medication alone is an imperfect treatment option for BN. In their meta-analysis, Nakash-Eisikovits et al. (2002) calculated the rate of post-treatment symptoms based on 10 RCTs: at treatment termination, bulimic patients still binged, on average, 4.3 times per week, and still purged 6.2 times per week. For those receiving both pharmacotherapy and psychotherapy, the average rates were 2.5 for both binge and purge frequency. Although these data indicate substantial improvement over conditions prior to treatment, they do not constitute a return to mental health, i.e. according to DSM–IV criteria, the average patient still has bulimia, even after an adequate trial of drug or combined treatment. According to Whittal et al. (1999), the ES of combined treatment was significantly better than that of medication alone (for binge frequency: 1.77 vs. 0.66; for purge frequency: 1.33 vs. 0.39), and significantly better than the ES of CBT for binge frequency (1.77 vs. 1.28) but not purge frequency (1.33 vs. 1.22). Nakash-Eisikovits et al. (2002) demonstrated a small advantage for combined treatment over medication for binge episodes, and a moderate advantage for purging episodes (d = 0.2 and 0.5, respectively). In the review by Bacaltchuk et al. (2000), remission rates were 23% for antidepressants alone vs. 42% when combined with psychotherapy (p = 0.06). Thus, there is consistent evidence for an increased response rate and/or enhanced improvement from combining psychotherapy with pharmacotherapy.

For BED, Carter et al. (2003) recommend the use of a SSRI at the upper dose approved for major depressive disorder; for patients unresponsive or intolerant to SSRIs, they suggest topiramate, starting at 25 mg nightly, then increased by 25 mg weekly. Reas & Grilo (2008) reviewed eight studies, including a total of 683 BED patients, studying the effects of pharmacotherapy combined with psychotherapy. Combined treatment failed to significantly enhance binge outcomes, although specific medications (orlistat, topiramate) enhanced weight loss achieved with CBT.

Conclusions and future directions for research

Despite significant progress over the past decades, pharmacotherapy research for EDs still has a long way to go. Methodological improvements are needed, notably to include a more comprehensive evaluation of the cognitive and emotional disturbances in EDs, to obtain both objective and subjective measures of change, and to assess non-purging as well as purging methods of weight control. Novel pharmacological compounds should target not only dietary restraint or binge eating, but also maladaptive weight and shape-related cognitions. Large-scale well-designed trials should investigate combination of treatments or treatment augmentations, in order to target both eating-related symptoms (eating behaviors, weight) and the underlying psychological and cognitive disturbances. Future research should also investigate the moderators and mediators of outcome, so that specific mechanisms of action can be enhanced. New trials should include patients with severe comorbid conditions, as frequently seen in clinical settings, and assess long-term outcomes. More research should be done on treatment of EDs during adolescence, in order to lower the likelihood of chronic disorders in adulthood. The effects of starvation or malnutrition on treatment resistance should be further investigated and corrected. Research into the factors (historical, clinical, biological) differentiating ED patients who achieve remission from those who remain symptomatic, might provide clues to elucidate which treatment(s) can best target specific components of these complex biopsychosocial disorders.

References

Allison KC, Lundgren JD, O'Reardon JP et al. (2010). Proposed diagnostic criteria for night eating syndrome. *International Journal of Eating Disorders* **43**, 241–247.

American Psychiatric Association (APA) (1994). *Diagnostic and Statistical Manual of Mental Disorders*, 4th edn. Washington, DC: American Psychiatric Association.

American Psychiatric Association (APA) (2006). Practice guideline for the treatment of patients with eating disorders (American Psychiatric Association). *American Journal of Psychiatry* **157**, 1–39.

Appolinario JC, Bacaltchuk J, Sichieri R et al. (2003). A randomized, double-blind, placebo-controlled study of sibutramine in the treatment of binge-eating disorder. *Archives of General Psychiatry* **60**, 1109–1116.

Arnold LM, McElroy SL, Hudson JI et al. (2002). A placebo-controlled, randomized trial of fluoxetine in the treatment of binge-eating disorder. *Journal of Clinical Psychiatry* **63**, 1028–1033.

Arterburn DE, Crane PK, Veenstra DL (2004). The efficacy and safety of sibutramine for weight loss: a systematic review. *Archives of Internal Medicine* **164**, 994–1003.

Attia E, Haiman C, Walsh BT (1998). Does fluoxetine augment the inpatient treatment of anorexia nervosa? *American Journal of Psychiatry* **155**, 144–151.

Bacaltchuk J, Hay P (2003). Antidepressants vs. placebo for people with bulimia nervosa. *Cochrane Database of Systematic Reviews* **4**, CD003391.

Bacaltchuk J, Trefiglio RP, Oliveira IR et al. (2000). Combination of antidepressants and psychological treatments for bulimia nervosa: a systematic review. *Acta Psychiatrica Scandinavica* **101**, 256–264.

Baranowska B, Rozbicka G, Jeske W, Abdel-Fattah MH (1984). The role of endogenous opiates in the mechanism of inhibited luteinizing hormone (LH) secretion in women with anorexia nervosa: the effect of endorphin secretion. *Journal of Clinical Endocrinology and Metabolism* **59**, 412–416.

Barbarich NC, McConaha CW, Gaskill J et al. (2004a). An open trial of olanzapine in anorexia nervosa. *Journal of Clinical Psychiatry* **65**, 1480–1482.

Barbarich NC, McConaha CW, Halmi KA et al. (2004b). Use of nutritional supplements to increase the efficacy of fluoxetine in the treatment of anorexia nervosa. *International Journal of Eating Disorders* **35**, 10–15.

Biederman J, Herzog DB, Rivinus TM et al. (1985). Amitriptyline in the treatment of anorexia nervosa: a double-blind, placebo-controlled study. *Journal of Clinical Psychopharmacology* **5**, 10–16.

Birmingham CL, Goldner EM, Bakan R (1994). Controlled trial of zinc supplementation in anorexia nervosa. *International Journal of Eating Disorders* **15**, 251–255.

Bissada H, Tasca G, Barber AM, Bradwejn J (2008). Olanzapine in the treatment of low body weight and obsessive thinking in women with anorexia nervosa: a randomized, double-blind, placebo-controlled trial. *American Journal of Psychiatry* **165**, 1281–1288.

Boachie A, Goldfield GS, Spettigue W (2003). Olanzapine use as an adjunctive treatment for hospitalized children with anorexia nervosa: case reports. *International Journal of Eating Disorders* **33**, 98–103.

Bosanac P, Kurlender S, Norman T *et al.* (2007). An open-label study of quetiapine in anorexia nervosa. *Human Psychopharmacology* **22**, 223–230.

Brambilla F, Garcia CS, Fassino S *et al.* (2007). Olanzapine therapy in anorexia nervosa: psychobiological effects. *International Clinical Psychopharmacology* **22**, 197–204.

Carter WP, Hudson JI, Lalonde JK *et al.* (2003). Pharmacologic treatment of binge eating disorder. *International Journal of Eating Disorders* **34**, S74–S88.

Claudino AM, de Oliveira IR, Appolinario JUC *et al.* (2007). Double-blind, randomized, placebo-controlled trial of topiramate plus cognitive-behavior therapy in binge-eating disorder. *Journal of Clinical Psychiatry* **68**, 1324–1332.

Claudino AM, Hay P, Lima MS *et al.* (2006). Antidepressants for anorexia nervosa. *Cochrane Database of Systematic Reviews* **1**, CD004365.

Crisp AH, Lacey JH, Crutchfield M (1987). Clomipramine and 'drive' in people with anorexia nervosa. *British Journal of Psychiatry* **150**, 355–358.

Crow SJ, James E, Mitchell JE *et al.* (2009). What potential role is there for medication treatment in anorexia nervosa? *International Journal of Eating Disorders* **42**, 1–8.

Dally P, Sargant W (1966). Treatment and outcome of anorexia nervosa. *British Medical Journal* **2**, 793–795.

Dennis K, Le Grange D, Bremer J (2006). Olanzapine use in adolescent anorexia nervosa. *Eating and Weight Disorders* **11**, e53–e56.

Fairburn CG, Harrison PJ (2003). Eating disorders. *Lancet* **361**, 407–416.

Fallon BA, Walsh BT, Sadik C *et al.* (1991). Outcome and clinical course in inpatient bulimic women: a 2-to-9-year follow-up study. *Journal of Clinical Psychiatry* **52**, 272–278.

Faris PL, Kim SW, Meller WH *et al.* (2000). Effect of decreasing afferent vagal activity with odansetron on symptoms of bulimia nervosa: a randomized double-blind trial. *Lancet* **355**, 792–797.

Fassino S, Leombruni P, Daga G *et al.* (2002). Efficacy of citalopram in anorexia nervosa: a pilot study. *European Neuropsychopharmacology* **12**, 453–459.

Fichter MM, Kruger R, Rieg W (1996). Fluvoxamine in prevention of relapse in bulimia nervosa: effects on eating-specific psychopathology. *Journal of Clinical Psychopharmacology* **16**, 9–18.

Fisman S, Steele M, Short J *et al.* (1996). Case study: anorexia nervosa and autistic disorder in an adolescent girl. *Journal of the American Academy of Child and Adolescent Psychiatry* **35**, 937–940.

Flament MF, Corcos M, Igoin L *et al.* (1994). Treatment of normal-weight bulimia nervosa with fluvoxamine: negative results from a controlled double-blind study with 103 outpatients. Presented at the European Regional Symposium of the World Psychiatric Association: Developmental Issues in Psychiatry, Lisbon, 10–14 July 1994.

Fluoxetine Bulimia Nervosa Collaborative Study Group (1992). Fluoxetine in the treatment of bulimia nervosa: a multicenter, placebo-controlled, double-blind trial. *Archives of General Psychiatry* **49**, 139–147.

Gadde KM, Franciscy DM, Wagner II HR *et al.* (2003). Zonisamide for weight loss in obese adults: a randomized controlled trial. *Journal of the American Medical Association* **289**, 1820–1825.

Garfinkel PE, Garner DM (1982). The hospital management. In *Anorexia Nervosa: A Multidimensional Perspective* (p. 248). New York, NY: Brunner/Mazel.

Golay A, Laurent-Jaccard A, Habicht F *et al.* (2005). Effect of orlistat in obese patients with binge eating disorder. *Obesity Research* **13**, 1701–1708.

Goldberg SC, Halmi KA, Eckert ED *et al.* (1979). Cyproheptadine in anorexia nervosa. *British Journal of Psychiatry* **134**, 67–70.

Golden NH, Iglesias EA, Jacobson MS *et al.* (2005). Alendronate for the treatment of osteopenia in anorexia nervosa: a randomized, double-blind, placebo-controlled trial. *Journal of Clinical Endocrinology and Metabolism* **90**, 3179–3185.

Goldstein DJ, Wilson MG, Thompson VL et al. (1995). Long-term fluoxetine treatment of bulimia nervosa. *British Journal of Psychiatry* **166**, 660–666.

Goodwin GM, Bowden CL, Calabrese JR et al. (2004). A pooled analysis of 2 placebo-controlled 18-month trials of lamotrigine and lithium maintenance in bipolar I disorder. *Journal of Clinical Psychiatry* **65**, 432–441.

Grinspoon S, Thomas E, Pitts S et al. (2000). Prevalence and predictive factors for regional osteopenia in women with anorexia nervosa. *Annals of Internal Medicine* **133**, 790–794.

Gross HA, Ebert MH, Faden VB et al. (1981). A double-blind controlled trial of lithium carbonate in primary anorexia nervosa. *Journal of Psychopharmacology* **1**, 376–381.

Gross HA, Ebert MH, Faden VB et al. (1983). A double-blind trial of delta9-tetrahydrocannabinol in primary anorexia nervosa. *Journal of Clinical Psychopharmacology* **3**, 165–171.

Grucza RA, Przybeck TR, Cloninger CR (2007). Prevalence and correlates of binge eating disorder in a community sample. *Comprehensive Psychiatry* **48**, 124–131.

Guerdjikova Al, McElroy SL, Kotwal R (2008). High-dose escitalopram in the treatment of binge-eating disorder with obesity: a placebo-controlled monotherapy trial. *Human Psychopharmacology: Clinical and Experimental* **23**, 1–11.

Guerdjikova Al, McElroy SL, Welge JA et al. (2009). Lamotrigine in the treatment of binge-eating disorder with obesity: a randomized, placebo-controlled monotherapy trial. *International Clinical Psychopharmacology* **24**, 150–158.

Halmi KA, Eckert E, LaDu TJ, Cohen J (1986). Anorexia nervosa: treatment efficacy of cyproheptadine and amitriptyline. *Archives of General Psychiatry* **43**, 177–181.

Halmi KA, Eckert E, Marchi P et al. (1991). Comorbidity of psychiatric diagnoses in anorexia nervosa. *Archives of General Psychiatry* **48**, 712–718.

Hoek HW (2006). Incidence, prevalence and mortality of anorexia nervosa and other eating disorders. *Current Opinion in Psychiatry* **19**, 389–394.

Hoek HW, Van Hoeken D (2003). Review of the prevalence and incidence of eating disorders. *International Journal of Eating Disorders* **34**, 383–396.

Holtkamp K, Konrad K, Kaiser N et al. (2005). A retrospective study of SSRI treatment in adolescent anorexia nervosa: insufficient evidence for efficacy. *Journal of Psychiatric Research* **39**, 303–310.

Hoopes SP, Reimherr FW, Hedges DW et al. (2003). Treatment of bulimia nervosa with topiramate in a randomized, double-blind, placebo-controlled trial, part 1: improvement in binge and purge measures. *Journal of Clinical Psychiatry* **64**, 1335–1341.

Home RL, Ferguson JM, Pope HG et al. (1988). Treatment of bulimia with bupropion: a multicenter controlled trial. *Journal of Clinical Psychiatry* **49**, 262–266.

Howell MJ, Schenck CH (2009). Treatment of nocturnal eating disorders. *Current Treatment Options in Neurology* **11**, 333–339.

Hsu LKG, Clement L, Santhouse Jun ESY (1991). Treatment of bulimia nervosa with lithium carbonate: a controlled study. *Journal of Nervous and Mental Disease* **179**, 351–355.

Hudson JI, Hiripi E, Pope HG, Kessler RC (2007). The prevalence and correlates of eating disorders in the national comorbidity survey replication. *Biological Psychiatry* **61**, 348–358.

Hudson JI, McElroy SL, Raymond NC et al. (1998). Fluvoxamine in the treatment of binge-eating disorder: a multicenter placebo-controlled, double-blind trial. *American Journal of Psychiatry* **155**, 1756–1762.

Hudson JI, Pope HG, Keck PE, McElroy SL (1989). Treatment of bulimia nervosa with trazodone: short-term response and long-term follow-up. *Clinical Neuropharmacology* **12**, S38–S46.

Igoin-Apfelbaum L, Apfelbaum M (1987). Naltrexone and bulimic symptoms. *Lancet* **7**, 1087–1088.

Jonas JM, Gold MS (1988). The use of opiate antagonists in treating bulimia: a study of low-dose *vs.* high-dose naltrexone. *Psychiatry Research* **24**, 195–199.

Kaplan AS, Garfinkel PE, Darby PL, Garner DM (1983). Carbamazepine in treatment of bulimia. *American Journal of Psychiatry* **140**, 1225–1226.

Katz RL, Keen CL, Litt IF *et al.* (1987). Zinc deficiency in anorexia nervosa. *Journal of Adolescent Health Care* **8**, 400–406.

Kaye WH, Nagata T, Weltzin TE *et al.* (2001). Double-blind placebo-controlled administration of fluoxetine in restricting and restricting-purging type anorexia nervosa. *Biological Psychiatry* **49**, 644–652.

Kennedy SH, Goldbloom DS, Ralevski E (1993). Is there a role for selective monoamine oxidase inhibitor therapy in bulimia nervosa? A placebo-controlled trial of brofaromine. *Journal of Clinical Psychopharmacology* **13**, 415–422.

Kennedy SH, Piran N, Warsh JJ *et al.* (1988). A trial of isocarboxazid in the treatment of bulimia nervosa. *Journal of Clinical Psychopharmacology* **8**, 391–396.

Kotler LA, Devlin MJ, Davies M, Walsh BT (2003). An open trial of fluoxetine for adolescents with bulimia nervosa. *Journal of Child and Adolescent Psychopharmacology* **13**, 329–335.

Lacey JH, Crisp AH (1980). Hunger, food intake and weight: the impact of clomipramine on a refeeding anorexia nervosa population. *Postgraduate Medicine Journal* **56** (Suppl. 1), S79–S85.

Langtry HD, Gillis JC, Davis R (2003). Topiramate: a review of its pharmacodynamic and pharmacokinetic properties and clinical efficacy in the management of epilepsy. *Drugs* **54**, 752–773.

Lask B, Fosson A, Rolfe U, Thomas S (1993). Zinc deficiency and childhood-onset anorexia nervosa. *Journal of Clinical Psychiatry* **54**, 63–66.

Machado PP, Machado BC, Goncalves S, Hoek HW (2007). The prevalence of eating disorders not otherwise specified. *International Journal of Eating Disorders* **40**, 212–217.

Malhotra S, King KH, Welge JA *et al.* (2002). Venlafaxine treatment of binge-eating disorder associated with obesity: a series of 35 patients. *Journal of Clinical Psychiatry* **63**, 802–806.

Marrazzi MA, Bacon JP, Kinzie J, Luby ED (1995). Naltrexone use in the treatment of anorexia nervosa and bulimia nervosa. *International Journal of Clinical Psychopharmacology* **10**, 163–172.

McElroy SL, Arnold LM, Shapira NA *et al.* (2003*b*). Topiramate in the treatment of binge eating disorder associated with obesity: a randomized, placebo-controlled trial. *American Journal of Psychiatry* **160**, 255–268.

McElroy SL, Casuto LS, Nelson EB *et al.* (2000). Placebo-controlled trial of sertraline in the treatment of binge eating disorder. *American Journal of Psychiatry* **157**, 1004–1006.

McElroy SL, Guerdjikova A, Kotwal R *et al.* (2007*a*). Atomoxetine in the treatment of binge-eating disorder: a randomized controlled trial. *Journal of Clinical Psychiatry* **68**, 390–398.

McElroy SL, Guerdjikova AL, Martens B *et al.* (2009). Role of antiepileptic drugs in the management of eating disorders. *CNS Drugs* **23**, 139–156.

McElroy SL, Hudson JI, Capece JA *et al.* (2007*b*). Topiramate for the treatment of binge eating disorder associated with obesity: a placebo-controlled study. *Biological Psychiatry* **61**, 1039–1048.

McElroy SL, Hudson JI, Malhotra S *et al.* (2003*a*). Citalopram in the treatment of binge-eating disorder: a placebo-controlled trial. *Journal of Clinical Psychiatry* **64**, 807–813.

McElroy SL, Kotwal R, Guerdjikova Al *et al.* (2006). Zonisamide in the treatment of binge eating disorder with obesity: a randomized controlled trial. *Journal of Clinical Psychiatry* **67**, 1897–1906.

McKnight RM, Park RJ (2010). Atypical antipsychotics and anorexia nervosa: a review. *European Eating Disorders Review* **18**, 10–21.

Mehler C, Wewetzer C, Schulze U *et al.* (2001). Olanzapine in children and adolescents with chronic anorexia nervosa. A study of five cases. *European Child and Adolescent Psychiatry* **10**, 151–157.

Mehler PS, Mackenzie TD (2009). The treatment of osteopenia and osteoporosis in anorexia nervosa: a systematic review of the literature. *International Journal of Eating Disorders* **42**, 195–201.

Mehler-Wex C, Romanos M, Kirchheiner J, Schulze UME (2008). Atypical antipsychotics in severe anorexia nervosa in children and adolescents: review and case reports. *European Eating Disorders Review* **16**, 100–108.

Milano W, Petrella C, Sabatino C, Capasso A (2004). Treatment of bulimia nervosa with sertraline: a randomized controlled trial. *Advances in Therapy* **21**, 232–237.

Mitchell JE, Christenson G, Jennings J et al. (1989). A placebo-controlled, double-blind crossover study of naltrexone hydrochloride in outpatients with normal weight bulimia. *Journal of Clinical Psychopharmacology* **9**, 94–97.

Mitchell JE, Crow S (2006). Medical complications of anorexia nervosa and bulimia nervosa. *Current Opinion in Psychiatry* **19**, 438–443.

Mitchell JE, Laine DE, Morley JE, Levine AS (1986). Naloxone but not CCK-8 may attenuate binge eating behavior in patients with the bulimia syndrome. *Biological Psychiatry* **21**, 1399–1406.

Mondraty N, Birmingham LC, Touyz S et al. (2005). Randomized controlled trial of olanzapine in the treatment of cognitions in anorexia nervosa. *Australasian Psychiatry* **13**, 72–75.

Nakash-Eisikovits O, Dierberger A, Westen D (2002). A multidimensional meta-analysis of pharmacotherapy for bulimia nervosa: summarizing the range of outcomes in controlled clinical trials. *Harvard Review of Psychiatry* **10**, 193–211.

Newman-Toker J (2000). Risperidone in anorexia nervosa. *Journal of the American Academy of Child and Adolescent Psychiatry* **39**, 941–942.

Nickel C, Tritt K, Muehlbacher M et al. (2005). Topiramate treatment in bulimia nervosa patients: a randomized, double-blind, placebo-controlled trial. *International Journal of Eating Disorders* **38**, 295–300.

Nielsen S (2001). Epidemiology and mortality of eating disorders. *Psychiatric Clinics of North America* **24**, 201–214.

Norris M, Spettigue W, Buchholz A et al. (2011). Olanzapine use for the adjunctive treatment of adolescents with anorexia nervosa. *Journal of Child and Adolescent Psychopharmacology* **21**, 213–220.

O'Reardon JP, Allison KC, Martino NS et al. (2006). A randomized, placebo-controlled trial of sertraline in the treatment of night eating syndrome. *American Journal of Psychiatry* **163**, 893–898.

Padwal RS, Rucker D, Li SK et al. (2003). Long-term pharmacotherapy for obesity and overweight. *Cochrane Database of Systematic Reviews* **4**, CD004094.

Powers PS, Bannon Y, Eubanks R, McCormick T (2007). Quetiapine in anorexia nervosa patients: an open label outpatient pilot study. *International Journal of Eating Disorders* **40**, 21–26.

Pyle R, Mitchell J, Eckert E, Hatsukami D (1990). Maintenance treatment and 6 month outcome for bulimic patients who respond to initial treatment. *American Journal of Psychiatry* **147**, 871–875.

Reas DL, Grilo CM (2008). Review and meta-analysis of pharmacotherapy for binge-eating disorder. *Obesity* **16**, 2024–2038.

Ricca V, Mannucci E, Mezzani B et al. (2001). Fluoxetine and fluvoxamine combined with individual cognitive-behaviour therapy in binge eating disorder: a one-year follow-up study. *Psychotherapy and Psychosomatics* **70**, 298–306.

Romano SJ, Halmi KA, Sarkar NP et al. (2002). A placebo-controlled study of fluoxetine in continued treatment of bulimia nervosa after successful acute fluoxetine treatment. *American Journal of Psychiatry* **159**, 96–102.

Rothschild R, Quitkin HM, Quitkin FM (1994). A double-blind placebo controlled comparison of phenelzine and imipramine in the treatment of bulimia in atypical depressives. *International Journal of Eating Disorders* **15**, 1–9.

Schüle C, Sighart C, Hennig J, Laakmann G (2006). Mirtazapine inhibits salivary cortisol concentrations in anorexia nervosa. *Progress in Neuro-Psychopharmacology & Biological Psychiatry* **30**, 1015–1019.

Simon J, Schmidt U, Pilling S (2005). The health service use and cost of eating disorders. *Psychological Medicine* **35**, 1543–1551.

Spitzer RL, Devlin MJ, Walsh BT et al. (1991). Binge eating disorder: to be or not to be in DSM-IV. *International Journal of Eating Disorders* **10**, 627–629.

Stacher G, Kiss A, Wiesnagrotzki S et al. (1986). Oesophageal and gastric motility disorders in patients categorized as having primary anorexia nervosa. *Gut* **27**, 1120–1126.

Stunkard A, Berkowitz R, Tanrikut C et al. (1996). D-fenfluramine treatment of binge eating disorder. *American Journal of Psychiatry* **153**, 1455–1459.

Trunko ME, Schwartz TA, Duvvuri V, Kaye WH (2010). Aripiprazole in anorexia nervosa and low-weight bulimia nervosa: case reports. *International Journal of Eating Disorders.* Published online: 22 February 2010. doi:10.1002/eat.20807.

Vandereycken W (1984). Neuroleptics in the short-term treatment of anorexia nervosa: a double-blind placebo-controlled trial with sulpiride. *British Journal of Psychiatry* **144**, 288–292.

Vandereycken W, Pierloot R (1982). Pimozide combined with behavior therapy in the short-term treatment of anorexia nervosa: a double-blind placebo-controlled crossover study. *Acta Psychiatrica Scandinavica* **66**, 445–450.

Walsh BT, Gladis M, Roose SP (1988). Phenelzine *vs.* placebo in 50 patients with bulimia. *Archives of General Psychiatry* **45**, 471–475.

Walsh BT, Kaplan AS, Attia E *et al.* (2006). Fluoxetine after weight restoration in anorexia nervosa; a randomized controlled trial. *Journal of the American Medical Association* **295**, 2605–2612.

Wermuth BM, Davis KL, Hollister E, Stunkard AJ (1977). Phenytoin treatment of the binge-eating syndrome. *American Journal of Psychiatry* **134**, 1249–1253.

Whittal ML, Agras WS, Gould RA (1999). Bulimia nervosa: a meta-analysis of psychosocial and pharmacological treatments. *Behavior Therapy* **30**, 117–135.

Wilfley DE, Crow SJ, Hudson JI *et al.* (2008). Efficacy of sibutramine for the treatment of binge eating disorder: a randomized multicenter placebo-controlled double-blind study. *American Journal of Psychiatry* **165**, 51–58.

Zhu AJ, Walsh BT (2002). Pharmacologic treatment of eating disorders. *Canadian Journal of Psychiatry* **47**, 227–234.

Evidence-based pharmacotherapy of nicotine and alcohol dependence

Wim van den Brink

Introduction

Substance use disorders (SUDs) are frequently occurring mental health problems that are associated with serious morbidity and excessive mortality, suffering of family and friends, societal damage, criminality, public nuisance, and in some instances destabilization of certain regions or even countries. According to the Global Burden of Disease (GBD) 2000 study, about 4% of the global burden, as measured in disability adjusted life years (DALYs), was attributable each to alcohol and tobacco, and 0.8% to illicit drugs. Tobacco use was found to be the most important of 25 risk factors for developed countries in the comparative risk assessment. It had the highest mortality risk of all the substance use categories, especially for the elderly. Alcohol use was also important in developed countries, but constituted the most important of all risk factors in emerging economies. The burden of disease attributable to the use of legal substances clearly outweighed the use of illegal drugs (Rehm *et al.*, 2006). Using slightly different terms, the European Brain Council estimated that about 37 million Europeans have a SUD (including nicotine and alcohol dependence) resulting in an annual 110 billion euros of societal costs, including healthcare, unemployment, and crime-related costs (Andlin-Sobocki & Rehm, 2005). The GBD study concluded by stating that a large part of the substance-attributable burden would be avoidable if known effective interventions were implemented (Rehm *et al.*, 2006).

Twin studies show that experimental and recreational use of alcohol and other drugs is mainly related to shared environmental risk factors such as socio-economic status, religion, and parental alcohol and drug use (45–70%), whereas continued alcohol and drug use and the development of alcohol and drug dependence are mainly related to genetic risk factors (40–80%) often in combination with unique environmental risk factors such as peer pressure or peer pulling (20–50%) (e.g. Agrawal & Lynskey, 2008; Fowler *et al.*, 2007). The best available data show that the genetic variance of different SUDs can best be explained by two separate, but highly correlated ($r = 0.82$), genetic risk profiles: one factor mainly involving illegal substances (e.g. cannabis and cocaine) and one mainly involving legal substances (e.g. alcohol, nicotine and caffeine) (Kendler *et al.*, 2003, 2007). These results suggest that the genetic variants that influence human drug dependence are likely to include psychological traits (e.g. impulsivity, anxiety) and/or brain systems that impact a wide range of substance classes. The latter include several brain structures often with their own neurotransmitters, including reward and motivational systems (e.g. nucleus accumbens; dopamine

Table 11.1. Functions, brain structures, and neurotransmitters involved in addiction.[a]

Function	Brain structure	Neurotransmitter
Motivation/reward	Ventral tegmental area Nucleus accumbens (shell)	Endorphins Dopamine
Conditioning/craving	Nucleus accumbens (core) Amygdala Thalamus Orbitofrontal cortex Anterior cingulate cortex	Dynorphins Dopamine CRH Glutamate GABA
Salience	Orbitofrontal cortex	Dopamine
Habit formation	Putamen Caudate nucleus	Dopamine
Conflict registration/inhibition	Anterior cingulate cortex Ventromedial prefrontal cortex Dorsolateral prefrontal cortex	Dopamine Serotonin Norepinephrine Glutamate GABA
Withdrawal	Locus ceruleus Amygdala	Norepinephrine CRH Glutamate

[a] This is a simplified summary of the neurobiology of addiction.

and endorphins), behavioral conditioning resulting in attentional bias, craving and salience (amygdala, thalamus, ortbitofrontal cortex: dopamine, glutamate, CRH), conflict monitoring and behavioral inhibition systems (anterior cingulate cortex, dorsolateral prefrontal cortex; norepinephrine, serotonin, GABA, glutamate), compulsivity like functions (dorsal striatum; dopamine), and finally the stress system following (repeated) withdrawal (locus ceruleus, amygdala; CRH, norpepineprine) (e.g. Koob & Volkow, 2010; also Table 11.1). Together, these findings indicate that two pharmacological approaches are possible for the treatment of patients with SUD: one strategy directed to the working mechanisms of specific substances (e.g. methadone in the case of opioid dependence treatment) and another strategy directed to general addiction mechanisms (e.g. bupropion in the treatment of nicotine dependence).

In the current review we discuss abstinence oriented treatments and stabilizing/harm reduction treatments. We decided to only discuss the evidence-based treatment of substance with the highest levels of personal and social harms according to experts in the field of toxicology, epidemiology, and addiction treatment (Nutt *et al.*, 2007, 2010; van Amsterdam *et al.*, 2010). In this chapter we cover nicotine and alcohol dependence, while in the following chapter we cover opioids, cocaine, methamphetamine, and cannabis.

In order to select the best available evidence and to make the best recommendations, we conducted a search mainly using existing Cochrane reviews, other statistical meta-analyses, high quality systematic reviews and electronic databases (PubMed, PsycINFO) if none of the above were available. In addition we always tried to update existing reviews with high-quality studies (mainly RCTs) from the previously mentioned electronic databases. In this review we try to provide evidence-based answers to the following three questions:

(1) What should be the best first-line pharmacological treatment for a certain SUD?
(2) How long should this treatment last?
(3) What strategies can be used if first-line treatment fails?

Nicotine dependence

Worldwide, there are 1.3 billion smokers, with 4.9 million tobacco-related deaths per year. Smoking a cigarette leads to a fast increase of nicotine in the arterial circulation and nicotine reaches the brain within 15 seconds. In the brain, nicotine binds to the $\alpha4/\beta2$ and $\alpha7$ nicotine acetylcholinergic receptors (nAchR) on the dopaminergic neurons at the ventral tegmental area and the nucleus accumbens resulting in the release of dopamine and glutamate.

Each year nearly 20 million smokers in the USA attempt to quit smoking. Only 6% will succeed long term (Jorenby et al., 1999).

Different proven-effective medications are currently available for the treatment of nicotine dependence with different treatment goals and different mechanisms of action. First, nAchR antagonist treatment and the use of anti-nicotine vaccines could make smoking ineffective and lead to total abstinence. Second, full and partial nAchR agonists are available to replace carcinogenic tar-containing cigarettes by safer forms of nAchR stimulation (e.g. nicotine gum and varenicline, respectively). Finally antidepressants are used to prevent nicotine withdrawal through norepinephrine reuptake inhibition in the locus ceruleus (e.g. nortriptyline and bupropion). However, it cannot be excluded that one of the antidepressants (bupropion) also has a direct anti-addiction effect through its dopamine reuptake inhibition in the mesolimbic system or its antagonistic effect on the nAchR, whereas partial nAchR agonists such as varenicline may have a direct anti-addiction effect through the increase in the number of dopamine D2 receptors in the striatum (Crunelle et al., 2010).

Full nAchR agonists: nicotine replacement therapy (NRT)

Nicotine replacement therapy is currently the most frequently used aid to stop smoking. In a Cochrane review, Stead et al. (2008) discuss the results of 132 RCTs of which 111 RCTs with over 40 000 participants contributed to the primary comparison between any type of NRT and a placebo or non-NRT control group. The risk ratio (RR) of abstinence for any form of NRT relative to control was 1.58 with no significant differences between the different types of administration: for nicotine gum RR = 1.43; for nicotine patch RR = 1.66; for nicotine inhaler RR = 1.90; for oral tablets/lozenges RR = 2.00; and for nicotine nasal spray RR = 2.02. The absolute effects of NRT use will depend on the baseline quit rate, which varies in different clinical settings. Studies of people attempting to quit on their own suggest that success rates after 6–12 months are 3–5%. Use of NRT might be expected to increase the rate by 2–3%, resulting in a number needed to treat (NNT) of 33–50. The effects were largely independent of the duration of therapy, the intensity of additional support provided or the setting in which the NRT was offered. In highly dependent smokers there was a significant benefit of 4 mg gum compared with 2 mg gum, but weaker evidence of a benefit from higher doses of patch. There was evidence that combining a nicotine patch with a rapid delivery form of NRT was more effective than a single type of NRT. The Cochrane review does not contain a systematic evaluation of side-effects, but from a rather extensive description it seems that side-effects are generally mild with no serious adverse events (see also Hays & Ebbert, 2010): nicotine gum use is associated with hiccoughs, jaw pain, gastrointestinal disturbances, and orodental problems; nicotine patches show skin sensitivity and irritation in up to 54% of the users, but this is usually mild and rarely leads to treatment discontinuation; nicotine inhaler and nasal spray are mainly related to local irritation at the site of administration; nicotine sublingual tablets have been reported to cause hiccoughs, burning and smarting sensation in the mouth, sore throat, coughing, dry lips, and mouth ulcers.

Only one study directly compared NRT to the antidepressant bupropion (Jorenby *et al.*, 1999). In this 9-week RCT ($n = 893$), abstinence at 6 months using a nicotine patch was significantly lower compared with bupropion: abstinence rates at 12 months were 16% in the placebo group, 16% in the nicotine-patch group, 30% in the bupropion group, and 36% in the group with a combination of bupropion and the nicotine patch, with no significant difference between the last two groups.

Two open-label RCTs directly compared NRT with varenicline (Aubin *et al.*, 2008; Tsukahara *et al.*, 2010). In the study of Aubin *et al.* (2008), participants were randomly assigned to 12 weeks titrated varenicline ($n = 376$) or 10 weeks NRT patch ($n = 370$). The 52-weeks continuous abstinence rate was significantly better for varenicline than for NRT (26% *vs.* 20%; OR 1.40). Varenicline also resulted in significantly less craving, withdrawal symptoms, and smoking satisfaction ($p < 0.001$) compared with NRT. However, varenicline more often caused nausea (37% *vs.* 10%). The much smaller study of Tsukahara *et al.* (2010; $n = 32$) did not show any difference between the two treatment conditions; gastrointestinal problems occurred more often in the varenicline group, whereas skin problems were more frequent in the NRT group.

The study of Jorenby *et al.* (1999 found a non-significant effect of bupropion addition to NRT. However, a meta-analysis of five RCTs (Shah *et al.*, 2008; $n = 2.204$) showed that combination therapy (NRT plus bupropion or varenicline) was more effective than NRT alone: $RR = 1.42, 1.54$, and 1.58 for abstinence at 3, 6, and 12 months, respectively. Adverse effects during combination treatment were minimal and similar to placebo or monotherapy.

Partial nAchR agonists (varenicline, cytisine)

A relatively new, but well-studied, treatment of nicotine dependence is the use of partial nAchR agonist, i.e. compounds that bind and activate the nAchR but have less than a full agonist effect. In a recently updated Cochrane review, Cahill *et al.* (2010) describe and analyze 11 trials comparing varenicline with placebo and one trial comparing cytisine with placebo. Three of the varenicline trials also included a bupropion experimental arm (Gonzales *et al.*, 2006; Jorenby *et al.*, 2006; Nides *et al.*, 2006). Finally the authors included two open-label RCTs comparing varenicline with NRT (Aubin *et al.*, 2008; Tsukahara *et al.*, 2010). Varenicline was more effective than placebo: pooled RR ($n = 4443$) for continuous abstinence at 6 months or longer for varenicline at standard dosage *vs.* placebo was 2.31. Varenicline at lower or variable doses ($n = 1272$) was also effective ($RR = 2.09$), but a direct comparison between standard and the next lowest dose of varenicline indicated a significant benefit for the standard regimen ($RR = 1.25$). These data indicate that for a typical clinical trial with a behavioral support quit rate of 7.5%, the NNT for varenicline is around 10. The main adverse effect of varenicline was nausea, which was mostly at mild to moderate levels and usually subsided over time. The authors discuss one maintenance trial in which a group of 12-weeks varenicline responders is randomized to another 12 weeks of varenicline or placebo (Tonstad *et al.*, 2006). The study shows a significant maintenance effect with 12 months continuous abstinence of 44% *vs.* 37% ($OR = 1.34$).

Initial post-marketing safety data raised questions about a possible association between varenicline and depressed mood, agitation, and suicidal behavior or ideation. However, subsequent studies have found little evidence to support these possible associations (e.g. Gunnell *et al.*, 2009).

In all three studies, varenicline was substantially more effective than bupropion: pooled RR at 12 months was 1.52 ($n = 1622$).

In the two available studies, varenicline was not significantly more effective than NRT: pooled RR ($n = 778$) for abstinence at 24 weeks was 1.13. However, there are a few studies directly comparing bupropion with NRT (Hughes *et al.*, 2007) showing some heterogeneity but these studies generally favor bupropion. Thus, if varenicline is more efficacious than bupropion, it is probably also more efficacious than NRT, which is consistent with the direction of effect found in the study of Aubin *et al.* (2008).

The one cytisine RCT included in this review (Scharfenberg *et al.*, 1971) found that significantly more participants taking cytisine stopped smoking compared with placebo at 6 months (RR = 1.91) and 2-year follow up (RR = 1.61).

For lobeline, another partial nAchR agonist, no high-quality studies (placebo-controlled RCT with long-term follow-up) were found and, therefore, no conclusion can be drawn on the effect of this medication for smoking cessation (Stead & Hughes, 1997).

nAchR antagonist (mecamylamine)

Mecamylamine is a nAchR antagonist that blocks the effect of nicotine. It has been marketed as an antihypertensive for many years. Studies examining the effects of short-term mecamylamine administration on smoking behavior have shown that low doses tend to increase smoking, probably in an attempt to overcome the nicotine blockade produced by mecamylamine. However, when much higher doses were administered, mecamylamine seemed to result in smoking reduction or cessation. However, the doses needed to stop smoking also produced side-effects including constipation, urinary retention, abdominal cramps, and weakness from the drug's hypotensive effects. In a Cochrane review by Lancaster & Stead (1998) two RCTs were identified using the combination of NRT and oral mecamylamine for smoking cessation. In the first study (Rose *et al.*, 1994), 48 volunteers were randomized to receive nicotine patch treatment plus mecamylamine capsules or nicotine patch plus placebo capsules. The addition of mecamylamine-containing capsules to nicotine patches led to a statistically significant increase in sustained abstinence at 6 and at 12 months. In the second study (Rose *et al.*, 1998), 80 volunteers were randomized to one of four groups: nicotine patch plus mecamylamine capsules; nicotine patch alone; mecamylamine alone; or no active drug. The reported rates of sustained abstinence at 6 months were 40% in the group treated with the combination of nicotine and mecamylamine, 20% in the group treated with nicotine alone, and 15% in the groups treated with mecamylamine alone, and with no drug treatment. However, the higher abstinence in the group treated with nicotine and mecamylamine was not statistically significant. In a recent RCT, 540 subjects were randomized to NRT plus placebo (0 mg mecamylamine), NRT plus low-dose mecamylamine (3 mg) or NRT plus high-dose mecamylamine (6 mg) (Glover *et al.*, 2007). No significant differences in 4-week abstinence rates were found and the authors, therefore, conclude that if adding mecamylamine to nicotine replacement therapy (NRT) improves the chances of success at stopping smoking, the effect is very small. In summary then, no promising data are available for mecamylamine alone or the combination of NRT plus mecamylamine. Moreover, varenicline, being a partial nAchR agonist, seems to represent a better alternative for this theoretical interesting option.

Antidepressants (nortriptyline, bupropion, St John's wort)

Two antidepressants have been extensively studied for smoking cessation: nortriptyline and bupropion. An updated Cochrane review (Hughes et al., 2007) describes and analyzes 49 RCTs with bupropion and nine trials of nortriptyline. When used as the sole pharmacotherapy, both bupropion ($n = 11 140$) and nortriptyline ($n = 975$) were significantly more effective than placebo: RR = 1.69 and 2.03 respectively. From the available data, bupropion and nortriptyline appear to be equally effective and of similar efficacy to NRT. There was insufficient evidence that adding bupropion or nortryptiline to NRT provides an additional benefit: RR = 1.23 (NS) and RR = 1.29 (NS), respectively.

As already mentioned before, pooling three trials comparing bupropion to varenicline showed significantly lower quitting rates with bupropion ($n = 1622$; RR = 0.66; also Johnson, 2010). There is a risk of about 1 in 1000 of seizures associated with bupropion use. As with varenicline, bupropion has been associated with suicide risk, but whether this is causal is unclear. Nortriptyline has the potential for serious side-effects, but none has been seen in the few small trials for smoking cessation.

Other antidepressants were studied less extensively: four trials of fluoxetine, three of selegiline, one of paroxetine, one of sertraline, and one of venlafaxine. As in most of the nortryptiline and bupropion studies, these studies excluded smokers with current depression but almost all included smokers with a past history of depression. There was no evidence of a significant effect of any of these medications: fluoxetine ($n = 1486$; RR = 0.92, n.s.); paroxetine ($n = 224$; RR = 1.08, n.s.); sertraline ($n = 134$; RR = 0.71, n.s.), moclobemide ($n = 88$, RR = 1.57, n.s.), selegiline ($n = 250$; RR = 1.49, n.s.) or venlafaxine ($n = 147$; RR = 1.22, n.s.).

Two recent RCTs ($n = 143$ and $n = 118$, respectively), showed that different dosages of St John's Wort (SJW) were not significantly more effective in smoking cessation than placebo (Parsons et al., 2009; Sood et al., 2010).

Other medications

Several other medications have been tried for the treatment of nicotine dependence, e.g. opioid antagonists (e.g. naltrexone), cannabis receptor antagonists (e.g. rimonabant), anxiolytics (e.g. diazepam), and α2-norepinephrine agonists (e.g. clonidine). Finally, several vaccinations against nicotine dependence have been tested.

Opioid receptor antagonists

In an updated Cochrane review David et al. (2006) described 20 studies with naltrexone and five with naloxone. Only four of the naltrexone RCTs (with or without additional NRT) could be used for a meta-analysis with long-term cessation as main outcome ($n = 582$). All four trials failed to detect a significant difference in quit rates between naltrexone and placebo (pooled RR = 1.26, n.s.). Most studies were performed with relatively low dosages of naltrexone (25–75 mg) and the study by O'Malley et al. (2006) suggested that higher dosages (100 mg or more) could be effective in long-term smoking cessation. In addition, two study reports (Covey et al., 1999; King et al., 2006) raised the possibility of a difference in effect by gender, with women showing more evidence of a benefit than men. In a recent RCT, Toll et al. (2010; $n = 172$) showed that adding 27 weeks of naltrexone (25 mg) to 8 weeks of NRT resulted in a non-significantly lower 6-month abstinence rate in the naltrexone group (RR = 0.81, n.s.). No trials of naloxone with a long-term follow-up were found.

Cannabinoid receptor antagonists

Cannabinoid receptor antagonists are interesting because they may not only be effective in smoking cessation, but also lead to weight reduction. Cahill & Ussher (2007) found three RCTs covering 1567 smokers looking for smoking cessation and 1661 quitters looking for relapse prevention. A significant 12-month effect was shown for rimonabant 20 mg (pooled RR = 1.50), but not for 5 mg (pooled RR = 1.12, n.s.). In the relapse prevention trial, quitters on 20 mg rimonabant were significantly more likely to remain abstinent than quitters on placebo on either 5 or 20 mg rimonabant: RR = 1.30 and 1.29, respectively. Weight gain was significantly lower among the 20 mg quitters than in the 5 mg or placebo quitters: overweight or obese smokers tended to lose weight, while normal-weight smokers did not. Adverse events included nausea and respiratory tract infections. In a recent study (Rigotti *et al.*, 2009), adding NRT to 20 mg rimonabant significantly improved 6-months abstinence (OR = 1.96). Meanwhile, post-marketing surveillance has led the European Medicines Agency (EMA) to require the manufacturers to withdraw rimonabant, because of links to mental disorders, including suicidal ideation and suicide attempts. Unfortunately, another cannabinoid receptor antagonist (taranabant) was shown not to be effective in smoking cessation during an 8-week RCT (Morrison *et al.*, 2010; $n = 317$; OR = 1.2., n.s.). Moreover, the study indicated significantly more psychiatric side-effects such as depression, affect lability, and irritability. It seems, therefore, unlikely that another cannabinoid receptor antagonist will become clinically available in the near future.

Anxiolytics

In an updated Cochrane review, Hughes *et al.* (2000) identified one trial each of the anxiolytics diazepam, meprobamate, metoprolol, and oxprenolol and two trials of the anxiolytic buspirone. With buspirone the pooled RR ($n = 201$) was 0.76 (n.s.) in favor of the placebo condition. None of the trials showed strong evidence of an effect on smoking cessation. However, some studies were rather small, confidence intervals were wide, and an effect of anxiolytics cannot be fully ruled out on current evidence.

Alpha$_2$-norepinephrine agonists

According to the updated Cochrane review of Gourley *et al.* (2004), in 2008 there were six trials meeting inclusion criteria: three with oral, and three with transdermal clonidine. Some behavioral counseling was offered to all participants in five of the six trials. There was only one trial with a statistically significant effect of clonidine on smoking cessation, but the pooled RR of clonidine versus placebo ($n = 776$) was significant and substantial: 1.63. However, the quality of the trials was rather poor and there was a high incidence of dose-dependent side-effects, particularly dry mouth, sedation, and hypotension. Together, this makes clonidine a less attractive first-line treatment option.

Nicotine vaccines

The idea behind nicotine vaccines is simple: attach an antibody to the nicotine molecule and nicotine will not be able to pass the blood–brain barrier; nicotine will thus not reach the nAchRs, smoking will not have a psychopharmacological effect any more and subsequently the patient will stop smoking. Currently, five different vaccines are in development, of which three have reached advanced stages of clinical evaluation (Cerny and Cerny, 2009). Currently, no overall significant effects have been reported. The main reason for this failure seems to be the large interindividual differences in the production of antibodies with positive effects only

Table 11.2. Effectiveness of pharmacological interventions in nicotine-dependent patients.

	Effect[a]	Effect size[b]	Side-effects
NRT vs. placebo	+	**1.54**	mild
Varenicline vs. placebo	++	**2.31**	debatable
Bupropion vs. placebo	+	**1.69**	mild
Nortriptiline vs. placebo	+	**2.03**	moderate
Clonidine vs. placebo	+	**1.63**	serious
Mecamylamine vs. placebo	0	–	serious
Naltrexone vs. placebo	0	1.26	mild
Rimonabant vs. placebo	+	**1.30**	very serious
Varenicline vs. NRT	0	1.40	NA
Bupropion vs. NRT	0	1.13	NA
Varenicline vs. bupropion	+	**1.52**	NA

NRT, nicotine replacement therapy.
[a] Effect indicates whether there is a substantial advantage of the first over the second compound.
[b] Bold numbers indicate statistically significant relative risks (RRs) or odds ratios (ORs).

in the subgroup of patients with high antibody levels (Cornuz et al., 2008). In addition, early studies showed high rates of (non-serious) side-effects such as flu-like symptoms during the first or the first few days after vaccination. Finally, it is not clear how many vaccinations are needed to reach adequate antibody levels and how often booster vaccinations are needed.

Conclusion: nicotine dependence treatment

There is clear evidence that the treatment of nicotine dependence can have great benefits. The rate of successful smoking cessation after 1 year is 3–5% when the patient simply tries to stop, 7–16% in the case of behavioral interventions, and up to 24% when receiving pharmacological treatment plus behavioral support (Laniado-Laborín, 2010). Table 11.2 provides a short summary of what has been presented so far regarding the effect of pharmacological interventions. Based on these data, first-line pharmacological interventions include varenicline as probably the most effective treatment, directly followed by NRT and bupropion. Second-line treatments include nortriptiline and clonidine with good effect sizes, but a higher probability of side-effects (see also Bader et al., 2009; Crain & Bhat, 2010; Frishman, 2009; Nides, 2008).

Combining different types of NRT and the combination of NRT with other effective medications may result in better outcomes (Shah et al., 2008). Most of the studies combined pharmacological treatment with behavioral support and this is important to know when applying these results in clinical practice. Most treatments were 7–12 weeks of active medication followed by 3–9 months medication-free follow-up. Based on a meta-analysis of 12 long-term follow-up studies, the effect of NRT remained at least 8 years with about 30% of the original quitters relapsing during follow-up (Etter & Stapleton, 2006). There are also indications that longer pharmacological treatments may result in better outcomes, but there are no exact data about the optimal treatment duration. A new development is the use of individual differences in the genetic make up of patients in order to improve patient–treatment matching and treatment success (e.g. Rose *et al.*, 2010; Uhl *et al.*, 2008, 2010). Finally it should be noted that nicotine dependence is a chronic relapsing disease and that more than one treatment episode might be needed to obtain an optimal final outcome (Gonzales *et al.*, 2001; Gourlay *et al.*, 1995; Han *et al.*, 2006).

Alcohol dependence

In the USA and Western Europe 10–20% of men and 5–10% of women at some point in their lives will meet criteria for alcohol abuse or dependence. The World Health Organization estimates that worldwide about 140 million people suffer from alcohol dependence, and excessive alcohol use is responsible for 4% of worldwide mortality (Rehm *et al.*, 2009). Following ingestion, alcohol is easily absorbed in the stomach, small intestine, and the colon. After absorption, alcohol is quickly distributed and 2–10% leaves the body unchanged through the lungs, kidneys, and the skin. The remaining 90–98% is metabolized in the liver: with the enzyme alcohol dehydrogenase (ADH) ethanol is oxidized to the toxic substance acetaldehyde, which in turn is transformed into harmless acetic acid with the help of aldehyde dehydrogenase (ALDH). Alcohol passes the blood–brain barrier and subsequently has an effect on a large number of receptors, e.g. stimulation of $GABA_A$ receptors, inhibition of glutamatergic NMDA, AMPA, and $mGluR_5$ receptors, stimulation of glycine receptors, stimulation of nAch receptors and probably indirectly stimulation of the dopamine (D2 and D3) and the adenosine receptors.

This review does not discuss detoxification, complications during detoxification (seizures, delirium), and the medications that can and in some cases should be used, but is restricted to the pharmacological treatment of alcohol dependence. Different kinds of medication are currently available for the treatment of alcohol dependence with different goals and different mechanisms of action, e.g. creation of aversive reaction to alcohol by blocking the metabolism of ethanol (disulfiram), by reducing the positive reinforcing effect of alcohol (e.g. naltrexone), or the reduction of craving and the negative reinforcing effect of alcohol (e.g. acamprosate).

Disulfiram

Disulfiram was the first medication that became available for the treatment of alcohol dependence (1947). Within 12 hours, disulfiram causes inhibition of ALDH resulting in high levels of acetaldehyde after (small amounts of) alcohol intake and a series of unpleasant symptoms such as nausea, vomiting, flushing, sweating, headaches, and palpitations. In order to prevent these aversive symptoms the patient has to stop using alcohol. In the first controlled trial, Fuller *et al.* (1986; $n = 605$ VA patients) were not able to show long-term efficacy of disulfiram over placebo. In a review of five other studies ($n = 1207$), Garbutt *et al.* (1999) showed that disulfiram was probably able to increase the number of non-drinking days and to reduce the total amount of alcohol intake, but that long-term abstinence was not better than placebo. Moreover, disulfiram has a number of rather frequent serious side-effects, such as epileptic seizures, cardiac problems, and neuropathic pains. There were, however, indications that the results were better if disulfiram was taken under daily supervision (e.g. Chick *et al.*, 1992). This is consistent with some recent studies indicating that supervised disulfiram might be more effective than other potentially effective medications for the treatment of alcohol dependence. In three open-label RCTs, the group of de Sousa et al. (de Sousa & de Sousa, 2004, 2005; de Sousa et al., 2008) in India found that family-supervised disulfiram was more effective in terms of 8–12 months abstinence than naltrexone (RR = 1.95), acamprosate (RR = 1.91), and topiramate (RR = 1.61). Similarly, Laaksonen et al. (2008) found that disulfiram was more effective than acamprosate and naltrexone during a 12-week RCT with all patients also receiving cognitive–behavior therapy ($n = 234$). In a recent naturalistic retrospective study, Diehl et al. (2010; $n = 353$) found that supervised disulfiram was more effective than acamprosate, especially in patients with a long duration of alcohol dependence. In summary, disulfiram seems to be an effective intervention only with intensive supervision and/or psychosocial support, with serious side-effects not only in the case of alcohol use (aversive effect) but also when no alcohol is being used.

Opioid receptor antagonists (naltrexone/nalmefene)

Naltrexone is a mu-opioid receptor antagonist that reduces the rewarding effect of alcohol and probably also reduces craving for alcohol. The effect occurs within hours. Nalmefene is a very similar compound, but also has affinity to the other opioid receptors. Moreover, nalmefene has a longer half-life, greater oral bioavailability, and no observed dose-dependent liver toxicity.

In a recent Cochrane review, Rösner et al. (2010a) described and analyzed 50 RCTs ($n = 7793$): 47 with oral or injectable extended-release naltrexone ($n = 3881$) and three with nalmefene ($n = 286$) vs. placebo ($n = 3626$). Active treatment varied between 4 and 52 weeks and follow-up after treatment discontinuation ranged from 3 to 17 months. The analyses unequivocally showed that naltrexone is an effective and safe medication for the treatment of alcohol dependence: significant reduction of the risk of a return to heavy drinking (RR = 0.83; NNT = 9.1), significant reduction in number of heavy drinking days (mean difference (MD) = –3.25 days), significant reduction in consumed amount of alcohol (MD = –10.83 grams), and a significant reduction in gamma-glutamyltransferase (MD = –10.37 units). However, naltrexone had no significant effect on continuous abstinence rates after treatment discontinuation (RR = 0.96). Between 3 and 12 months after treatment was discontinued, patients who were in the naltrexone group had a significant 14% lower risk to return to heavy drinking (RR = 0.86), but only a non-significant 6% lower risk to return to any drinking. Side-effects of naltrexone were mild and mainly restricted to gastrointestinal problems and sedative effects.

The four RCTs with monthly injections with extended release naltrexone indicate that this formulation significantly reduced the risk of any drinking after detoxification to 92% of the placebo (RR = 0.92), significantly reduced the percentage of drinking days (MD = –8.54%), but only reduced the percentage of heavy drinking days by a non-significant 3% (MD = –3.05%). No direct comparisons between oral and injectable naltrexone are currently available and, therefore, no conclusions can be drawn about the effectiveness of extended release naltrexone regarding the improvement of treatment compliance and the related improvement of treatment outcome (see also Roozen et al., 2007).

Based on only three RCTs ($n = 396$), positive but no significant results were obtained for the effect of nalmefene in treating alcohol dependence: risk to return to heavy drinking (RR = 0.85, n.s.), risk to return to any drinking after detoxification (RR = 0.92, n.s.), 5%

reduction of heavy drinking days (MD = −4.70 days, n.s.), and a decrease of the amount of alcohol consumed per drinking day at about 4 grams (MD = −4.16, n.s.). Some of the side-effects, however, were statistically more prevalent in the nalmefene compared with the placebo condition, e.g. nausea, insomnia, and dizziness.

In a meta-analysis of three studies (Rösner et al., 2010a; n = 800), the effects of naltrexone were similar to those of acamprosate: return to heavy drinking (RR = 0.96, n.s.), return to any drinking (RR = 097, n.s.); patients on naltrexone reported significantly more nausea, whereas patients on acamprosate complained significantly more about diarrhea. However, in a single blind RCT, naltrexone was superior to acamprosate in terms of the return to both heavy drinking and any drinking (Rubio et al., 2001).

In single studies, naltrexone was non-significantly inferior in its effect on some alcohol outcomes to the anti-epileptics oxcarbazepine (Martinotti et al., 2007) and topiramate (Baltieri et al., 2008), the second generation antipsychotic (partial dopamine D2 receptor agonist) aripiprazole (Martinotti et al., 2009), and the serotonergic antidepressant nefazodone (Kranzler et al., 2000).

In a meta-analysis of only two studies (Anton et al., 2006; Kiefer et al., 2003; N = 614 and N = 80 respectively), the effect of the combination of naltrexone plus acamprosate was non-significantly better compared with naltrexone alone: return to heavy drinking (RR = 0.97; n.s.), and any drinking (RR = 0.88; n.s.). The combination treatment induced diarrhea and nausea significantly more often than naltrexone alone. Similar findings were observed in a non-randomized matched study (Feeney et al., 2006; n = 236).

In all the studies reported so far, naltrexone was administered daily for 4–52 weeks. An alternative approach is "targeted" or "as needed" use of naltrexone or nalmefene, i.e. patients taking the medication only in anticipation of a high-risk drinking situation or even the early phase of a drinking situation. This strategy has proven to be effective in at least three RCTs in heavy drinkers, problem drinkers, and alcohol-dependent subjects (Heinälä et al., 2001; Karhuvaara et al., 2007; Kranzler et al., 2009).

A number of studies indicate that naltrexone and nalmefene are most effective in patients with a specific genetic variation of the mu-opioid receptor. However, other studies were not able to replicate this intriguing finding.

In summary, naltrexone is a proven-effective treatment that prevents relapse to heavy drinking, limited compliance, and mild but rather frequent side-effects. The effect seems very similar to that of some other medications, including the well-studied glutaminergic compound acamprosate. A new development is the targeted use of medication in risk situations only.

Glutamatergic medications (acamprosate, topiramate)

Acamprosate

The principal neurochemical effects of acamprosate have been attributed to antagonism of NMDA glutamate receptors that restores the balance between excitatory and inhibitory neurotransmission, which has become dysregulated following chronic alcohol consumption. Recently, it has been proposed that acamprosate also modulates glutamate neurotransmission at metabotropic-5 glutamate receptors (mGluR5), in addition to its effect on acute withdrawal, acamprosate also attenuates conditioned reactions ("pseudo-withdrawal") and opponent processes associated with drinking-related cues, the latter explaining the potency of the substance to prevent a relapse after physical symptoms of withdrawal have disappeared. The onset of effect is assumed to take 1–2 weeks and most studies required at least 1–2 weeks of continuous abstinence before the start of the medication.

Rösner et al. (2010a) described and analyzed 24 RCTs ($n = 6915$). Compared with placebo, acamprosate was significantly more effective than placebo in reducing the risk of any drinking (RR = 0.86; NNT 9.1) and in cumulative abstinence duration (MD = 10.94 days), but secondary outcomes such as return to heavy drinking (RR = 0.99, n.s.) and gamma-glutamyltransferase (MD = – 11.91, n.s.) were not significantly better than placebo. Diarrhea was the only side-effect that was more frequently reported under acamprosate than placebo. Post-treatment return to any drinking was significantly better for the acamprosate group (RR = 0.91; NNT = 12.5), but return to heavy drinking was not (RR = 0.97).

In two RCTs (Anton et al., 2006; Kiefer et al., 2003), the combination acamprosate plus naltrexone tended to be more effective than acamprosate alone, but the difference in effect was not significant: return to any drinking (RR = 0.80, n.s.) and return to heavy drinking (RR = 0.81, n.s.). However, the combination treatment was associated with significantly more side-effects such as nausea and vomiting.

Finally, Besson et al. (1998) performed an open-label RCT ($n = 118$) comparing 12 months disulfiram plus acamprosate with 12 months disulfiram plus placebo and found a significant additional effect of acamprosate at least during the active treatment phase.

In summary, acamprosate is a proven-effective treatment of patients that are at least abstinent for 1–2 weeks and then promotes full abstinence even after treatment discontinuation, has limited treatment compliance and mild side-effects.

Topiramate

Topiramate, an anticonvulsant that augments GABA by binding to a non-benzodiazepine site on $GABA_A$ receptors and by antagonizing the AMPA subtype of the glutamate receptor, has demonstrated efficacy in the treatment of alcohol dependence in three placebo-controlled RCTs. In the first two studies (Johnson et al., 2003, $n = 150$; Johnson et al., 2007, $n = 371$), 12–14 weeks of topiramate (up to 300 mg/day) was significantly more effective than placebo at the end of the active treatment period in terms of the percentage drinking days, the percentage heavy drinking days and gamma-GT. In both studies, patients reported significantly more side-effects such as dizziness, paresthesia, weight loss, and memory/concentration problems. Both studies indicate that lower dosages of topiramate might also be effective and produce fewer side-effects. In the third RCT ($n = 155$), topiramate was significantly more effective than placebo and was non-significantly superior to naltrexone (Baltieri et al., 2008). Among alcohol-dependent smokers ($n = 103/155$), topiramate was (unintentionally) associated with reduced smoking, whereas naltrexone and placebo were not (Baltieri et al., 2009). In a 6-month open-label non-placebo controlled RCT ($n = 102$), topiramate was non-significantly superior to naltrexone in terms of alcohol craving, alcohol consumption outcomes, and reduction of smoking (Flórez et al., 2008). However, in India, topiramate was less effective than family-supervised disulfiram (de Sousa et al., 2008).

In summary, topiramate is a promising new treatment for alcohol dependence with unknown optimal dosing, but with frequent unpleasant side-effects in the dose that has been studied so far (see also Arbaizar et al., 2010). Currently, no long-term studies are available.

Other medications

In addition to the three registered medications for the treatment of alcohol dependence, a series of new potentially effective medications have been studied. Here we briefly discuss the findings regarding baclofen, GHB, and various types of antidepressants.

Baclofen

Baclofen is a $GABA_B$ agonist that is indicated for the treatment of spasticity and is currently under study for the treatment of alcohol dependence. Baclofen has been studied as a compound to support withdrawal and as a compound to prevent relapse after detoxification. Currently, there are three RCTs on relapse prevention: two studies with a positive and one study with a negative outcome. The first RCT ($n = 39$) showed that 4 weeks baclofen was more effective than placebo in reducing state anxiety, craving, and alcohol outcomes such as abstinence duration and reduced alcohol consumption (Addolorato et al., 2002). In a second RCT among chronic alcohol-dependent patients with liver cirrhosis ($n = 84$), 12 weeks of baclofen was significantly more effective than placebo: less craving, higher percentage with continued abstinence (71% vs. 29%; OR = 6.3) and cumulative abstinence duration (63 days vs. 31 days). No hepatic side-effects were recorded. However, in a recent RCT ($n = 80$), both craving in alcohol consumption outcomes for 12 weeks baclofen were very similar and not significantly different from those of 12 weeks placebo (Garbutt et al., 2010). According to the authors, a possible explanation for the difference between the last and the first two studies might be the fact the dependence severity in the positive trials was much higher than in the negative trial. No long-term studies are currently available.

In summary, baclofen seems a promising new treatment for patients with severe alcohol dependence, high levels of craving and state anxiety (see also Tyacke et al., 2010).

Gamma hydroxybutyric acid (GHB)

Gamma hydroxybutyric acid (GHB) is an agonist at the newly characterized excitatory GHB receptor and a weak agonist at the inhibitory $GABA_B$ receptor.

In a recent Cochrane review (Leone et al., 2010), 13 RCTs were described and analyzed, six about the effect of GHB on withdrawal symptoms and seven about the effect of GHB on preventing relapse and maintaining abstinence. In the two studies comparing GHB with placebo over a period of 3 and 6 months, GHB was significantly more effective than placebo in terms of craving (RD = −4.20 and RD = −4.30, respectively), maintaining total abstinence (RR = 5.35 and RR = 1.33, respectively), and relapse to heavy drinking (RR = 0.36 and RR = 0.34, respectively). Overall, the number of patients with GHB-related side-effects was quite low with dizziness, diarrhea, headache, rhinitis, and nausea being most frequently reported. Craving and the risk of GHB dependence seem to be higher in patients with polysubstance dependence than in patients with pure alcohol dependence (Caputo et al., 2009) and when used outside the medical context (e.g. van Amsterdam et al., 2010).

Three studies compared GHB with naltrexone: two studies at 3- and one study at 12-months follow-up. At 3 months, GHB treatment resulted in significantly better rates of total abstinence (RR = 2.59) and in non-significant lower rates of relapse to heavy drinking (RR = 3.23, n.s.). At 6 months there were no significant differences between the two treatment conditions.

The only study comparing GHB with disulfiram in maintaining abstinence at 12-months follow-up showed conflicting and mainly non-significant findings (Nava *et al.*, 2006).

In summary, GHB is a promising candidate for the treatment of alcohol dependence. It should be noted that almost all studies were performed in one country (Italy) and samples were generally rather small. Moreover, GHB is only licensed in a few countries and is listed as a narcotic drug in many other countries.

Gabapentin

There are only two small RCTs examining the effect of gabapentin on relapse prevention in alcohol-dependent patients. The first 4 weeks RCT ($n = 60$) showed that gabapentin was significantly more effective than placebo in terms of a greater reduction of craving, longer cumulative abstinence duration and fewer heavy drinking days (Furieri & Nakamura-Palacios, 2007). In the second RCT with 6 weeks active treatment and 6 weeks follow-up of alcohol-dependent patients with insomnia ($n = 21$), gabapentin was significantly more effective than placebo in the prevention of relapse to heavy drinking both at 6 and 12 weeks (70% *vs.* 18% and 40% *vs.* 0% respectively), but not more effective in the reduction of insomnia (Anton *et al.*, 2008). No long-term treatment studies are currently available.

Antidepressants

Despite the promise of pre-clinical research, there is generally little support for the effectiveness of antidepressants in the treatment of alcohol dependence (e.g. Johnson, 2008; Kenna, 2010), including SSRIs, the partial 5-HT$_1$ receptor agonist buspirone, and the 5-HT$_2$ receptor antagonist ritanserin. The 5-HT$_3$ antagonist ondansetron is still promising, especially in patients with early-onset alcohol-dependence (Johnson *et al.*, 2000; Kranzler *et al.*, 2003; Sellers *et al.*, 1994).

Conclusion: alcohol dependence treatment

Table 11.3 provides a brief summary of the current state of the art and clearly shows that there are a number of proven-effective and registered medications for the treatment of alcohol dependence (supervised disulfiram, naltrexone, acamprosate) and some other medications that have shown great promise, mainly in short-term studies (topiramate, GHB, baclofen, and gabapentin). Given the fact that alcohol dependence is a chronic relapsing disorder, first-line treatments are currently restricted to disulfiram, naltrexone, and acamprosate. There is renewed attention to disulfiram in cases where intensive (family) supervision can be organized. It should be noted, however, that treatment compliance is also a serious issue with the other medications and, therefore, pharmacological treatment should always be combined with good clinical management.

In general, effect sizes are modest and there is no treatment that seems to fit all patients. In search for an individualized approach, various researchers have been looking both at the phenotypic and the genetic level to match certain patients with certain medications in order to obtain better outcomes. What follows is some of the preliminary findings regarding this search for patient–treatment matching. Naltrexone seems to be more effective in alcohol-dependent patients with early-onset alcohol dependence (Kiefer *et al.*, 2005), in patients with a positive family history and low sociability (Krishnan-Sarin *et al.*, 2007; Rohsenow *et al.*, 2007), in patients with a certain variation of the mu-opioid receptor gene (e.g. Anton

Table 11.3. Effectiveness of pharmacological interventions in alcohol-dependent patients.

	Return to drinking	Return to heavy drinking	Number of HDD[a]	Side-effects	Remarks[b]
Disulfiram (D)	+	+	+	serious	D > NTX/ACA/TOP
Naltrexone (NTX$_{oral}$)	RR = 0.96	**RR = 0.83**[c]	−3.25	mild	NTX = ACA
Naltrexone (NTX $_{inj}$)	?	**RR = 0.92**	−3.05	moderate	
Nalmefene (NAL)	RR = 0.92	RR = 0.85	−4.70	few	
Acamprosate (ACA)	**RR = 0.86**	RR = 0.99	?	mild	
Comb NTX + ACA	?	?	?	moderate	Comb > NTX (n.s.) Comb > ACA (n.s.)
Topiramate (TOP)	+	+	+	frequent	TOP = NTX no long term trials
Baclofen	+	?	+	mild	no long term trials
GHB	**RR = 0.19**	**RR = 0.34**	?	few	GHB > NTX GHB = D no long term trials
Gabapentin	+	+	+	mild	no long term trials
Antidepressants	−	−	−	moderate	ondansetron?

[a] HDD, Heavy drinking days.
[b] Relative efficacy of the various medications compared with each other and absence of long-term trials.
[c] Bold numbers indicate statistically significant relative risks (RRs), odds ratios (ORs), or mean differences (MDs). n.s., not significant.

et al., 2008; Oslin *et al.*, 2003), and in patients with a certain variation of the dopmaine D4 receptor (Tidey *et al.*, 2008). Similarly, efficacy of acamprosate seems not to be predicted by phenotypical/clinical characteristics (Verheul *et al.*, 2005), but this medication might be more effective in patients with certain genetic variations of the dopamine D2 and certain glutamate receptor genes (Ooteman *et al.*, 2009), or in patients with a specific transcription factor (GATA4; Kiefer *et al.*, 2011). Finally, certain antidepressants might be effective only in patients with a certain age of onset.

References

Addolorato G, Caputo F, Capristo E *et al.* (2002). Baclofen efficacy in reducing alcohol craving and intake: a preliminary double-blind randomized controlled study. *Alcohol and Alcoholism* 37, 504–508.

Agrawal A, Lynskey MT (2008). Are there genetic influences on addiction: evidence from family, adoption and twin studies. *Addiction* 103, 1069–1081.

Andlin-Sobocki P, Rehm J (2005). Cost of addiction in Europe. *European Journal of Neurology* 12 (Suppl. 1), 28–33.

Anton RF, O'Malley SS, Ciraulo DA *et al.* (2006). COMBINE Study Research Group. Combined pharmacotherapies and behavioral interventions for alcohol dependence: the COMBINE study: a randomized controlled trial. *Journal of the American Medical Association* 295(17), 2003–2017.

Anton RF, Oroszi G, O'Malley S *et al.* (2008). An evaluation of mu-opioid receptor (OPRM1) as a predictor of naltrexone response in the treatment of alcohol dependence: results from the Combined Pharmacotherapies and

Behavioral Interventions for Alcohol Dependence (COMBINE) study. *Archives of General Psychiatry* **65**(2), 135–144.

Arbaizar B, Diersen-Sotos T, Gómez-Acebo I, Llorca J (2010). Topiramate in the treatment of alcohol dependence: a meta-analysis. *Actas Espanolas de Psiquiatria* **38**(1), 8–12.

Aubin HJ, Bobak A, Britton JR et al. (2008). Varenicline versus transdermal nicotine patch for smoking cessation: results from a randomised open-label trial. *Thorax* **63**(8), 717–724.

Bader P, McDonald P, Selby P (2009). An algorithm for tailoring pharmacotherapy for smoking cessation: results from a Delphi panel of international experts. *Tobacco Control* **18**, 34–42.

Baltieri DA, Daró FR, Ribeiro PL, de Andrade AG (2008). Comparing topiramate with naltrexone in the treatment of alcohol dependence. *Addiction* **103**, 2035–2044.

Baltieri DA, Daró FR, Ribeiro PL, Andrade AG (2009). Effects of topiramate or naltrexone on tobacco use among male alcohol-dependent outpatients. *Drug and Alcohol Dependence* **105**(1–2), 33–41.

Besson J, Aeby F, Kasas A, Lehert P, Potgieter A (1998). Combined efficacy of acamprosate and disulfiram in the treatment of alcoholism: a controlled study. *Alcoholism: Clinical & Experimental Research* **22**, 573–579.

Cahill K, Ussher MH (2007). Cannabinoid type 1 receptor antagonists (rimonabant) for smoking cessation. *Cochrane Database of Systematic Reviews* **4**, D005353.

Cahill K, Stead LF, Lancaster T (2010). Nicotine receptor partial agonists for smoking cessation. *Cochrane Database of Systematic Reviews* **12**, CD006103.

Caputo F, Francini S, Stoppo M et al. (2009). Incidence of craving for and abuse of gamma-hydroxybutyric acid (GHB) in different populations of treated alcoholics: an open comparative study. *Journal of Psychopharmacology* **23**, 883–890.

Cerny EH, Cerny T (2009). Vaccines against nicotine. *Human Vaccines* **5**, 200–205.

Chick J, Gough K, Falkowski W et al. (1992). Disulfiram treatment of alcoholism. *British Journal of Psychiatry* **161**, 84–89.

Cornuz J, Zwahlen S, Jungi WF et al. (2008). A vaccine against nicotine for smoking cessation: a randomized controlled trial. *PLoS One* **3**(6), e2547.

Covey LS, Glassman AH, Stetner F (1999). Naltrexone effects on short-term and long-term smoking cessation. *Journal of Addictive Diseases* **18**, 31–40.

Crain D, Bhat A (2010). Current treatment options in smoking cessation. *Hospital Practice (Minneapolis)* **38**(1), 53–61.

Crunelle CL, Miller ML, Booij J, van den Brink W (2010). The nicotinic acetylcholine receptor partial agonist varenicline and the treatment of drug dependence: a review. *European Neuropsychopharmacology* **20**(2), 69–79.

David SP, Lancaster T, Stead LF, Evins AE, Cahill K (2006). Opioid antagonists for smoking cessation. *Cochrane Database of Systematic Reviews* **4**, CD003086.

de Sousa A, De Sousa A (2004). A one-year pragmatic trial of naltrexone vs. disulfiram in the treatment of alcohol dependence. *Alcohol and Alcoholism* **39**(6), 528–531.

de Sousa A, de Sousa A (2005). An open randomized study comparing disulfiram and acamprosate in the treatment of alcohol dependence. *Alcohol and Alcoholism* **40**(6), 545–548.

de Sousa AA, De Sousa J, Kapoor H (2008). An open randomized trial comparing disulfiram and topiramate in the treatment of alcohol dependence. *Journal of Substance Abuse Treatment* **34**(4), 460–463.

Diehl A, Ulmer L, Mutschler J et al. (2010). Why is disulfiram superior to acamprosate in the routine clinical setting? A retrospective long-term study in 353 alcohol-dependent patients. *Alcohol and Alcoholism* **45**(3), 271–277.

Etter JF, Stapleton JA (2006). Nicotine replacement therapy for long-term smoking cessation: a meta-analysis. *Tobacco Control* **15**(4), 280–285.

Feeney GF, Connor JP, Young RM, Tucker J, McPherson A (2006). Combined acamprosate and naltrexone, with cognitive behavioural therapy is superior to either medication alone for alcohol abstinence: a single centres' experience with pharmacotherapy. *Alcohol and Alcoholism* **41**(3), 321–327.

Flórez G, García-Portilla P, Alvarez S et al. (2008). Using topiramate or naltrexone for the treatment of alcohol-dependent patients. *Alcoholism: Clinical & Experimental Research* **32**(7), 1251–1259.

Fowler T, Lifford K, Shelton K et al. (2007). Exploring the relationship between genetic and environmental influences on initiation and progression of substance use. *Addiction* **102**(3), 413–422.

Frishman WH (2009). Smoking cessation pharmacotherapy. *Therapeutic Advances in Cardiovascular Disease* **3**(4), 287–308.

Fuller RK, Branchey L, Brightwell DR et al. (1986). Disulfiram treatment of alcoholism. A Veterans Administration cooperative study. *Journal of the American Medical Association* **256**(11), 1449–1455.

Furieri FA, Nakamura-Palacios EM (2007). Gabapentin reduces alcohol consumption and craving: a randomized, double-blind, placebo-controlled trial. *Journal of Clinical Psychiatry* **68**(11), 1691–1700.

Garbutt JC, Kampov-Polevoy AB, Gallop R, Kalka-Juhl L, Flannery BA (2010). Efficacy and safety of baclofen for alcohol dependence: a randomized, double-blind, placebo-controlled trial. *Alcoholism: Clinical and Experimental Research* **34**, 1849–1857.

Garbutt JC, West SL, Carey TS, Lohr KN, Crews FT (1999). Pharmacological treatment of alcohol dependence: a review of the evidence. *Journal of the American Medical Association* **281**(14), 1318–1325.

Glover ED, Laflin MT, Schuh KJ et al. (2007). A randomized, controlled trial to assess the efficacy and safety of a transdermal delivery system of nicotine/mecamylamine in cigarette smokers. *Addiction* **102**, 795–802.

Gonzales D, Rennard SI, Nides M et al. (2006). Varenicline Phase 3 Study Group. Varenicline, an alpha4beta2 nicotinic acetylcholine receptor partial agonist, vs. sustained-release bupropion and placebo for smoking cessation: a randomized controlled trial. *Journal of the American Medical Association* **296**(1), 47–55.

Gonzales DH, Nides MA, Ferry LH et al. (2001). Bupropion SR as an aid to smoking cessation in smokers treated previously with bupropion: a randomized placebo-controlled study. *Clinical Pharmacology & Therapeutics* **69**(6), 438–444.

Gourlay SG, Forbes A, Marriner T, Pethica D, McNeil JJ (1995). Double blind trial of repeated treatment with transdermal nicotine for relapsed smokers. *British Medical Journal* **311**(7001), 363–366.

Gourlay SG, Stead LF, Benowitz N. (2004). Clonidine for smoking cessation. *Cochrane Database of Systematic Reviews* **3**, CD000058.

Gunnell D, Irvine D, Wise L, Davies C, Martin RM (2009). Varenicline and suicidal behaviour: a cohort study based on data from the General Practice Research Database. *British Medical Journal* **339**, b3805. doi: 10.1136/bmj.b3805.

Han ES, Foulds J, Steinberg MB et al. (2006). Characteristics and smoking cessation outcomes of patients returning for repeat tobacco dependence treatment. *International Journal of Clinical Practice* **60**(9), 1068–1074.

Hays JT, Ebbert JO (2010). Adverse effects and tolerability of medications for the treatment of tobacco use and dependence. *Drugs* **70**(18), 2357–2372.

Heinälä P, Alho H, Kiianmaa K et al. (2001). Targeted use of naltrexone without prior detoxification in the treatment of alcohol dependence: a factorial double-blind, placebo-controlled trial. *Journal of Clinical Psychopharmacology* **21**(3), 287–292.

Hughes JR, Stead LF, Lancaster T (2000). Anxiolytics for smoking cessation. *Cochrane Database of Systematic Reviews* **4**, CD002849.

Hughes JR, Stead LF, Lancaster T (2007). Antidepressants for smoking cessation. *Cochrane Database of Systematic Reviews* **1**, CD000031.

Johnson BA (2008). Update on neuropharmacological treatments for alcoholism: scientific basis and clinical findings. *Biochemical Pharmacology* **75**(1), 34–56.

Johnson BA, Ait-Daoud N, Bowden CL et al. (2003). Oral topiramate for treatment of alcohol dependence: a randomised controlled trial. *Lancet* **361**(9370), 1677–1685.

Johnson BA, Roache JD, Javors MA *et al.* (2000). Ondansetron for reduction of drinking among biologically predisposed alcoholic patients: a randomized controlled trial. *Journal of the American Medical Association* **284**, 963–971.

Johnson BA, Rosenthal N, Capece JA *et al.* (2007). Topiramate for treating alcohol dependence: a randomized controlled trial. *Journal of the American Medical Association* **298**(14), 1641–1651.

Johnson TS (2010). A brief review of pharmacotherapeutic treatment options in smoking cessation: bupropion versus varenicline. *Journal of the American Academy of Nurse Practitioners* **22**, 557–563.

Jorenby DE, Hays JT, Rigotti NA *et al.* (2006). Varenicline Phase 3 Study Group. Efficacy of varenicline, an alpha4beta2 nicotinic acetylcholine receptor partial agonist, vs. placebo or sustained-release bupropion for smoking cessation: a randomized controlled trial. *Journal of the American Medical Association* **296**(1), 56–63.

Jorenby DE, Leischow SJ, Nides MA *et al.* (1999). A controlled trial of sustained-release bupropion, a nicotine patch, or both for smoking cessation. *New England Journal of Medicine* **340**(9), 685–691.

Karhuvaara S, Simojoki K, Virta A *et al.* (2007). Targeted nalmefene with simple medical management in the treatment of heavy drinkers: a randomized double-blind placebo-controlled multicenter study. *Alcoholism: Clinical & Experimental Research* **31**(7), 1179–1187.

Kastelic A, Dubajic G, Strbad E (2008). Slow-release oral morphine for maintenance treatment of opioid addicts intolerant to methadone or with inadequate withdrawal suppression. *Addiction* **103**(11), 1837–1846.

Kendler KS, Myers J, Prescott CA (2007). Specificity of genetic and environmental risk factors for symptoms of cannabis, cocaine, alcohol, caffeine, and nicotine dependence. *Archives of General Psychiatry* **64**, 1313–1320.

Kendler KS, Prescott CA, Myers J, Neale MC (2003). The structure of genetic and environmental risk factors for common psychiatric and substance use disorders in men and women. *Archives of General Psychiatry* **60**(9), 929–937.

Kenna GA (2010). Medications acting on the serotonergic system for the treatment of alcohol dependent patients. *Current Pharmaceutical Design* **16**(19), 2126–2135.

Kiefer F, Helwig H, Tarnaske T *et al.* (2005). Pharmacological relapse prevention of alcoholism: clinical predictors of outcome. *European Journal of Addiction Research* **11**(2), 83–91.

Kiefer F, Jahn H, Tarnaske T *et al.* (2003). Comparing and combining naltrexone and acamprosate in relapse prevention of alcoholism: a double-blind, placebo-controlled study. *Archives of General Psychiatry* **60**, 92–99.

Kiefer F, Witt SH, Frank J *et al.* (2011). Involvement of the atrial natriuretic peptide transcription factor GATA4 in alcohol dependence, relapse risk and treatment response to acamprosate. *Pharmacogenomics Journal* **11**(5), 368–374.

King A, de Wit H, Riley RC *et al.* (2006). Efficacy of naltrexone in smoking cessation: a preliminary study and an examination of sex differences. *Nicotine and Tobacco Research* **8**(5), 671–682.

Koob GF, Volkow ND (2010). Neurocircuitry of addiction. *Neuropsychopharmacology* **35**(1), 217–238.

Kranzler HR, Modesto-Lowe V, Van Kirk J (2000). Naltrexone vs. nefazodone for treatment of alcohol dependence. A placebo-controlled trial. *Neuropsychopharmacology* **22**, 493–503.

Kranzler HR, Pierucci-Lagha A, Feinn R, Hernandez-Avila C (2003). Effects of ondansetron in early- versus late-onset alcoholics: a prospective, open-label study. *Alcoholism: Clinical & Experimental Research* **27**(7), 1150–1155.

Kranzler HR, Tennen H, Armeli S *et al.* (2009). Targeted naltrexone for problem drinkers. *Journal of Clinical Psychopharmacology* **29**(4), 350–357.

Krishnan-Sarin S, Krystal JH, Shi J, Pittman B, O'Malley SS (2007). Family history of alcoholism influences naltrexone-induced reduction in alcohol drinking. *Biological Psychiatry* **62**(6), 694–697.

Laaksonen E, Koski-Jännes A, Salaspuro M, Ahtinen H, Alho H (2008). A randomized, multicentre, open-label, comparative trial of disulfiram, naltrexone and acamprosate in the treatment of alcohol dependence. *Alcohol and Alcoholism* **43**(1), 53–61.

Lancaster T, Stead LF (1998). Mecamylamine (a nicotine antagonist) for smoking cessation. *Cochrane Database of Systematic Reviews* **2**, CD001009.

Laniado-Laborín R (2010). Smoking cessation intervention: an evidence-based approach. *Postgraduate Medicine* **122**(2), 74–82.

Leone MA, Vigna-Taglianti F, Avanzi G, Brambilla R, Faggiano F (2010). Gamma-hydroxybutyrate (GHB) for treatment of alcohol withdrawal and prevention of relapses. *Cochrane Database of Systematic Reviews* **2**, CD006266.

Martinotti G, Di Nicola M, Di Giannantonio M, Janiri L (2009). Aripiprazole in the treatment of patients with alcohol dependence: a double-blind, comparison trial vs. naltrexone. *Journal of Psychopharmacology* **23**(2), 123–129.

Martinotti G, Di Nicola M, Romanelli R et al. (2007). High and low dosage oxcarbazepine versus naltrexone for the prevention of relapse in alcohol-dependent patients. *Human Psychopharmacology* **22**(3), 149–156.

Morrison MF, Ceesay P, Gantz I, Kaufman KD, Lines CR (2010). Randomized, controlled, double-blind trial of taranabant for smoking cessation. *Psychopharmacology (Berlin)* **209**(3), 245–253.

Nava F, Premi S, Manzato E, Lucchini A (2006). Comparing treatments of alcoholism on craving and biochemical measures of alcohol consumption. *Journal of Psychoactive Drugs* **38**(3), 211–217.

Nides M (2008). Update on pharmacologic options for smoking cessation treatment. *American Journal of Medicine* **121**(4 Suppl. 1), S20–S31.

Nides M, Oncken C, Gonzales D et al. (2006). Smoking cessation with varenicline, a selective alpha4beta2 nicotinic receptor partial agonist: results from a 7-week, randomized, placebo- and bupropion-controlled trial with 1-year follow-up. *Archives of Internal Medicine* **166**(15), 1561–1568.

Nutt DJ, King LA, Phillips LD (2010). Independent Scientific Committee on Drugs. Drug harms in the UK: a multicriteria decision analysis. *Lancet* **376**(9752), 1558–1565.

Nutt DJ, King LA, Saulsbury W, Blakemore C (2007). Development of a rational scale to assess the harm of drugs of potential misuse. *Lancet* **369**(9566), 1047–1053.

O'Malley SS, Cooney JL, Krishnan-Sarin S et al. (2006). A controlled trial of naltrexone augmentation of nicotine replacement therapy for smoking cessation. *Archives of Internal Medicine* **166**(6), 667–674.

Ooteman W, Naassila M, Koeter MW et al. (2009). Predicting the effect of naltrexone and acamprosate in alcohol-dependent patients using genetic indicators. *Addiction Biology* **14**(3), 328–337.

Orman JS, Keating GM (2009). Buprenorphine/ naloxone: a review of its use in the treatment of opioid dependence. *Drugs* **69**(5), 577–607.

Oslin DW, Berrettini W, Kranzler HR et al. (2003). A functional polymorphism of the mu-opioid receptor gene is associated with naltrexone response in alcohol-dependent patients. *Neuropsychopharmacology* **28**(8), 1546–1552.

Parsons A, Ingram J, Inglis J et al. (2009). A proof of concept randomised placebo controlled factorial trial to examine the efficacy of St John's wort for smoking cessation and chromium to prevent weight gain on smoking cessation. *Drug and Alcohol Dependence* **102**(1–3), 116–122.

Rehm J, Mathers C, Popova S et al. (2009). Global burden of disease and injury and economic cost attributable to alcohol use and alcohol-use disorders. *Lancet* **373**(9682), 2223–2233.

Rehm J, Taylor B, Room R (2006). Global burden of disease from alcohol, illicit drugs and tobacco. *Drug and Alcohol Reviews* **25**, 503–513.

Rigotti NA, Gonzales D, Dale LC, Lawrence D, Chang Y; CIRRUS Study Group. (2009). A randomized controlled trial of adding the nicotine patch to rimonabant for smoking cessation: efficacy, safety and weight gain. *Addiction* **104**(2), 266–276.

Rohsenow DJ, Miranda R Jr, McGeary JE, Monti PM (2007). Family history and antisocial traits moderate naltrexone's effects on heavy drinking in alcoholics. *Experimental and Clinical Psychopharmacology* 15(3), 272–281.

Roozen HG, de Waart R, van den Brink W (2007). Efficacy and tolerability of naltrexone in the treatment of alcohol dependence: oral versus injectable delivery. *European Addiction Research* 13(4), 201–206.

Rose JE, Behm FM, Drgon T, Johnson C, Uhl GR (2010). Personalized smoking cessation: interactions between nicotine dose, dependence and quit-success genotype score. *Molecular Medicine* 16(7–8), 247–253.

Rose JE, Behm FM, Westman EC (1998). Nicotine-mecamylamine treatment for smoking cessation: the role of pre-cessation therapy. *Experimental and Clinical Psychopharmacology* 6(3), 331–343.

Rose JE, Behm FM, Westman EC et al. (1994). Mecamylamine combined with nicotine skin patch facilitates smoking cessation beyond nicotine patch treatment alone. *Clinical Pharmacology & Therapeutics* 56(1), 86–99.

Rösner S, Hackl-Herrwerth A, Leucht S et al. (2010a). Opioid antagonists for alcohol dependence. *Cochrane Database of Systematic Reviews* 12, CD001867.

Rösner S, Hackl-Herrwerth A, Leucht S et al. (2010b). Acamprosate for alcohol dependence. *Cochrane Database of Systematic Reviews* 9, CD004332.

Rubio G, Jiménez-Arriero MA, Ponce G, Palomo T (2001). Naltrexone versus acamprosate: one year follow-up of alcohol dependence treatment. *Alcohol and Alcoholism* 36(5), 419–425.

Scharfenberg G, Benndorf S, Kempe G (1971). [Cytisine (Tabex) as a pharmaceutical aid in stopping smoking]. *Das Deutsche Gesundheitswesen* 26(10), 463–465.

Sellers EM, Toneatto T, Romach MK et al. (1994). Clinical efficacy of the 5-HT3 antagonist ondansetron in alcohol abuse and dependence. *Alcoholism: Clinical & Experimental Research* 18(4), 879–885.

Shah SD, Wilken LA, Winkler SR, Lin SJ (2008). Systematic review and meta-analysis of combination therapy for smoking cessation. *Journal of the American Pharmaceutical Association* 48(5), 659–665.

Sood A, Ebbert JO, Prasad K et al. (2010). A randomized clinical trial of St. John's wort for smoking cessation. *Journal of Alternative and Complementary Medicine* 16(7), 761–767.

Stead LF, Hughes JR (1997). Lobeline for smoking cessation. *Cochrane Database of Systematic Reviews* 3, CD000124.

Stead LF, Perera R, Bullen C, Mant D, Lancaster T (2008). Nicotine replacement therapy for smoking cessation. *Cochrane Database of Systematic Reviews* 1, CD000146.

Tidey JW, Monti PM, Rohsenow DJ et al. (2008). Moderators of naltrexone's effects on drinking, urge, and alcohol effects in non-treatment-seeking heavy drinkers in the natural environment. *Alcoholism: Clinical & Experimental Research* 32(1), 58–66.

Toll BA, White M, Wu R et al. (2010). Low-dose naltrexone augmentation of nicotine replacement for smoking cessation with reduced weight gain: a randomized trial. *Drug and Alcohol Dependence* 111(3), 200–206.

Tonstad S, Tønnesen P, Hajek P et al. (2006). Varenicline Phase 3 Study Group. Effect of maintenance therapy with varenicline on smoking cessation: a randomized controlled trial. *Journal of the American Medical Association* 296, 64–71.

Tsukahara H, Noda K, Saku K (2010). A randomized controlled open comparative trial of varenicline vs. nicotine patch in adult smokers: efficacy, safety and withdrawal symptoms (the VN-SEESAW study). *Circulation Journal* 74(4), 771–778.

Tyacke RJ, Lingford-Hughes A, Reed LJ, Nutt DJ (2010). GABAB receptors in addiction and its treatment. *Advances in Pharmacology* 58, 373–396.

Uhl GR, Liu QR, Drgon T et al. (2008). Molecular genetics of successful smoking cessation: convergent genome-wide association study results. *Archives of General Psychiatry* 65(6), 683–693.

Unger A, Jung E, Winklbaur B, Fischer G (2010). Gender issues in the pharmacotherapy of opioid-addicted women: buprenorphine.

Journal of Addictive Diseases **29**(2), 217–230.

van Amsterdam J, Opperhuizen A, Koeter M, van den Brink W (2010). Ranking the harm of alcohol, tobacco and illicit drugs for the individual and the population. *European Journal of Addiction Research* **16**(4), 202–207.

Verheul R, Lehert P, Geerlings PJ, Koeter MW, van den Brink W (2005). Predictors of acamprosate efficacy: results from a pooled analysis of seven European trials including 1485 alcohol-dependent patients. *Psychopharmacology* (Berlin) **178**(2–3), 167–173.

Chapter 12

Evidence-based pharmacotherapy of illicit substance use disorders

Wim van den Brink

Introduction

According to the United Nation Office on Drugs and Crime and the World Health Organization (UNODC-WHO), the number of people dependent on illegal drugs worldwide amounts to 26 million, with only 5 million people receiving some kind of treatment (UNODC-WHO, 2009). According to the same report, different continents have different drug use patterns and different treatment needs for addiction to illegal drugs, with the highest treatment demand in Europe being opioid and cannabis dependence (60% and 19%, respectively); North America: cocaine and cannabis dependence (35% and 31%, respectively); South America: cocaine and cannabis dependence (54% and 31%, respectively); Africa: cannabis and opioid dependence (64% and 16%, respectively); Asia: opioid and (meth)amphetamine dependence (63 and 19%, respectively), and Australia: cannabis and opioid dependence (47 and 33%, respectively). It should be noted that many of the treatment-seeking people are polydrug users and that these percentages indicate the primary drug of abuse or the primary reason for treatment seeking.

The natural course of SUDs is varied, ranging from very positive outcomes reported in general population samples meeting alcohol abuse or dependence criteria (e.g. Dawson et al., 2005; de Bruijn et al., 2006) to very negative outcomes in treatment-seeking patients in criminal justice settings (e.g. Hser et al., 2001). In general, it takes years before patients with SUD are recognized, get motivated to address their substance disorder, and enter treatment. By this time, natural recovery is rare and most treatment-seeking patients have a chronic relapsing disorder often with periods of partial or full recovery followed by serious episodes of partial or full relapse. In addition, many SUD patients experience crisis situations due to drug intoxication (e.g. drug-induced psychosis), life-threatening overdose (e.g. respiratory depression and coma due to heroin overdose), or complications during withdrawal (e.g. delirium tremens in alcohol-dependent patients). In general, crisis intervention takes precedence over the treatment of the addiction itself and often needs hospitalization and a multidisciplinary treatment. If the patient is stabilized, treatment motivation directed at full detoxification and stable abstinence is initiated and pharmacological treatments (often in combination with psychosocial interventions and rehabilitation) are initiated. However, many patients (repeatedly) fail to remain abstinent and keep relapsing into serious drug use. For these patients, it might be better to discontinue abstinence-oriented treatments and to direct treatment at reduction of illegal drug use and at reduction of harm associated with drug use and related behaviors (such as drug injection and the related risk of

Essential Evidence-Based Psychopharmacology, Second Edition, ed. Dan J. Stein, Bernard Lerer, and Stephen M. Stahl. Published by Cambridge University Press. © Cambridge University Press.

blood-borne infection). Finally, there are patients with a chronic SUD, a negative treatment career and only a limited time to live. In these cases, interventions directed towards palliation might be indicated (van den Brink and van Ree, 2003; van den Brink & Haasen, 2006). In the current review we only discuss abstinence-oriented treatments and stabilizing/harm-reduction treatments. The following illicit substances are the most harmful: heroin, cocaine, (meth)amphetamine, and cannabis. Substances such as ecstasy, LSD, and hallucinogenic mushrooms are not very likely to be addictive, whereas substances like GHB, ketamine, khat, and anabolic steroids are not very likely to produce a high level of population harm. Moreover, there are very few high-quality studies about the treatment of patients with these addictions.

In order to select the best available evidence and to make the best recommendations, we conducted a search mainly using existing Cochrane reviews, other statistical meta-analyses, high-quality systematic reviews, and electronic databases (PubMed, PsycINFO) if none of the above were available. In addition we always tried to update existing reviews with high-quality studies (mainly RCTs) from the previously mentioned electronic databases. In this review we try to provide evidence-based answers to the following three questions:

(1) What should be the best first-line pharmacological treatment for a certain SUD?
(2) How long should this treatment last?
(3) What strategies can be used if first-line treatment fails?

Opioid dependence

Of all opioids, heroin is the most popular among addicts, although in some areas (especially in North America) prescription opioids (e.g. oxycodon) have almost completely replaced heroin (Brands et al., 2004; Canfield et al., 2010; Sproule et al., 2009). Heroin, also known as diamorphine, is a semi-synthetic opioid synthesized from morphine, a derivative of the opium poppy. The United Nations estimates that there are currently between 13 and 22 million opioid dependent people worldwide (UNODC, 2010). In most countries, heroin is injected intravenously, but there are some countries where heroin is mainly inhaled after vaporization ("chasing the dragon") (Blanken et al., 2010). After heroin, or its metabolite morphine, reaches the brain, it activates the (mu) opioid receptor, which in turn causes inhibition of the GABA-ergic neurons leading to an increased activity of dopamine neurons in the ventral tegmental area and the nucleus accumbens. The effect of taking opioids are multiple, including euphoria, analgesia, respiratory depression, indifference to anticipated distress, drowsiness, decreased concentration, and constipation.

Again, this review does not discuss detoxification and the medications that can and in some cases should be used, but is restricted to the pharmacological treatment of opioid dependence. Different kinds of medication are currently available for the treatment of opioid dependence (van den Brink & Haasen, 2006): (a) medications directed at total abstinence from all opioid agonists (abstinence-oriented treatment), and (b) medications replacing illegal opioids with medically prescribed oral opioids with a long half-life (substitution treatment). This latter form of treatment is sometimes referred to as harm reduction. However, harm reduction is a much broader term and includes, next to substitution treatment, needle and syringe exchange programs, safe sex education, and the implementation of safe user rooms.

Medication directed at total abstinence

Treatments directed at continued total abstinence are preceded by motivation and detoxification. Several strategies have been used in the detoxification process, such as opioid agonist reduction schemes (methadone, buprenorphine), symptomatic treatment of withdrawal symptoms (clonidine/lofexidine) or an opioid antagonist (naltrexone with or without sedation or full anesthesia). A description and discussion of these different strategies is beyond the scope of this review. However, most reviews indicate that the use of opioid reduction schemes is probably the most effective and the safest heroin detoxification strategy (Davoli et al., 2007; Gowing et al., 2009a, 2009b, 2010; Meader, 2010; van den Brink and Haasen, 2006).

In order to promote continued total abstinence from heroin or any other opioid agonist, the potent opioid receptor antagonist naltrexone has been applied and studied most frequently. In a Cochrane review, Minozzi et al. (2006) described and discussed the results of 10 RCTs ($n = 696$) using oral naltrexone. According to the reviewers, the results show that naltrexone maintenance therapy alone or associated with psychosocial therapy is significantly more efficacious than placebo alone or associated with psychosocial therapy in limiting the use of heroin during the treatment (RR $= 0.72$) and in the prevention phase during the study period (RR $=0.50$). However, no statistically significant benefit was shown for relapse at follow-up for any of the considered comparisons. In their evaluation of the evidence, the reviewers are rather reserved due to the heterogeneity of the studies and the high dropout rates in most studies (average about 70% during 3–6 months treatment). They suggest that naltrexone might be an efficacious adjuvant in therapy for participants who fear severe consequences in case they do not stop taking opioids, e.g. healthcare professionals, who might lose their job or parolees who risk re-incarceration. The same could be true for other regions in the world, i.e. outside North America, Western Europe or Australia or in places where other opioids are the main addictive substance. For example, a relatively small retrospective study from Iran ($n = 45$) showed that 80% of the opium- and/or heroin-dependent patients remained in oral naltrexone maintenance treatment and remained abstinent for at least 9 months after naltrexone supported (rapid) detoxification (Naderi-Heiden et al., 2010). However, this is an exceptional finding and treatment compliance remains a very serious problem with oral naltrexone maintenance treatment. Moreover, oral naltrexone treatment is associated with a significantly higher mortality than methadone maintenance treatment (e.g. Gibson & Degenhardt, 2007).

A possible solution to non-compliance is the use of extended-release formulations using either naltrexone intramuscular injections or naltrexone subcutaneous implants. Currently several extended-release injections and implants are available using different techniques and different assumed durations of protection (injections: 1–2 months, implants: 3–6 months). In a Cochrane review, Lobmaier et al. (2008) identified only one RCT for the evaluation of effectiveness and safety. In this trial, Comer et al. (2006; $n = 60$) showed that heroin-dependent patients with two monthly injections of high and low doses of extended-release naltrexone compared with patients with two monthly placebo injections had significant better treatment retention (68%, 60%, and 39%, respectively) and significantly fewer positive urine samples (23%, 47%, and 67%, respectively). It is important to note that the percentage of positive urine samples for cocaine, cannabis, benzodiazepines, and amphetamine also tended to be lower in the naltrexone groups compared with the placebo group. The most frequently reported treatment-related adverse events included fatigue and injection-site induration and injection-site pain. In a recent quasi-experimental study, the data of Comer et al.

(2006) were compared with existing data from an RCT using oral naltrexone (Brooks *et al.*, 2010). The study showed superior retention and a significantly higher percentage with negative urine samples for heroin in the naltrexone injection compared with the oral naltrexone group (52% *vs.* 37%). In an unpublished study (*n* = 250), Gastfriend *et al.* (2010) found that six monthly injections with extended-release naltrexone was significantly more effective than monthly placebo injections in relatively young (mean age 29–30 years) Russian heroin-dependent patients: median percentage of drug-free urine samples was 90% *vs.* 35%, and 6-month total abstinence of heroin use was 36% *vs.* 23%. However, in another unpublished safety trial (*n* = 121), Kampman (2008) showed that long-term (48 weeks) treatment dropout was high and similar (about 70%) for heroin-dependent patients with monthly injections of extended-release naltrexone and patients with daily use of oral naltrexone.

In the first open-label RCT (*n* = 56), Kunøe *et al.* (2009) showed that an extended-release naltrexone implant with an expected protective effect of 6 months was significantly more effective in the treatment of detoxified heroin-dependent patients than treatment as usual: on the 180-day timeline follow-up, the implant group reported heroin use on 18 days and opioid use on 37 days compared with 64 and 97 days for controls: difference 46 days and 60 days respectively. The naltrexone group was also significantly better on secondary outcomes, e.g. polydrug use, craving, treatment satisfaction, and quality of life. It should be noted, however, that only 56 out of the 667 (8%) of the patients that were assessed for suitability were randomized and that 480 (72%) failed to meet inclusion criteria and 131 (20%) refused the naltrexone implant. In the discussion, the authors admit that the study population might have been especially well motivated for this specific treatment and that results in a less selected population might be less positive. In a follow-up of this study, only 51% of the patients receiving treatment with an extended-release naltrexone implant accepted a second implant, 21% expressed a wish for a re-implant but failed to attend for the re-implantation session repeatedly, and 28% declined re-implantation (Kunøe *et al.*, 2010). In the second RCT (Hulse *et al.*, 2009), 70 patients were randomized to 6 months oral naltrexone (plus one placebo implant) or to a single naltrexone extended-release implant (plus daily oral placebo tablets). Significantly more participants in the oral compared with the implant group had blood naltrexone levels below 1 ng/mL in month 1 to month 4, and significantly more oral group participants had returned to regular heroin use by 6 months (62% *vs.* 17%; HR = 4.49) and at an earlier stage (115 versus 158 days after randomization). Unexpectedly, naltrexone blood levels in implant recipients were maintained above 1 ng/mL for only 101 (men) and 124 (women) days, and above 2 ng/mL for 56 (men) and 43 (women) days, indicating that the potential effective protection was considerably shorter than the assumed 6 months. In a small trial, 46 prisoners were randomized to an extended release naltrexone implant or methadone before release. Intention to treat analysis showed similar reductions in both groups in the frequency of heroin and benzodiazepine use and in criminality six months after prison release (Lobmaier *et al.*, 2010). Finally, three non-randomized studies suggested that naltrexone implants are associated with reduced overdose rates compared with oral naltrexone treatment (Hulse *et al.*, 2005), to similar mortality rates as patients treated with buprenorphine (Reece, 2010), and to a reduced overall mortality compared with methadone maintenance (Tait *et al.*, 2008).

In summary, oral naltrexone maintenance treatment seems to be a treatment option only for a small group of well-integrated patients with a strong motivation to become fully abstinent of all opioid agonists, whereas extended-release naltrexone maintenance could be helpful in less well-integrated patients with a strong motivation to become totally abstinent.

However, even in these selected populations there are serious questions and no convincing answers regarding the long-term efficacy. More studies are needed before a strong recommendation in favor of these new and promising treatment options is possible. Finally, it should be noted that patients on extended-release naltrexone should carry a medical alert device indicating that these patients need higher dosages of opioid analgesics, non-opioid painkillers (e.g. NSAIDs), or local anesthesia in the case of severe pain.

Substitution treatment

Substitution treatment with long-acting opioid agonists, such as methadone, buprenorphine, or the combination of buprenorphine/naloxone, is available in a growing number of countries and has become the main treatment in many of these countries. Unfortunately, there are also countries where these medications are strictly forbidden and regarded as illegal narcotics.

Methadone maintenance treatment (MMT)

Methadone maintenance treatment has been applied for the treatment of patients with opioid dependence since the 1960s. Methadone is a synthetic full mu-opioid agonist (and a glutamate NMDA receptor antagonist). In a recent Cochrane review, Mattick *et al.* (2009) evaluated the existing data comparing methadone with treatments not using opioid substitution. In their description and analysis of 11 RCTs ($n = 1969$) with a mean methadone dose ranging from 50 to 100 mg/day, methadone was significantly more effective than non-pharmacological approaches in treatment retention (RR = 4.44) and in the suppression of heroin use measured by self-report and urine/hair analysis (RR = 0.66), but methadone only showed a non-significant trend in terms of the reduction in criminal activity (RR = 0.39; n.s.) or mortality (RR = 0.48; n.s.). However, the authors indicate that these RCTs were not designed and thus not powered to study criminal activities and mortality and they refer to large-scale cohort studies showing a substantial and significant effect of methadone on the prevention of criminality (e.g. Lind *et al.*, 2005) and the reduction of mortality (e.g. Clausen *et al.*, 2008; Gibson & Degenhardt, 2007). Finally, MMT has shown to reduce HIV risk-taking behavior (specifically reduction in needle sharing) and thereby has achieved a reduction in the transmission of HIV (Gowing *et al.*, 2008). It is important to emphasize that methadone dosages between 60–100 mg/day are associated with significantly better treatment retention and greater reductions in heroin and cocaine use during treatment (Faggiano *et al.*, 2003).

It should be noted that methadone has some potentially serious side-effects such as (fatal) respiratory depression during intoxication and ECG QT-interval prolongation with the related risk of life threatening ventricular arrhythmias (Torsades de Pointes: TdP). With regard to overdose deaths, several studies have indicated that the period of treatment initiation is especially risky and that methadone titration should be carefully monitored (Buster *et al.*, 2002; Cornish *et al.*, 2010; Davoli *et al.*, 2007; Degenhardt *et al.*, 2009). With regard to QT-prolongation and TdP, (randomized) controlled studies have consistently shown that methadone increases the duration of the QT-interval even to clinically relevant and potentially harmful levels (e.g. Wedam *et al.*, 2007). However, findings on the relationship between methadone dose and QT-prolongation are not consistent and even in studies that show a dose–response relation, the association is rather weak (e.g. Anchersen *et al.*, 2009; Ehret *et al.*, 2006; Martell *et al.*, 2005). Finally, very little is known about the risk of a (fatal) case of TdP and clinically prolonged QT-intervals. Based on the current lack of consistent data, different guidelines have been proposed, some very restrictive (mainly by internal medicine representatives) and some rather lenient (mainly by addiction experts). For example, Krantz *et al.* (2009) recommend an ECG before the start of any methadone prescription, 30 days after prescription has started, annual control ECGs, and an ECG in the case of a methadone dose higher than 100 mg/day. In contrast, Byrne *et al.* (2010) recommend an ECG only on clinical indication (presence of a cardiac disease or a history with syncope) or when methadone is combined with medications that are likely to increase the QT-interval such as most antipsychotics.

In summary, MMT is a broadly accepted, effective, and safe treatment for patients with heroin dependence provided that some minimal safety measures are taken into account.

Buprenorphine with or without naloxone

Buprenorphine is a thebaine derivative with high binding affinities at the mu- and kappa-opioid receptors. It has partial agonist activity at the mu-opioid receptor, partial or full agonist activity at the ORL1/nociceptin and the delta-opioid receptors, and antagonist activity at the kappa-opioid receptors. Buprenorphine shows a very high first-pass metabolism and is therefore generally used sublingually.

In a Cochrane review, Mattick *et al.* (2008) compared buprenorphine maintenance treatment with placebo and methadone maintenance treatment using a total of 24 RCTs ($n = 4497$). Buprenorphine was significantly more effective than placebo in retention of patients in treatment at low doses (RR = 1.50), medium doses (RR = 1.74), and at high doses (RR = 1.74). However, only medium- and high-dose buprenorphine suppressed heroin use significantly better than placebo. Buprenorphine given in flexible doses was significantly less effective than methadone in retaining patients in treatment (RR = 0.80), but not different in the suppression of illegal opioid use for those who remained in treatment. Low-dose methadone is more likely to retain patients than low-dose buprenorphine (RR = 0.67). Medium-dose buprenorphine does not retain more patients than low-dose methadone, but may suppress heroin use better. There was no advantage for medium-dose buprenorphine over medium-dose methadone in retention (RR = 0.79) and medium-dose buprenorphine was inferior in suppression of heroin use. Based on these data, the authors conclude that buprenorphine maintenance is an effective intervention for the treatment of heroin dependence, but it is less effective than methadone delivered at adequate dosages. In a recent review and economic analysis Connock *et al.* (2007) reach similar conclusions: both flexible-dose methadone and buprenorphine maintenance treatment are more effective and more cost-effective than no drug therapy and flexible-dose methadone is somewhat more effective than a flexible dose of buprenorphine resulting in slightly higher health gains and lower costs. However, they also note that these findings need to be balanced by the more recent experience of clinicians in the use of buprenorphine, the possible risk of higher mortality of MMT, and individual patient preferences. For example, low retention rates in some of the studies may have been caused by slow induction strategies. In addition, several studies have shown that buprenorphine might be safer than methadone with lower mortality rates during treatment induction (Bell *et al.*, 2009a, 2009b). However, Gibson *et al.* (2007) and Degenhardt *et al.* (2009) showed that initial reductions in mortality with buprenorphine compared with methadone were offset by a somewhat higher mortality in buprenorphine-treated patients due to longer out-of-treatment periods. Both treatments resulted in a similar reduction of mortality compared with non-treated heroin-dependent patients. A possibly important advantage of buprenorphine over methadone is that buprenorphine has no effect on the QT-interval or on the risk of TdP (Wedam *et al.*, 2007). It should be noted, however, that QT prolongation might be more likely in patients on a high dose of methadone and that buprenorphine, a partial mu-opioid receptor agonist, might not be the best alternative in these cases.

In order to prevent diversion and abuse of buprenorphine, naloxone has been added to buprenorphine. Naloxone, a short-acting mu-opioid receptor antagonist, is badly absorbed sublingually and has no effect when the combination of bupronorphine plus naloxone (4:1) is taken sublingually as prescribed. However, when taken intravenously, both compounds will enter the brain very quickly and naloxone will cause serious withdrawal symptoms in heroin-dependent patients thus preventing intravenous abuse. The effect of buprenorphine/naloxone has been studied in three RCTs: one trial comparing 4 weeks buprenorphine/naloxone with buprenorphine alone and placebo (Fudala *et al.*, 2003: $n = 323$), one trial comparing 17 weeks buprenorphine/naloxone with methadone (Kamien *et al.*, 2008: $n = 268$), and one stepped care trial comparing 6 months buprenorphine/naloxone with methadone (Kakko *et al.*, 2007: $n = 96$). The results of these trials suggest that buprenorphine/naltrexone is more effective than placebo and equally effective as methadone (see also Orman & Keating, 2009).

Unfortunately, treatment retention in methadone, buprenorphine and the combination of buprenorphine/naloxone is far from perfect and, despite previous expectations, the combination of buprenorphine/naloxone can still be abused (Alho *et al.*, 2007; Bruce *et al.*, 2009). In order to address these problems, a buprenorphine implant was developed delivering a steady level of buprenorphine over a period of 6 months. In the first RCT with this new formulation ($n = 108$), buprenorphine implants were more effective than placebo implants: a median of 41% *vs.* 21% of negative urine samples for illicit opioids during the first 16 weeks in the experimental and the control condition, respectively (Ling *et al.*, 2010). It should be noted that (minor) implant site reactions were rather common (57%) possibly limiting the willingness to have additional implants. No direct comparisons between oral and implant buprenorphine are currently available.

In summary, buprenorphine maintenance is a safe and effective treatment for heroin-dependent patients and new formulations are being developed to improve treatment retention and to prevent abuse and diversion.

Heroin-assisted treatment (HAT)

Methadone and buprenorphine maintenance are effective treatments with moderate effect sizes and a substantial fraction of heroin-dependent patients do not respond to these treatments. In order, to create a better outcome for these treatment-refractory patients, heroin-assisted treatment (HAT) was developed in the 1990s and tested in the last two decades. HAT consists of an offer to use pharmaceutical grade heroin three times per day in a special polyclinic with close supervision to prevent abuse and diversion, and is generally combined with a standard offer of psychosocial support.

Efficacy and safety of HAT has now been tested in six RCTs in six countries ($n = 2055$) and effectiveness has been studied in two long-term cohort studies ($n = 2314$) in two countries (Blanken *et al.*, 2010). All RCTs showed a significantly positive effect on their primary outcome variable. In a Cochrane review (Ferri *et al.*, 2010), including eight studies comparing HAT with MMT ($n = 2007$), the authors concluded that HAT is significantly more effective than MMT in preventing relapse to the use of street heroin (RR $= 0.70$), in reducing the

use of other illicit substances (RR = 0.63), in the prevention of incarceration and impris-
onment (RR = 0.64) and marginally more effective in the reduction of criminal activities
(RR = 0.80). However, HAT is also significantly associated with more (serious) adverse events
(RR = 1.61). In their summary, Ferri *et al.* (2010) conclude that the available evidence suggests a small added value of heroin prescribed alongside flexible doses of methadone for long-
term, treatment-refractory opioid users, but that due to the higher rate of serious adverse
events, heroin prescription should remain a treatment of last resort for people who are currently or have in the past failed in maintenance treatment. Meanwhile, this overall conclusion
of the Cochrane review has been seriously questioned (e.g. Blanken *et al.*, 2010), and a probably more positive update of this review is being prepared (personal communication with Dr.
Ferri, December 2010). Currently, heroin is registered as a medicinal product for the treatment of treatment-refractory heroin-dependent patients in Switzerland, Germany, and the
Netherlands.

Other medications

Recently two other opioid agonists have been tested in trials: (1) slow-release oral morphine
(SROM) and (2) oral heroin.

In a cross-over study, patients intolerant to methadone (*n* = 39) or patients with inadequate withdrawal suppression on adequate doses of methadone (*n* = 28) were switched to
SROM (1:8) resulting in significant reductions in side-effects, withdrawal symptoms, and
craving (Kastelic *et al.*, 2008). In a similar cross-over study (Mitchell *et al.*, 2004), replacement of methadone by SROM resulted in improved social functioning, weight loss, fewer
and less troublesome side-effects, greater drug liking, reduced heroin craving, an enhanced
sense of feeling 'normal' and similar outcomes for unsanctioned drug use, depression, and
health. The majority of subjects preferred SROM (78%) over methadone (22%). Positive
findings were also reported in two non-controlled studies (Kraigher *et al.*, 2005; Vasilev
et al., 2006).

In an open-label, prospective cohort study with two non-randomly assigned treatment
arms 128 heroin-dependent patients on oral heroin were compared with 237 patients receiving oral heroin plus HAT (Frick *et al.*, 2010): retention rates were high and very similar for
both groups (> 70% after 4 years and > 50% after 8 years).

Conclusion: opioid-dependence treatment

Based on the data that were presented and taking into account treatment retention, treatment
effectiveness and safety aspects (see Table 12.1), the first-line treatment for most patients
is opioid maintenance with adequate doses of methadone or with buprenophine (with
or without naloxone). Buprenorphine might be preferred in cases with QT prolongation
and in cases with a historically increased risk of opioid overdose. Whether buprenorphine
implants are better than oral buprenorphine remains to be seen. Patients that (repeatedly) fail
in methadone or buprenorphine maintenance treatment may benefit from heroin-assisted
treatment. Finally, naltrexone should be reserved as a first-line treatment for patients with an
extraordinarily strong motivation and a stable social network and as an extended treatment
option for patients that achieved stable abstinence from illegal opioids, restored their social
network during opioid maintenance treatment, and have a strong motivation to become
abstinent from all opioids. Whether extended-release formulations of naltrexone are more
effective and safer than oral naltrexone still needs to be proven (see also WHO, 2009).

Table 12.1. Effectiveness of pharmacological interventions in opioid-dependent patients.

	Compliance	Effect size	Population effect compliance × ES	Overdose risk	Overall rating
Oral naltrexone	Very Low	Good	Low	Discontinuation	Low
Naltrexone XR	High	Good	Good(?)	Low	Moderate
Methadone (MMT)	Moderate	Good	Good	Initiation	Good
Buprenorphine	Moderate	Good	Good	Low	Good
Buprenorphine/ naloxone	Moderate	Good	Good	Low	Good
Buprenorphine XR	High	Good	Unknown	Low	Unknown
Heroin-Assisted Tx (HAT)	High	Good	Good	During Tx	Good

ES, Effect size.
Naltrexone XR, Extended release (intramuscular injection or implant).
Buprenorphine XR, Extended release (implant).

Cocaine dependence

Cocaine is becoming one of the most frequently used illicit drugs with 15–20 million last-year users and a substantial treatment demand especially in North America, South America, and Europe (UNODC, 2010). Cocaine is snorted, smoked (crack) or injected with the latter two routes of administration probably being more addictive than snorting. The effect is almost immediate and very short-lasting with a maximum of 45–60 minutes. This short effect seems to be responsible for the tendency in many cocaine abusers to engage in bingeing episodes with repeated use of cocaine within a very short period, resulting in the dangerous situation of intoxication. In the brain, cocaine causes inhibition of dopamine, serotonin, and norepinephrine receptor transporters, which indirectly affects the opioid, the glutamatergic, and the cholinergic brain systems. Therefore, it comes as no surprise that many different kinds of medications affecting very different neurotransmitter systems have been studied as potential treatments for cocaine dependence. In this review, we subsequently review the evidence for anticonvulsants, antidepressants, antipsychotics and dopamine agonists, stimulant-like medications, disulfiram, opioid agonists, and some miscellaneous medications.

Anticonvulsants

In a Cochrane review, Minozzi et al. (2006), identified 15 RCTs ($n = 1066$), including studies with carbamazepine (six studies), gabapentin (three studies), tiagabine (three studies), phenytoin (two studies), lamotrigine (one study), topiramate (one study), and valproate (one study). In an overall analysis including all studies, no significant differences were found for any of the efficacy measures comparing any anticonvulsants with placebo. Moreover, placebo was found to be superior to gabapentin in diminishing the number of dropouts and superior to phenytoin for side-effects. Also, none of the single anticonvulsant–placebo comparisons was significantly in favor of the anticonvulsant. It should be noted, however, that the effect of topiramate was not significant over the total study period, but significant effects in favor of topiramate occurred after titration to full dose was established, i.e. after week 8 (Kampman et al., 2004). Since the publication of the Cochrane review, two other RCTs have been published. In a large RCT ($n = 140$), Winhusen *et al.* (2005) confirmed the negative conclusion regarding tiagabine. Recently, Brodie *et al.* (2009) finished the first RCT ($n = 103$) with vigabatrin (gamma-vinyl gamma-aminobutyric acid = GVG). The study showed a significant positive effect of vigabatrin compared with placebo on treatment retention (62% *vs.* 42%) and all cocaine-related outcomes (abstinence during treatment: 28% *vs.* 8%; abstinence during follow-up: 24% *vs.* 4%). It should be noted, however, that vigabatrin is known for its risk of severe visual-field defects and this risk needs to be taken into account when prescribing this medication. In the USA, the use of vigabatrin is restricted to treatment-refractory partial seizure disorders in adults and infantile spasm of sufficient severity that benefits are determined to outweigh the potential risk of vision loss. However, visual-field deficits have been reported only with chronic use of vigabatrin (i.e. more than 12 months). While both cocaine and alcohol dependence are chronic and relapsing disorders, it is likely that a shorter duration of treatment can be helpful in facilitating long-term abstinence.

In summary, the results of the currently available studies generally do not support the use of anticonvulsants in the treatment of cocaine dependence. The only compounds that deserve further study are topiramate and time-limited treatment with vigabatrin (see also Alvarez *et al.*, 2010).

Antidepressants

In the latest Cochrane review, Silva de Lima *et al.* (2003) described and analyzed 17 RCTs and one quasi-randomized study ($n = 1177$), including desipramine (12 studies), fluoxetine (four studies), ritanserin (one study) and imipramine (one study). The findings suggest that antidepressants as a group are not more effective than placebo in all of the drug-related outcomes. Most of the individual trials showed a similar decrease in cocaine use and craving with placebo and the active drug. When relapse in cocaine-free patients was evaluated, the same pattern of response was found. Only three trials (all desipramine) showed statistical significant differences favoring the intervention when compared with placebo. In a separate meta-analysis including only desipramine trials, this medication showed a favorable trend in terms of a reduction in cocaine-positive urine samples ($RR = 0.82$; n.s.), but desipramine did not differ from placebo on other drug-related measures. Since the Cochrane review was rather old, we searched the literature for more recent trials examining the effect of antidepressants on cocaine dependence. Five additional RCTs were identified (Ciraulo *et al.*, 2005; Johnson *et al.*, 2006; Moeller *et al.*, 2007; Passos *et al.*, 2005; Winhusen *et al.*, 2005). These studies showed that sertraline, paroxetine, venlafvaxine, and nefazodone are probably not effective in the treatment of cocaine dependence. However, Johnson *et al.* (2006; $n = 63$) showed that high doses of ondansetron were significantly more effective in the reduction of cocaine-positive urine samples than low dosages of ondansetron and placebo. Finally, the study of Moeller *et al.* (2007; $n = 76$) showed that citalopram leads to a significant reduction in cocaine-positive urine samples compared with placebo.

In summary, current research generally does not support the use of antidepressants in the treatment of cocaine dependence, although further studies are justified to test the possible effects of ondansetron and citalopram. However, it is not very likely that citalopram is going to be an effective medication against cocaine dependence, because many other SSRIs have already failed to show significant benefits. The $5\text{-}HT_3$ receptor antagonist ondansetron is probably the most promising medication for the treatment of cocaine dependence and other substance-use disorders.

Antipsychotics

In a Cochrane review, Amato et al. (2007) described and analyzed seven small studies ($n =$ 293), including the following antipsychotics: risperidone (three studies), olanzapine (three studies), and haloperidol (two studies). Only a few studies reported on dependence-related outcome; in the few cases that studies did report on such outcomes no significant differences were found for any of the efficacy measures comparing any antipsychotic medication with placebo. Since this Cochrane review was published, at least three additional studies were published. In a 16-week RCT ($n = 48$), olanzapine and placebo did not differ on any outcome measure (Hamilton et al., 2009). Similarly, in a 12-week RCT ($n = 31$), weekly long-acting risperidone injections were not more effective than weekly placebo injections in active cocaine users in terms of a reduction in cocaine use or craving and active treatment was associated with worsening of depressive symptoms and weight gain (Loebl et al., 2008). In a small ($n = 22$) open-label, uncontrolled study, Kennedy et al. (2008) showed some promise for quetiapine (at the expense of sedation and weight gain). Finally, an open-label, uncontrolled study among 10 non-schizophrenic cocaine addicts showed some promise for treatment with the partial dopamine agonist aripiprazole (Vorspan et al., 2008).

In summary, neither classical nor atypical antipsychotics seem to be effective in the treatment of cocaine dependence. Moreover, all antipsychotics have side-effects resulting in premature treatment discontinuation.

Dopamine agonists

In a Cochrane review, Soares et al. (2003) reviewed 17 RCTs ($n = 1224$), including the following opioid agonists: amantadine, bromocriptine, and pergolide. There were no significant differences between the various dopamine agonists and placebo in trials where participants had primary cocaine dependence or in trials where patients had an additional diagnosis of opioid dependence or when patients were in methadone maintenance treatment. Since this Cochrane review was last updated (2003), three RCTs on the effectiveness of dopamine agonist for the treatment of cocaine dependence were published. In a single blind, placebo-controlled RCT ($n = 42$), Focchi et al. (2005) confirmed that pergolide is not more effective than placebo. Similarly, in a large RCT ($n = 199$), Kampman et al. (2006) found that amantadine with or without propranolol was not more effective than placebo in the treatment of cocaine-dependent patients. In a screening trial, 60 cocaine-dependent patients were randomized to 8 weeks treatment with the dopamine agonist cabergoline, the dopamine precursor levodopa/carbidopa, the cognitive enhancer hydergine or placebo (Shoptaw et al., 2005). Cabergoline was significantly more effective in the reduction of cocaine-positive urine samples than placebo (42% vs. 25%) with no significant difference in adverse events. Finally, two RCTs are available on the effect of the dopamine precursor levodopa/carbidopa (Shoptaw et al., 2005, Mooney et al., 2007). These RCTs did not show a significant effect of levodopa/carbidopa on cocaine craving and did not significantly reduce cocaine use.

In summary, it seems that dopamine agonists are not effective in the treatment of cocaine dependence. However, the possible effect of cabergoline needs to be studied in a larger RCT.

Stimulant-like medications

In a Cochrane review (Castells et al., 2010), a meta-analysis of 16 high-quality RCTs was presented ($n = 1345$), including seven stimulant-like medications or medications with a stimulant metabolite: bupropion (three studies), dexamphetamine (three studies), methylphenidate (three studies), modafinil (one study), mazindol (four studies), methamphetamine (one study), and selegiline (one study). Overall, psychostimulants did not reduce cocaine use (standardized mean difference (SMD) = 0.11, n.s.), but there was a statistical trend for improving sustained cocaine abstinence (RR = 1.41; p = 0.07). The proportion of adverse event-induced dropouts was similar for psychostimulants and placebo. When the type of drug was included as a moderating variable, the proportion of patients achieving sustained cocaine abstinence was significantly higher for bupropion (RR = 1.64) and dextroamphetamine (RR = 2.12), whereas modafinil showed a statistical trend with better outcomes than placebo (RR = 2.67, n.s.). In addition, psychostimulants appeared to increase the proportion of patients achieving sustained cocaine (RR = 1.84) and heroin abstinence (RR = 1.77) amongst methadone-maintained dual heroin/cocaine addicts. This review found mixed results with very promising results for methadone-maintained dual heroin-cocaine addicts and for some specific drugs such as dextroamphetamine, bupropion, and possibly modafinil. Unfortunately, the review failed to mention the positive results of the study with methamphetamine (Mooney et al., 2009). This study (n = 82) found significantly fewer cocaine-positive urine samples for sustained-release methamphetamine compared with immediate release methamphetamine and placebo (29% vs. 66% and 60%, respectively). One recent study on modafinil in cocaine dependence was not included in this Cochrane review (Anderson et al., 2009). In the multi-center RCT of Anderson et al., 210 patients were randomized to different doses of modafinil or placebo. Modafinil was not significantly more effective than placebo on the primary outcome (weekly percentage of cocaine non-use days), but it was significantly better than placebo on the maximum number of consecutive non-use days of cocaine. Moreover, all outcome variables were significantly better for modafinil in the subgroup without alcohol-dependence comorbidity. These findings are consistent with other reviews on stimulant-like medications (Herin et al., 2010) and modafinil (Martínez-Raga et al., 2008). Many of the stimulant-like medications have abuse and diversion liability. It is, therefore, recommended to use sustained release formulations and to actively control the intake of the medication. In addition, innovative formulations have been developed that reduce the risk of abuse, e.g. lisdexamphetamine. Lisdexamphetamine is a pro-drug in which dexamphetamine is coupled to the essential amino acid L-lysine which makes it inactive when injected and has a sustained effect only if used as an oral medication, with decoupling of the two components in the gastrointestinal tract (Blick & Keating, 2007).

In summary, some stimulant-like medications are a promising strategy in the treatment of patients with cocaine dependence.

Disulfiram

Disulfiram is an effective medication for the treatment of alcohol dependence because it inhibits aldehyde dehydrogenase, an enzyme which is involved in the metabolism of alcohol. However, disulfiram also inhibits dopamine-beta-hydroxylase, resulting in an excess of dopamine and decreased synthesis of norepinephrine and this has been proposed to favorably influence the functioning of the meso-limbic circuits disrupted by cocaine addiction

In a Cochrane review including seven RCTs (n = 492), Pani et al. (2010) were not able to draw confident conclusions about the effectiveness of disulfiram in the treatment of cocaine dependence due to the heterogeneity of the included studies and the impossibility to perform meta-analyses on the efficacy and safety of disulfiram compared with placebo. However, in most individual studies, there was at least a trend towards a positive effect of disulfiram compared with placebo on at least one of the cocaine outcome parameters. In one study (Pettinati *et al.*, 2008), the combination of disulfiram plus naltrexone was significantly more effective than naltrexone alone, disulfiram alone, and placebo. Overall, these studies did not show statistically significant differences in the number of patients reporting side-effects. However, these studies did not specifically investigate the potential toxicity resulting from the interaction between disulfiram and cocaine. In a very recent study among 161 cocaine/opioid-dependent patients in methadone maintenance treatment, Oliveto *et al.* (2011) found no effect of disulfiram 250 mg/day on cocaine-use parameters, but they did find a significant negative effect of disulfiram doses lower than 250 mg/day, indicating that low doses of disulfiram are contraindicated in cocaine-dependent patients.

In summary, disulfiram is a promising treatment for cocaine dependence, but better and larger trials are needed to firmly establish efficacy and safety, especially the effect of dosing and safety in terms of the potential interaction between cocaine and disulfiram.

Opioid agonists

It has been suggested repeatedly that (a) higher doses of agonist treatment in heroin-dependent patients with comorbid cocaine dependence would result in higher cocaine reduction and abstinence rates (e.g. Peles *et al.*, 2006) and (b) that buprenorphine would be more effective in this respect than methadone. In the most recent Cochrane review on the effect of methadone dose on treatment outcome, Faggiano *et al.* (2003) showed that higher methadone doses were associated with significantly higher rates of at least 3 weeks cocaine abstinence (RR = 1.81). However, in a recent RCT ($n = 252$) no differences in cocaine-negative urine samples were observed between patients treated with 70 or 100 mg methadone (Epstein *et al.*, 2009). Findings on the effect of buprenorphine are also inconsistent, with some studies showing a better effect of high compared with low doses of buprenorphine on cocaine abstinence (Montoya *et al.*, 2004) and other studies failing to find an effect of buprenorphine dose (Schottenfeld *et al.*, 1997). Inconsistent results were also found with regard to the relative effectiveness of buprenorphine and methadone in achieving cocaine abstinence: in a small RCT ($n = 51$), Strain *et al.* (1994) found no significant differences between the two treatments, whereas Schottenfeld *et al.* (2005), in a larger RCT ($n = 116$) found methadone to be superior to buprenorphine. In a recent meta-analysis including 37 RCTs ($n = 3029$), Castells *et al.* (2009) concluded that high doses of opioid-maintenance treatment were significantly more efficacious than lower ones in the achievement of sustained heroin abstinence (RR = 2.24), but had no effect on cocaine abstinence. At equivalent doses, methadone was significantly more efficacious than buprenorphine on cocaine abstinence (RR = 1.63). Finally, the recent Cochrane review on heroin-assisted treatment in treatment-refractory heroin-dependent patients shows that this novel treatment also results in a significant reduction of other illicit drugs (RR = 0.63), including cocaine (Ferri *et al.*, 2010).

Opioid antagonists

Opioid antagonists have been used in many different addictions (smoking, alcohol dependence, opioid dependence, amphetamine dependence) and several addiction-like disorders (pathological gambling, obesity). It is, therefore, understandable that opioid antagonists have also been tested for the treatment of cocaine dependence. Currently, there are four RCTs, one positive study in cocaine-dependent patients (Schmitz *et al.*, 2001) and three negative studies in patients dependent on both cocaine and alcohol (Schmitz *et al.*, 2004, 2009; Pettinati *et al.*, 2008). In a secondary analysis, the combination naltrexone plus disulfiram was significantly more effective than disulfiram or naltrexone alone or placebo in achieving at least 3 weeks abstinence of both alcohol and cocaine (Pettinati *et al.*, 2008).

In summary, the available RCTs do not support the use of naltrexone in treating cocaine-dependent patients. Combination treatments need further study.

Vaccination

In the first and only placebo-controlled RCT testing a novel cocaine vaccine (five injections over a period of 12 weeks) in opioid and cocaine-dependent patients enrolled in a methadone maintenance program ($n = 115$), only 38% of the vaccinated patients attained effective serum IgG anticocaine antibody levels (Martell *et al.*, 2009). Serum IgG levels went up rather slowly, but between weeks 9 through 16, the percentage of cocaine-free urine samples was significantly greater in the high IgG compared with the low IgG and placebo groups (45% *vs.* 35%). However, soon after vaccination stopped, antibody levels began to fall off and the frequency of cocaine-free urine samples was no longer significantly different between the vaccinated and placebo groups. All of the reported adverse events were considered mild or moderate in intensity. Adverse events that were more frequent in the vaccinated compared with the placebo group were: injection site induration (3% *vs.* 0%), site tenderness (10% *vs.* 6%), feeling cold (12% *vs.* 7%), hot flushes (19% *vs.* 12%), hyperhydrosis (15% *vs.* 10%) and nausea (14% *vs.* 2%). Together these findings indicate that vaccination only results in relapse prevention 6–8 weeks after the first vaccination and that long-term effects are not likely to occur with the currently available vaccines.

Miscellaneous medications

In the first and only RCT comparing the $GABA_B$ receptor agonist baclofen with placebo ($n = 70$), there was no significant overall difference between groups in cocaine-free urine samples, but baclofen did significantly reduce cocaine use in the subgroup of patients with heavier cocaine use at baseline.

Meanwhile, a series of other medications were tested in placebo-controlled RCTs for their potential reduction of cocaine use in cocaine-dependent patients with no significant effect, including the NMDA glutamate receptor antagonists acamprosate and memantine (Kampman *et al.*, 2011 and Bisaga *et al.*, 2010, respectively), acetylcholinesterase inhibitor donepezil (Winhusen *et al.*, 2005), the sulfa non-steroidal anti-inflammatory (NSAID) drug celecoxib (Reid *et al.*, 2005), the nicotinic acetylcholine receptor antagonist mecamylamine (Reid *et al.*, 2005), the calcium channel antagonist amlodipine (Malcolm *et al.*, 2005), the cortisol synthesis inhibitor ketoconazole (Kosten *et al.*, 2002), and the herbal product ginkgo biloba (Kampman *et al.*, 2003). Moreover, the AMPA glutamate receptor modulator piracetam was associated with increased cocaine use (Kampman *et al.*, 2003).

Conclusions: cocaine-dependence treatment

Currently, a large number of compounds have been tested in (small) RCTs, but only a few of them show enough promise to justify further testing and none of the medications has been registered for the treatment of cocaine dependence. Table 12.2 provides a short summary of the findings. Based on these findings, potential first-line treatments include: bupropion,

Table 12.2. Effectiveness of pharmacological interventions in cocaine-dependent patients.

Type of medication	Effectiveness	Remarks
Anticonvulsants	Generally not effective (carbamazepine, gabapentin, tiagabine, phenytoin, lamotrigine)	Further study needed (topiramate, vigabatrin)
Antidepressants	Generally not effective (desipramine, fluoxetine, ritanserin, imipramine)	Further study needed (ondansetron, citalopram?)
Antipsychotics	Generally not effective (risperidon, olanzapine, haloperidol)	Further study needed (quetiapine?, aripiprazole)
Dopamine agonists	Generally not effective (amantadine, bromocriptine, pergolide, levodopa/carbidopa)	Further study needed (cabergoline)
Stimulant-like medications	Some very promising (bupropion, dexamphetamine, modafinil) Some not effective (methylphenidate[a], mazindol, selegiline)	Further study needed (methamphetamine SR)
Disulfiram	Probably effective	Further study needed
Opioid agonists (high dose)	Findings inconclusive (methadone, buprenorphine, heroin)	Further study needed (all partial) agonists)
Opioid antagonists	Generally not effective (naltrexone)	Further study needed (naltrexone+disulfiram)
Vaccination	Not enough data available	Further study needed
Miscellaneous	Generally not effective (acamprosate, memantine, donepezil, celecoxib, mecamylamine, amlodipine, ketoconazole, piracetam, ginkgo biloba)	Further study needed (baclofen)

[a] Mainly studied in cocaine-dependent patients with comorbid ADHD.
?, indications but no proof of efficacy.

dexamphetamine, and disulfiram. In cocaine-dependent patients without a comorbid diagnosis of alcohol dependence, modafinil is likely to become a first-line treatment. Finally, cocaine-dependent patients with a comorbid diagnosis of opioid dependence are likely to benefit from high dosages of methadone. Other, second-line, promising medications involve topiramate, vigabatrin, baclofen, ondansetron, aripiprazole, cabergoline, and methamphetamine. However, it should be emphasized that for almost none of these medications long-term treatment and outcomes are yet available and that currently none of all these medications has been registered for the treatment of cocaine dependence. Moreover, most of these medications have substantial side-effects and certain of these medications have an addictive potential, thus prescription of these medications should be combined with supervision and control.

Cannabis dependence
Worldwide, cannabis is the most frequently consumed illicit drug with a last-year prevalence of 129–191 million users. It is now well-established that cannabis can cause withdrawal, and that cannabis dependence develops in approximately 9% of all subjects that ever used cannabis. Cannabis-dependent patients constitute an increasing percentage of all patients seeking help for a substance-use disorder (UNODC, 2010). Cannabis contains approximately

60 different cannabinoids, including delta-9-tetrahydrocannabinol (THC) and cannabidiol (CBD). The most important psychoactive ingredient in cannabis is THC. After inhalation, THC quickly reaches the brain where it binds to the type-1 cannabinoid (CB1) and the type-1 vanilloid (VR1) pain receptors. The effects are mild analgesia, appetite stimulation, muscle relaxation, euphoria, changes in time–space perception, and changes in visual, auditory, and olfactory perceptions. In a minority of cases, anxiety or psychosis occur. The latter is often thought to be related to the increased concentration of THC together with a decreased concentration of CBD in cultivated new subtypes of cannabis plants.

To date, several medications have been investigated for different indications, e.g. reduced withdrawal, attenuation of subjective or reinforcing effects, and reduced relapse. Medications that have been studied for the treatment of cannabis dependence include: (a) those that may attenuate the reinforcing effects of cannabis and (b) those that directly prevent relapse to cannabis use after initial abstinence. Although the literature on this issue is still rather small we do not discuss single case reports, but restrict our review to controlled laboratory studies, case-series, small open-label clinical studies, and RCTs when available.

Medications for the treatment of cannabis dependence
Several human laboratory studies have tested the CB1 receptor antagonist rimonabant (Gorelick et al., 2006; Huestis et al., 2001, 2007) and the opioid receptor antagonist naltrexone (Greenwald & Stitzer, 2000; Haney, 2007; Haney et al., 2003a; Wachtel & de Wit, 2000) on the reduction of subjective effects of cannabis. Findings were inconsistent and probably related to dose differences. No clinical trials are available for these medications. Effects of other medications on the reduction of subjective cannabis effects were examined only in single human laboratory studies: oral THC formulation dronabinol (Hart et al, 2002; effect doubtful), alpha$_2$-adrenoreceptor agonist clonidine (Cone et al., 1988; no effect), the antidepressant bupropion (Haney et al., 2001; reduced subjective high, but increased withdrawal), the antidepressant nefazodone (Haney et al., 2003b; no effect), and the mood stabilizer divalproex (Haney et al., 2004; increased subjective effects).

In a human laboratory study the effects of dronabinol, lofexidine, and the combination of both medications on relapse were tested. In this study, neither dronabinol nor lofexidine alone reduced the number of participants that elected to smoke any amount of cannabis compared with placebo during a 4-day maintenance period, but the combination of the two drugs doubled the rate of complete abstinence (Haney et al., 2008).

In an open-label clinical study ($n = 13$), the noradrenergic ADHD medication atomoxetine showed a non-significant reduction of cannabis use (Tirado et al., 2008). In another open-label study ($n = 10$), the 5-HT1$_A$ receptor agonist buspirone resulted in a significant reduction of craving, irritability, and cannabis use (McRae et al., 2006). However, several adverse events were reported and only two patients finished the 12-week trial. In yet another open-label study ($n = 20$), 7 days of lithium treatment resulted in relatively high rates of cannabis abstinence in 12 treatment completers: 64%, 65%, and 41% at 10, 24, and 90 days post-treatment follow-up, respectively (Winstock et al., 2009). In a case series ($n = 6$), the GABA$_B$ agonist baclofen was associated with mild withdrawal and high long-term abstinence (Nanjayya et al., 2010).

Currently, there are only two placebo-controlled RCTs. In the first RCT with a cross-over design ($n = 25$), divalproex treatment was associated with an increase in adverse events, low treatment compliance and no significant reduction in cannabis use (Levin et al., 2004). In the second RCT ($n = 106$), 13 weeks of nefazodone or sustained-release bupropion demonstrated no significant effects in withdrawal or abstinence compared with 13 weeks of placebo (Carpenter *et al.*, 2009).

Conclusion: cannabis-dependence treatment

Currently there are no proven-effective medications for the treatment of cannabis dependence. So far, antidepressants (bupropion, nefazodone) and mood stabilizers (lithium, divalproex) are not very promising. Among the more promising medications are naltrexone, buspirone, atomoxetine, and dronabinol (see also Vandrey & Haney, 2009). A recently developed combination of THC and CBD (ratio 1:1) might be an interesting alternative for future trials since CBD does not alter the main effect of THC, but might reduce the probability of (serious) adverse effects of THC (Vann *et al.*, 2008).

Overall conclusion

Despite the availability of and use of disulfiram since the late 1940s in the treatment of alcohol dependence and the extensive studies of methadone in the treatment of opioid dependence since the late 1960s, substance-use disorders were often seen as amoral behaviors of weak-willed individuals and subsequently addicts were seriously stigmatized. In the last three decades, addictive behaviors have been redefined as brain diseases (Leshner, 1997). More recently, pathological gambling has been conceptualized as a non-chemical or behavioral addiction with similar underlying neurobiological mechanisms as the ones involved in substance-use disorders (e.g. Petry, 2006; Potenza, 2006). As a direct consequence of these changes, new treatments are being developed and tested, including pharmacological interventions and more recently different forms of neuromodulation (e.g. transcranial magnetic stimulation and deep brain stimulation). In this review, the status of currently available pharmacological interventions is summarized using mainly data from RCTs and meta-analyses of different RCTs. This does not imply that studies using other designs are not relevant, but placebo-controlled RCTs provide the best strategy to distinguish between interventions that are effective for a certain target population and interventions that are most likely not going to be beneficial. In contrast, non-controlled studies might be better for the study of the effect of certain medication in routine practice and for the study of infrequent (serious) adverse events.

This review shows that great progress has been made, but it also shows that no magic bullets are available. Table 12.3 shows that a series of proven-effective pharmacological interventions is now available for patients with nicotine dependence (NRT, bupropion, varenicline), alcohol-dependent patients (naltrexone, acamprosate, disulfiram, topiramate), patients with opioid dependence (methadone, buprenorphine, heroin), and pathological gamblers (nalrexone, nalmefene). With regard to cocaine dependence, the findings are less conclusive, but promising results have been obtained with stimulant-like medications and disulfiram. The general recognition of cannabis dependence as an important addiction that needs treatment, including pharmacological treatment, is quite recent, and as a consequence relatively few studies have been performed and currently no proven-effective or promising pharmacological interventions are available. Overall, it seems that agonist-like treatments take a very prominent role in the treatment of smoking, opioid dependence and probably also in cocaine dependence, whereas antagonist-like treatments tend to be less successful. In addition to these established treatments, many new compounds are tested and more effective

Table 12.3. First- and second-line pharmacological treatments in addictive disorders.

Disorder	First-line treatment	Second-line treatment
Nicotine dependence	Varenicline Bupropion Nrt	Nortryptiline Clonidine
Alcohol dependence	Naltrexone Acamprosate Disulfiram	Topiramate Baclofen?
Opioid dependence	Methadone Buprenorphine Heroin	Naltrexone (XR)
Cocaine dependence	Bupropion Dexamphetamine Disulfiram? Modafinil? Methadone High Dose?	Topiramate? Vigabatrin? Baclofen? Ondansetron? Cabergoline? Aripiprazole? Methamphetamine?
Cannabis dependence	Naltrexone? Buspirone? Atomoxetine? Dronabinol?	
Pathological gambling	Naltrexone Nalmefene	Paroxetine??

?, indications but no proof of efficacy.
XR, extended release.
??, inconsistent findings.

medications are expected to become available in the next decade. It should be noted, however, that many of the non-registered but promising medications have not been tested in long-term treatment and follow-up studies and that more studies are needed to show long term effectiveness in most of the novel compounds. As a consequence it is also not always known how long active treatment should be continued.

Despite the enormous progress, it should also be recognized that effect-sizes for proven-effective medications are generally quite modest and many patients do not respond to certain medications. Different strategies have been used to improve this situation, including (a) combination of different medications at the same time in the same patient, (b) combination of pharmacotherapy with psychosocial interventions, (c) stimulation of treatment compliance with treatment-adherence stimulation strategies, (d) matching of certain patients to certain treatment-based and phenotypic, endophenotypic, or genetic differences between patients. In some instances these kinds of strategies have been quite successful. For example, combining acamprosate with naltrexone (Kiefer *et al.*, 2003) or disulfiram with acamprosate (Besson *et al.*, 1998) in alcohol-dependent patients has shown to be a promising strategy. Also, combining medication with psychological interventions such as contingency management in the treatment of cocaine dependence seems to be rather promising (e.g. Kampman, 2010). However, combining acamprosate with psychotherapeutic interventions was not more effective than acamprosate alone and therefore patients that do not want to participate in psychotherapy should still be offered acamprosate (e.g. de Wildt *et al.*, 2002). In general, psychotherapeutic interventions directed just at medication compliance have not been very effective, but new pharmacological formulations, including sustained-release tablets and injections and subcutaneous implants, are rather promising. Finally, patient–treatment matching seems to be the most promising strategy; coupling certain patients to certain medications may result in larger effect sizes, lower numbers needed to treat, fewer unnecessary side-effects and better cost-effectiveness. Unfortunately, phenotypic (clinical) characteristics have not been very useful in the prediction of treatment effectiveness of medications, probably due to the fact that these characteristics have a complex and often weak or non-existing relationship with the underlying addictive processes and the mechanism of action of pharmacological interventions (e.g. Ooteman et al. 2005; Verheul et al., 2005). One interesting exception is the matching power of the presence of a family history of alcoholism or the (also genetically related) presence of antisocial behavior. It has been shown, for example, that alcohol-dependent patients with a positive family history or low sociability respond better to naltrexone than patients without such a family history and without antisocial traits (Rohsenow et al., 2007). Similarly, pathological gamblers with a family history of alcoholism respond better to naltrexone than pathological gamblers without such a family history (Grant et al., 2008b). Better results are likely to be obtained with endophenotypic and genetic patient characteristics since these patient variables are closer to the neurobiological basis of addiction and the mechanism of action of the medication. Meanwhile, substantial progress has been made in the prediction of medication effects by genetic patient characteristics (pharmacogenomics). For example, a variation in a single candidate gene (mu-opioid receptor gene) can predict the effect of a single pharmacological intervention (naltrexone) in alcohol-dependent patients (e.g. Anton et al., 2008; Oslin et al., 2003). Even more interestingly, a combination of different candidate genes (mu-opioid receptor, dopamine receptor, GABA receptor, glutamate receptor) can successfully predict the effect of different medications (naltrexone, acamprosate) simultaneously in alcohol dependence (e.g. Ooteman et al., 2009). Finally, a genetic profile, based on multiple genes obtained through genome-wide scanning, can predict the effect of different pharmacological strategies (NRT, bupropion) in nicotine-dependent patients (Uhl et al., 2008, 2010).

Finally, it should be noted that this review was restricted to the pharmacological treatment of substance dependence and that treatment of acute intoxication and withdrawal were not included. Moreover, this review focused in the pharmacological treatment of single drug dependence and polydrug dependence was not systematically addressed. For a review on the pharmacotherapy of dual substance abuse and dependence, the reader is referred to Kenna et al. (2007). This review is also restricted to the pharmacological treatment of adult patients with substance-use disorders or pathological gambling. However, there is an increasing interest in the (pharmacological) treatment of children and adolescents. For a preliminary review, the reader is referred to Simkin & Grenoble (2010). Similarly, there is great interest in the role of pharmacotherapy in the treatment of pregnant substance-dependent patients. Available studies and reviews are informative but rarely conclusive and more work needs to be done in this field (e.g. NRT in smoking cessation: Coleman et al., 2011; methadone dose in opioid dependence: Cleary et al., 2011; methadone vs. buprenorphine in opioid dependence: Jones et al., 2010, Unger et al., 2010). Finally, the review did not systematically address the role of psychotherapy and psychosocial interventions. It should be noted, however, that many of the pharmacological RCTs included routine or standardized psychotherapy in all treatment arms. This means that the results of proven-effective pharmacological interventions can not always be generalized to treatment conditions where no psychosocial support is available. However, it also does not automatically indicate that pharmacological interventions are only effective in the presence of psychosocial support or psychotherapy (e.g. de Wildt et al., 2002).

In conclusion, great progress has been made in the treatment of patients with substance-use disorders and pathological gambling, but more refined studies in different populations are needed taking into account the stage of the disease and the genetic, endophenotypic, and genetic profile of individual patients. In addition, new studies are needed to examine the optimal combination of pharmacotherapy, psychotherapy, and social rehabilitation. Together, these studies will provide a more optimistic outcome for patients, families, and societies suffering from addictive disorders.

References

Alho H, Sinclair D, Vuori E, Holopainen A (2007). Abuse liability of buprenorphine-naloxone tablets in untreated IV drug users. *Drug and Alcohol Dependence* **88**, 75–78.

Alvarez Y, Farré M, Fonseca F, Torrens M (2010). Anticonvulsant drugs in cocaine dependence: a systematic review and meta-analysis. *Journal of Substance Abuse Treatment* **38**, 66–73.

Amato L, Minozzi S, Pani PP, Davoli M (2007). Antipsychotic medications for cocaine dependence. *Cochrane Database of Systematic Reviews* **3**, CD006306.

Anchersen K, Clausen T, Gossop M, Hansteen V, Waal H (2009). Prevalence and clinical relevance of corrected QT interval prolongation during methadone and buprenorphine treatment: a mortality assessment study. *Addiction* **104**, 993–999.

Anderson AL, Reid MS, Li SH et al. (2009). Modafinil for the treatment of cocaine dependence. *Drug and Alcohol Dependence* **104**, 133–139.

Anton RF, Oroszi G, O'Malley S et al. (2008). An evaluation of mu-opioid receptor (OPRM1) as a predictor of naltrexone response in the treatment of alcohol dependence: results from the Combined Pharmacotherapies and Behavioral Interventions for Alcohol Dependence (COMBINE) study. *Archives of General Psychiatry* **65**(2), 135–144.

Bell J, Trinh L, Butler B, Randall D, Rubin G (2009a). Comparing retention in treatment and mortality in people after initial entry to methadone and buprenorphine treatment. *Addiction* **104**, 1193–1200.

Bell JR, Butler B, Lawrance A, Batey R, Salmelainen P (2009b). Comparing overdose mortality associated with methadone and buprenorphine treatment. *Drug and Alcohol Dependence* **104**, 73–77.

Besson J, Aeby F, Kasas A, Lehert P, Potgieter A (1998). Combined efficacy of acamprosate and disulfiram in the treatment of alcoholism: a controlled study. *Alcoholism: Clinical & Experimental Research* **22**, 573–579.

Bisaga A, Aharonovich E, Cheng WY et al. (2010). A placebo-controlled trial of memantine for cocaine dependence with high-value voucher incentives during a pre-randomization lead-in period. *Drug and Alcohol Dependence* **111**, 97–104.

Blanken P, van den Brink W, Hendriks VM et al. (2010). Heroin-assisted treatment in the Netherlands: History, findings, and international context. *European Neuropsychopharmacology* **20** (Suppl. 2), S105–S158.

Blick SK, Keating GM (2007). Lisdexamfetamine. *Paediatric Drugs* **9**(2), 129–35; discussion 136–138.

Brands B, Blake J, Sproule B, Gourlay D, Busto U (2004). Prescription opioid abuse in patients presenting for methadone maintenance treatment. *Drug and Alcohol Dependence* **73**(2), 199–207.

Brodie JD, Case BG, Figueroa E et al. (2009). Randomized, double-blind, placebo-controlled trial of vigabatrin for the treatment of cocaine dependence in Mexican parolees. *American Journal of Psychiatry* **166**, 1269–1277.

Brooks AC, Comer SD, Sullivan MA et al. (2010). Long-acting injectable versus oral naltrexone maintenance therapy with psychosocial intervention for heroin dependence: a quasi-experiment. *Journal of Clinical Psychiatry* **71**, 1371–1378.

Bruce RD, Govindasamy S, Sylla L, Kamarulzaman A, Altice FL (2009). Lack of reduction in buprenorphine injection after introduction of co-formulated buprenorphine/naloxone to the Malaysian market. *American Journal of Drug and Alcohol Abuse* 35(2), 68–72.

Buster MC, van Brussel GH, van den Brink W (2002). An increase in overdose mortality during the first 2 weeks after entering or re-entering methadone treatment in Amsterdam. *Addiction* 97, 993–1001.

Byrne A, Hallinan R, Newman RG (2010). Does electrocardiography improve methadone safety? *American Journal of Health-System Pharmacy* 67(12), 968–969.

Canfield MC, Keller CE, Frydrych LM et al. (2010). Prescription opioid use among patients seeking treatment for opioid dependence. *Journal of Addiction Medicine* 4(2), 108–113.

Carpenter KM, McDowell D, Brooks DJ, Cheng WY, Levin FR (2009). A preliminary trial: double-blind comparison of nefazodone, bupropion-SR, and placebo in the treatment of cannabis dependence. *American Journal of Addiction* 18, 53–64.

Castells X, Casas M, Pérez-Mañá C et al. (2010). Efficacy of psychostimulant drugs for cocaine dependence. *Cochrane Database of Systematic Reviews* 2, CD007380.

Castells X, Kosten TR, Capellà D et al. (2009). Efficacy of opiate maintenance therapy and adjunctive interventions for opioid dependence with comorbid cocaine use disorders: a systematic review and meta-analysis of controlled clinical trials. *American Journal of Drug and Alcohol Abuse* 35(5), 339–349.

Ciraulo DA, Sarid-Segal O, Knapp CM et al. (2005). Efficacy screening trials of paroxetine, pentoxifylline, riluzole, pramipexole and venlafaxine in cocaine dependence. *Addiction* 100 (Suppl. 1), 12–22.

Clausen T, Anchersen K, Waal H (2008). Mortality prior to, during and after opioid maintenance treatment (OMT): a national prospective cross-registry study. *Drug and Alcohol Dependence* 94(1–3), 151–157.

Cleary BJ, Donnelly J, Strawbridge J et al. (2010). Methadone dose and neonatal abstinence syndrome – systematic review and meta-analysis. *Addiction* 105(12), 2071–2084.

Coleman T, Chamberlain C, Cooper S, Leonardi-Bee J (2011). Efficacy and safety of nicotine replacement therapy for smoking cessation in pregnancy: systematic review and meta-analysis. *Addiction* 106(1), 52–61.

Comer SD, Sullivan MA, Yu E et al. (2006). Injectable, sustained-release naltrexone for the treatment of opioid dependence: a randomized, placebo-controlled trial. *Archives of General Psychiatry* 63, 210–218.

Cone EJ, Welch P, Lange WR (1988). Clonidine partially blocks the physiologic effects but not the subjective effects produced by smoking marijuana in male human subjects. *Pharmacology, Biochemistry & Behavior* 29(3), 649–652.

Connock M, Juarez-Garcia A, Jowett S et al. (2007). Methadone and buprenorphine for the management of opioid dependence: a systematic review and economic evaluation. *Health Technology Assessment* 11(9), 1–171, iii–iv.

Cornish R, Macleod J, Strang J, Vickerman P, Hickman M (2010). Risk of death during and after opiate substitution treatment in primary care: prospective observational study in UK General Practice Research Database. *British Medical Journal* 341, c5475.

Davoli M, Bargagli AM, Perucci CA et al. (2007). VEdeTTE Study Group. Risk of fatal overdose during and after specialist drug treatment: the VEdeTTE study, a national multi-site prospective cohort study. *Addiction* 102(12), 1954–1959.

Dawson DA, Grant BF, Stinson FS et al. (2005). Recovery from DSM-IV alcohol dependence: United States, 2001–2002. *Addiction* 100, 281–292.

de Bruijn C, van den Brink W, de Graaf R, Vollebergh WA (2006). The three year course of alcohol use disorders in the general population: DSM-IV, ICD-10 and the Craving Withdrawal Model. *Addiction* 101(3), 385–392.

Degenhardt L, Randall D, Hall W et al. (2009). Mortality among clients of a state-wide opioid pharmacotherapy program over 20 years: risk factors and lives saved. *Drug and Alcohol Dependence* 105(1–2), 9–15.

De Wildt WA, Schippers GM, Van Den Brink W et al. (2002). Does psychosocial treatment enhance the efficacy of acamprosate in patients with alcohol problems? *Alcohol and Alcoholism* 37, 375–382.

Ehret GB, Voide C, Gex-Fabry M et al. (2006). Drug-induced long QT syndrome in injection drug users receiving methadone: high frequency in hospitalized patients and risk factors. *Archives of Internal Medicine* **166**(12), 1280–1287.

Epstein DH, Schmittner J, Umbricht A *et al.* (2009). Promoting abstinence from cocaine and heroin with a methadone dose increase and a novel contingency. *Drug and Alcohol Dependence* **101**(1–2), 92–100.

Faggiano F, Vigna-Taglianti F, Versino E, Lemma P (2003). Methadone maintenance at different dosages for opioid dependence. *Cochrane Database of Systematic Reviews* **3**, CD002208.

Ferri M, Davoli M, Perucci CA (2010). Heroin maintenance for chronic heroin-dependent individuals. *Cochrane Database of Systematic Reviews* **8**, CD003410.

Focchi GR, Leite MC, Andrade AG, Scivoletto S (2005). Use of dopamine agonist pergolide in outpatient treatment of cocaine dependence. *Substance Use and Misuse* **40**(8), 1169–1177.

Frick U, Rehm J, Zullino D *et al.* (2010). Long-term follow-up of orally administered diacetylmorphine substitution treatment. *European Journal of Addiction Research* **16**(3), 131–138.

Fudala PJ, Bridge TP, Herbert S *et al.* (2003). Buprenorphine/Naloxone Collaborative Study Group. Office-based treatment of opiate addiction with a sublingual-tablet formulation of buprenorphine and naloxone. *New England Journal of Medicine* **349**, 949–958.

Gastfriend DR. (2010). http://www.medscape. com/viewarticle/722907

Gibson AE, Degenhardt LJ (2007). Mortality related to pharmacotherapies for opioid dependence: a comparative analysis of coronial records. *Drug and Alcohol Review* **26**(4), 405–410.

Gorelick DA, Heishman SJ, Preston KL *et al.* (2006). The cannabinoid CB1 receptor antagonist rimonabant attenuates the hypotensive effect of smoked marijuana in male smokers. *American Heart Journal* **151**(3), 754.e1–754.e5.

Gowing L, Ali R, White JM (2009a). Opioid antagonists with minimal sedation for opioid withdrawal. *Cochrane Database of Systematic Reviews* **4**, CD002021.

Gowing L, Ali R, White JM (2009b). Buprenorphine for the management of opioid withdrawal. *Cochrane Database of Systematic Reviews* **3**, CD002025.

Gowing L, Ali R, White JM (2010). Opioid antagonists under heavy sedation or anaesthesia for opioid withdrawal. *Cochrane Database of Systematic Reviews* **1**, CD002022.

Gowing L, Farrell M, Bornemann R, Sullivan LE, Ali R (2008). Substitution treatment of injecting opioid users for prevention of HIV infection. *Cochrane Database of Systematic Reviews* **2**, CD004145.

Grant JE, Kim SW, Hollander E, Potenza MN (2008b). Predicting response to opiate antagonists and placebo in the treatment of pathological gambling. *Psychopharmacology (Berlin)* **200**(4), 521–527.

Greenwald MK, Stitzer ML (2000). Antinociceptive, subjective and behavioral effects of smoked marijuana in humans. *Drug and Alcohol Dependence* **59**(3), 261–275.

Hamilton JD, Nguyen QX, Gerber RM, Rubio NB (2009). Olanzapine in cocaine dependence: a double-blind, placebo-controlled trial. *American Journal of Addiction* **18**(1), 48–52.

Haney M (2007). Opioid antagonism of cannabinoid effects: differences between marijuana smokers and nonmarijuana smokers. *Neuropsychopharmacology* **32**(6), 1391–1403.

Haney M, Bisaga A, Foltin RW (2003a). Interaction between naltrexone and oral THC in heavy marijuana smokers. *Psychopharmacology (Berlin)* **166**(1), 77–85.

Haney M, Hart CL, Vosburg SK *et al.* (2004). Marijuana withdrawal in humans: effects of oral THC or divalproex. *Neuropsychopharmacology* **29**(1), 158–170.

Haney M, Hart CL, Vosburg SK *et al.* (2008). Effects of THC and lofexidine in a human laboratory model of marijuana withdrawal and relapse. *Psychopharmacology (Berlin)* **197**(1), 157–168.

Haney M, Hart CL, Ward AS, Foltin RW (2003b). Nefazodone decreases anxiety during marijuana withdrawal in humans. *Psychopharmacology (Berlin)* **165**(2), 157–165.

Haney M, Ward AS, Comer SD *et al.* (2001). Bupropion SR worsens mood during marijuana withdrawal in humans.

Psychopharmacology (Berlin) **155**(2), 171–179.

Hart CL, Haney M, Ward AS, Fischman MW, Foltin RW (2002). Effects of oral THC maintenance on smoked marijuana self-administration. *Drug and Alcohol Dependence* **67**(3), 301–309.

Herin DV, Rush CR, Grabowski J (2010). Agonist-like pharmacotherapy for stimulant dependence: preclinical, human laboratory, and clinical studies. *Annals of the New York Academy of Sciences* **1187**, 76–100.

Hser YI, Hoffman V, Grella CE, Anglin MD (2001). A 33-year follow-up of narcotics addicts. *Archives of General Psychiatry* **58**, 503–508.

Huestis MA, Boyd SJ, Heishman SJ et al. (2007). Single and multiple doses of rimonabant antagonize acute effects of smoked cannabis in male cannabis users. *Psychopharmacology (Berlin)* **194**, 505–515.

Huestis MA, Gorelick DA, Heishman SJ et al. (2001). Blockade of effects of smoked marijuana by the CB1-selective cannabinoid receptor antagonist SR141716. *Archives of General Psychiatry* **58**, 322–328.

Hulse GK, Morris N, Arnold-Reed D, Tait RJ (2009). Improving clinical outcomes in treating heroin dependence: randomized, controlled trial of oral or implant naltrexone. *Archives of General Psychiatry* **66**, 1108–1115.

Hulse GK, Tait RJ, Comer SD et al. (2005). Reducing hospital presentations for opioid overdose in patients treated with sustained release naltrexone implants. *Drug and Alcohol Dependence* **79**(3), 351–357.

Johnson BA, Roache JD, Ait-Daoud N et al. (2006). A preliminary randomized, double-blind, placebo-controlled study of the safety and efficacy of ondansetron in the treatment of cocaine dependence. *Drug and Alcohol Dependence* **84**(3), 256–263.

Jones HE, Kaltenbach K, Heil SH et al. (2010). Neonatal abstinence syndrome after methadone or buprenorphine exposure. *New England Journal of Medicine* **363**(24), 2320–2331.

Kakko J, Grönbladh L, Svanborg KD et al. (2007). A stepped care strategy using buprenorphine and methadone versus conventional methadone maintenance in heroin dependence: a randomized controlled trial. *American Journal of Psychiatry* **164**, 797–803.

Kamien JB, Branstetter SA, Amass LA (2008). Buprenorphine-naloxone versus methadone maintenance therapy: a randomised double-blind trial with opioid dependent patients. *Heroin Addiction and Related Clinical Problems* **10**(4), 5–18.

Kampman KM (2008) http://www.medpagetoday.com/MeetingCoverage/APA/9373

Kampman KM (2010). What's new in the treatment of cocaine addiction? *Curr Psychiatry Rep.* Oct; **12**(5), 441–447.

Kampman KM, Dackis C, Lynch KG, et al. (2006). A double-blind, placebo-controlled trial of amantadine, propranolol, and their combination for the treatment of cocaine dependence in patients with severe cocaine withdrawal symptoms. *Drug Alcohol Depend.* Nov 8; **85**(2), 129–137.

Kampman KM, Dackis C, Pettinati HM et al. (2011). A double-blind, placebo-controlled pilot trial of acamprosate for the treatment of cocaine dependence. *Addictive Behaviors* **36**(3), 217–221.

Kampman K, Majewska MD, Tourian K et al. (2003). A pilot trial of piracetam and ginkgo biloba for the treatment of cocaine dependence. *Addictive Behaviors* **28**, 437–448.

Kampman KM, Pettinati H, Lynch KG et al. (2004). A pilot trial of topiramate for the treatment of cocaine dependence. *Drug and Alcohol Dependence* **75**(3), 233–240.

Kenna GA, Nielsen DM, Mello P, Schiesl A, Swift RM (2007). Pharmacotherapy of dual substance abuse and dependence. *CNS Drugs* **21**(3), 213–237.

Kennedy A, Wood AE, Saxon AJ et al. (2008). Quetiapine for the treatment of cocaine dependence: an open-label trial. *Journal of Clinical Psychopharmacology* **28**(2), 221–224.

Kiefer F, Jahn H, Tarnaske T et al. (2003). Comparing and combining naltrexone and acamprosate in relapse prevention of alcoholism: a double-blind, placebo-controlled study. *Archives of General Psychiatry* **60**, 92–99.

Kosten TR, Oliveto A, Sevarino KA, Gonsai K, Feingold A (2002). Ketoconazole increases cocaine and opioid use in methadone maintained patients. *Drug and Alcohol Dependence* **66**, 173–180.

Kraigher D, Jagsch R, Gombas W *et al.* (2005). Use of slow-release oral morphine for the treatment of opioid dependence. *European Journal of Addiction Research* **11**(3), 145–151.

Krantz MJ, Martin J, Stimmel B, Mehta D, Haigney MC (2009). QTc interval screening in methadone treatment. *Annals of Internal Medicine* **150**(6), 387–395.

Kunøe N, Lobmaier P, Vederhus JK *et al.* (2009). Naltrexone implants after in-patient treatment for opioid dependence: randomised controlled trial. *British Journal of Psychiatry* **194**, 541–546.

Kunøe N, Lobmaier P, Vederhus JK *et al.* (2010). Retention in naltrexone implant treatment for opioid dependence. *Drug and Alcohol Dependence* **111**(1–2), 166–169.

Leshner AI (1997). Addiction is a brain disease, and it matters. *Science* **278**(5335), 45–47.

Levin FR, McDowell D, Evans SM *et al.* (2004). Pharmacotherapy for marijuana dependence: a double-blind, placebo-controlled pilot study of divalproex sodium. *American Journal of Addiction* **13**(1), 21–32.

Lind B, Chen S, Weatherburn D, Mattick R (2005). The effectiveness of methadone maintenance treatment in controlling crime. An Australian aggregate-level analysis. *Journal of Criminology* **45**, 201–211.

Ling W, Casadonte P, Bigelow G *et al.* (2010). Buprenorphine implants for treatment of opioid dependence: a randomized controlled trial. *Journal of the American Medical Association* **304**, 1576–1583.

Lobmaier P, Kornor H, Kunoe N, Bjørndal A (2008). Sustained-release naltrexone for opioid dependence. *Cochrane Database of Systematic Reviews* **2**, CD006140.

Lobmaier PP, Kunøe N, Gossop M, Katevoll T, Waal H (2010). Naltrexone implants compared to methadone: outcomes six months after prison release. *European Addiction Research* **16**(3), 139–145.

Loebl T, Angarita GA, Pachas GN *et al.* (2008). A randomized, double-blind, placebo-controlled trial of long-acting risperidone in cocaine-dependent men. *Journal of Clinical Psychiatry* **69**(3), 480–486.

Malcolm R, LaRowe S, Cochran K *et al.* (2005). A controlled trial of amlodipine for cocaine

dependence: a negative report. *Journal of Substance Abuse Treatment* **28**, 197–204.

Martell BA, Arnsten JH, Krantz MJ, Gourevitch MN (2005). Impact of methadone treatment on cardiac repolarization and conduction in opioid users. *American Journal of Cardiology* **95**(7), 915–918.

Martell BA, Orson FM, Poling J *et al.* (2009). Cocaine vaccine for the treatment of cocaine dependence in methadone-maintained patients: a randomized, double-blind, placebo-controlled efficacy trial. *Archives of General Psychiatry* **66**, 1116–1123.

Martínez-Raga J, Knecht C, Cepeda S (2008). Modafinil: a useful medication for cocaine addiction? Review of the evidence from neuropharmacological, experimental and clinical studies. *Current Drug Abuse Reviews* **1**(2), 213–221.

Mattick RP, Breen C, Kimber J, Davoli M (2009). Methadone maintenance therapy versus no opioid replacement therapy for opioid dependence. *Cochrane Database of Systematic Reviews* **3**, CD002209.

Mattick RP, Kimber J, Breen C, Davoli M (2008). Buprenorphine maintenance versus placebo or methadone maintenance for opioid dependence. *Cochrane Database of Systematic Reviews* **2**, CD002207.

McRae AL, Brady KT, Carter RE (2006). Buspirone for treatment of marijuana dependence: a pilot study. *American Journal of Addiction* **15**(5), 404.

Meader N (2010). A comparison of methadone, buprenorphine and alpha(2) adrenergic agonists for opioid detoxification: a mixed treatment comparison meta-analysis. *Drug and Alcohol Dependence* **108**(1–2), 110–114.

Minozzi S, Amato L, Vecchi S *et al.* (2006). Oral naltrexone maintenance treatment for opioid dependence. *Cochrane Database of Systematic Reviews* **1**, CD001333.

Mitchell TB, White JM, Somogyi AA, Bochner F (2004). Slow-release oral morphine versus methadone: a crossover comparison of patient outcomes and acceptability as maintenance pharmacotherapies for opioid dependence. *Addiction* **99**(8), 940–945.

Moeller FG, Schmitz JM, Steinberg JL *et al.* (2007). Citalopram combined with behavioral therapy reduces cocaine use: a double-blind, placebo-controlled trial.

American Journal of Drug and Alcohol Abuse 33, 367–378.

Montoya ID, Gorelick DA, Preston KL et al. (2004). Randomized trial of buprenorphine for treatment of concurrent opiate and cocaine dependence. *Clinical Pharmacology & Therapeutics* 75, 34–48.

Mooney ME, Herin DV, Schmitz JM et al. (2009). Effects of oral methamphetamine on cocaine use: a randomized, double-blind, placebo-controlled trial. *Drug and Alcohol Dependence* 101(1–2), 34–41.

Mooney ME, Schmitz JM, Moeller FG, Grabowski J (2007). Safety, tolerability and efficacy of levodopa-carbidopa treatment for cocaine dependence: two double-blind, randomized, clinical trials. *Drug and Alcohol Dependence* 88(2–3), 214–223.

Naderi-Heiden A, Naderi A, Naderi MM et al. (2010). Ultra-rapid opiate detoxification followed by nine months of naltrexone maintenance therapy in Iran. *Pharmacopsychiatry* 43(4), 130–137.

Nanjayya SB, Shivappa M, Chand PK, Murthy P, Benegal V (2010). Baclofen in cannabis dependence syndrome. *Biological Psychiatry* 68(3), e9–10.

Oliveto A, Poling J, Mancino MJ et al. (2011). Randomized, double blind, placebo-controlled trial of disulfiram for the treatment of cocaine dependence in methadone-stabilized patients. *Drug and Alcohol Dependence* 113(2–3), 184–191.

Ooteman W, Naassila M, Koeter MW et al. (2009). Predicting the effect of naltrexone and acamprosate in alcohol-dependent patients using genetic indicators. *Addiction Biology* 14(3), 328–337.

Ooteman W, Verheul R, Naassila M et al. (2005). Patient-treatment matching with anti-craving medications in alcohol dependent patients: a review on phenotypic, endophenotypic and genetic indicators. *Journal of Substance Use* 10, 75–96.

Oslin DW, Berrettini W, Kranzler HR et al. (2003). A functional polymorphism of the mu-opioid receptor gene is associated with naltrexone response in alcohol-dependent patients. *Neuropsychopharmacology* 28(8), 1546–1552.

Pani PP, Trogu E, Vacca R et al. (2010). Disulfiram for the treatment of cocaine dependence. *Cochrane Database of Systematic Reviews* 1, CD007024.

Passos SR, Camacho LA, Lopes CS, dos Santos MA (2005). Nefazodone in out-patient treatment of inhaled cocaine dependence: a randomized double-blind placebo-controlled trial. *Addiction* 100(4), 489–494.

Peles E, Kreek MJ, Kellogg S, Adelson M (2006). High methadone dose significantly reduces cocaine use in methadone maintenance treatment (MMT) patients. *Journal of Addictive Diseases* 25(1), 43–50.

Petry NM (2006). Should the scope of addictive behaviors be broadened to include pathological gambling? *Addiction* 101(Suppl. 1), 152–160.

Pettinati HM, Kampman KM, Lynch KG et al. (2008). A double blind, placebo-controlled trial that combines disulfiram and naltrexone for treating co-occurring cocaine and alcohol dependence. *Addictive Behaviors* 33(5), 651–667.

Potenza MN (2006). Should addictive disorders include non-substance-related conditions? *Addiction* 101(Suppl. 1), 142–51.

Reece AS (2010). Favorable mortality profile of naltrexone implants for opiate addiction. *Journal of Addictive Diseases* 29, 30–50.

Reid MS, Angrist B, Baker S et al. (2005). A placebo-controlled screening trial of celecoxib for the treatment of cocaine dependence. *Addiction* 100 (Suppl. 1), 32–42.

Rohsenow DJ, Miranda R Jr, McGeary JE, Monti PM (2007). Family history and antisocial traits moderate naltrexone's effects on heavy drinking in alcoholics. *Experimental and Clinical Psychopharmacology* 15(3), 272–281.

Schmitz JM, Lindsay JA, Green CE et al. (2009). High-dose naltrexone therapy for cocaine-alcohol dependence. *American Journal of Addiction* 18(5), 356–362.

Schmitz JM, Stotts AL, Rhoades HM, Grabowski J (2001). Naltrexone and relapse prevention treatment for cocaine-dependent patients. *Addictive Behaviors* 26(2), 167–180.

Schmitz JM, Stotts AL, Sayre SL, DeLaune KA, Grabowski J (2004). Treatment of cocaine-alcohol dependence with naltrexone and relapse prevention therapy. *American Journal of Addiction* 13(4), 333–341.

Schottenfeld RS, Chawarski MC, Pakes JR et al. (2005). Methadone versus buprenorphine with contingency management or performance feedback for cocaine and opioid dependence. *American Journal of Psychiatry* **162**(2), 340–349.

Schottenfeld RS, Pakes JR, Oliveto A, Ziedonis D, Kosten TR (1997). Buprenorphine vs. methadone maintenance treatment for concurrent opioid dependence and cocaine abuse. *Archives of General Psychiatry* **54**(8), 713–720.

Shoptaw S, Watson DW, Reiber C et al. (2005). Randomized controlled pilot trial of cabergoline, hydergine and levodopa/carbidopa: Los Angeles Cocaine Rapid Efficacy Screening Trial (CREST). *Addiction* **100**(Suppl. 1), 78–90.

Silva de Lima M, Farrell M, Lima Reisser AARL, Soares B (2003). Antidepressants for cocaine dependence. *Cochrane Database of Systematic Reviews* **2**, CD002950.

Simkin DR, Grenoble S (2010). Pharmacotherapies for adolescent substance use disorders. *Child and Adolescent Psychiatry Clinics of North America* **19**(3), 591–608.

Soares B, Lima Reisser AARL, Farrell M, Silva de Lima M (2003). Dopamine agonists for cocaine dependence. *Cochrane Database of Systematic Reviews* **2**, CD003352.

Sproule B, Brands B, Li S, Catz-Biro L (2009). Changing patterns in opioid addiction: characterizing users of oxycodone and other opioids. *Canadian Family Physician* **55**(1), 68–69, 69.e1–5.

Tait RJ, Ngo HT, Hulse GK (2008). Mortality in heroin users 3 years after naltrexone implant or methadone maintenance treatment. *Journal of Substance Abuse Treatment* **35**(2), 116–124.

Tirado CF, Goldman M, Lynch K, Kampman KM, O'Brien CP (2008). Atomoxetine for treatment of marijuana dependence: a report on the efficacy and high incidence of gastrointestinal adverse events in a pilot study. *Drug and Alcohol Dependence* **94**(1–3), 254–257.

Uhl GR, Drgon T, Johnson C et al. (2010). Genome-wide association for smoking cessation success in a trial of precessation nicotine replacement. *Molecular Medicine* **16**(11–12), 513–526.

Uhl GR, Liu QR, Drgon T et al. (2008). Molecular genetics of successful smoking cessation: convergent genome-wide association study results. *Archives of General Psychiatry* **65**(6), 683–693.

Unger A, Jung E, Winklbaur B, Fischer G (2010). Gender issues in the pharmacotherapy of opioid-addicted women: buprenorphine. *Journal of Addictive Diseases* **29**(2), 217–230.

UNODC-WHO (2009). *UNODC-WHO Joint Program on Drug Dependence Treatment and Care.* Vienna/Geneva: UNODC-WHO.

UNODC (2010). *World Drug Report 2010* (United Nations Publication, Sales No. E.10.XI.13).

Van den Brink W, Haasen C (2006). Evidence-based treatment of opioid-dependent patients. *Canadian Journal of Psychiatry* **51**(10), 635–646.

van den Brink W, van Ree JM. (2003) Pharmacological treatments for heroin and cocaine addiction. *European Journal of Neuropsychopharmacology* **13**, 476–487.

Vandrey R, Haney M (2009). Pharmacotherapy for cannabis dependence: how close are we? *CNS Drugs* **23**(7), 543–553.

Vann RE, Gamage TF, Warner JA et al. (2008). Divergent effects of cannabidiol on the discriminative stimulus and place conditioning effects of Delta(9)-tetrahydrocannabinol. *Drug and Alcohol Dependence* **94**(1–3), 191–198.

Vasilev GN, Alexieva DZ, Pavlova RZ (2006). Safety and efficacy of oral slow release morphine for maintenance treatment in heroin addicts: a 6-month open noncomparative study. *European Addiction Research* **12**(2), 53–60.

Verheul R, Lehert P, Geerlings PJ, Koeter MW, van den Brink W (2005). Predictors of acamprosate efficacy: results from a pooled analysis of seven European trials including 1485 alcohol-dependent patients. *Psychopharmacology* (Berlin) **178**(2–3), 167–173.

Vorspan F, Bellais L, Keijzer L, Lépine JP (2008). An open-label study of aripiprazole in nonschizophrenic crack-dependent patients. *Journal of Clinical Psychopharmacology* **28**(5), 570–572.

Wachtel SR, de Wit H (2000). Naltrexone does not block the subjective effects of oral

Delta(9)-tetrahydrocannabinol in humans. *Drug and Alcohol Dependence* **59**(3), 251–260.

Wedam EF, Bigelow GE, Johnson RE, Nuzzo PA, Haigney MC (2007). QT-interval effects of methadone, levomethadyl, and buprenorphine in a randomized trial. *Archives of Internal Medicine* **167**(22), 2469–2475.

Winhusen TM, Somoza EC, Harrer JM *et al.* (2005). A placebo-controlled screening trial of tiagabine, sertraline and donepezil as cocaine dependence treatments. *Addiction* **100**(Suppl. 1), 68–77.

Winstock AR, Lea T, Copeland J (2009). Lithium carbonate in the management of cannabis withdrawal in humans: an open-label study. *Journal of Psychopharmacology* **23**, 84–93.

WHO (2009). *Guidelines for the Psychosocially Assisted Pharmacological Treatment of Opioid Dependence.* Geneva: WHO.

Evidence-based pharmacotherapy of Alzheimer's disease

13

Darren Cotterell and Martin Brown

Introduction

Dementia is defined as an acquired global impairment of cognitive capacities sufficient to impact on normal functioning. There are a number of recognized causes of dementia but the most prevalent is Alzheimer's disease (AD) which accounts for 50–70% of diagnoses. In the UK, where approximately 700 000 people are thought to have a diagnosable dementia, it has been estimated that the annual cost of dementia-related care is £17 billion (Dementia UK, 2007). This reflects the combined cost of informal care, care funded both by social services and the National Health Service, and accommodation. Approximately two-thirds of people with dementia will continue to live in private households. In North America, 5.3 million people are estimated to have Alzheimer's disease, with annual healthcare costs of $172 billion (Hebert *et al.*, 2003). These figures are expected to treble by 2050.

Early onset AD (before the age of 65) accounts for a small minority of cases with roughly 0.1% in total arising from mutations in one of three genes, Presenilin 1, Presenilin 2 and amyloid precursor protein (APP), or a duplication of the APP gene (Campion *et al.*, 1999; Rovelet-Lecrux *et al.*, 2006) – seen most commonly in Down syndrome. The vast majority of cases are of a late-onset or sporadic form. The prevalence of the condition increases with age, with an approximate doubling with every 5-year increase across the age range such that one in five will satisfy diagnostic criteria above the age of 80. In addition to increasing age the most consistent risk factor is one of family history, with the only established genetic risk factor for the development of late-onset AD (LOAD) being the possession of an apolipoprotein (ApoE) ε4 allele. The ApoE ε4 allele has been demonstrated to lower the age of onset of LOAD in a dose-dependent manner, with a three times increased risk in heterozygotes and 15 times risk in homozygotes (Corder *et al.*, 1993).

Alzheimer's disease is characterized by an insidious onset and gradual progression. Aphasia, executive dysfunction, apraxia, and agnosia can occur at an early stage; using the *Diagnostic and Statistical Manual Version IV* (DSM–IV) and *International Classification of Diseases Version 10* (ICD-10) criteria to make a diagnosis of Alzheimer's dementia requires at least one of these four features to be present in combination with impairment of memory, with co-existing functional impairment. Whilst all these features may lead to a tentative diagnosis of AD, this can only be confirmed definitively by post-mortem examination of brain tissue. The illness is often associated with mood and behavioral symptoms, known as the "Behavioral and Psychological Symptoms of Dementia" (BPSD), which can be particularly challenging for carers to manage and often precipitate the need for institutional care.

Essential Evidence-Based Psychopharmacology, Second Edition, ed. Dan J. Stein, Bernard Lerer, and Stephen M. Stahl. Published by Cambridge University Press. © Cambridge University Press.

Neuropathology and neurochemistry

In the last 10 years our understanding of the neuropathology of AD has advanced greatly and has certainly vastly outstripped the development of new pharmaceutical approaches to its management for the practising clinician. A brief overview of this area is relevant to understanding therapeutic approaches, and particularly drugs in development.

In his original description of the pathological findings Alzheimer described both senile plaques and neurofibrillary tangles (NFT). It has been discovered that the principal components of plaques are varying lengths of amyloid-beta (Aβ) peptide, one of the proteolytically cleaved products of amyloid precursor protein (APP). Whilst found in many parts of the body, little is known about the physiological function of APP, though it is hypothesized to have a role in cell–cell adhesion and in maintaining synaptic integrity (Chen, 2007). APP cleavage by β- or γ-secretase generates Aβ peptide of between 39 and 42 amino acids in length and these are the predominant constituents of Aβ plaques. Aβ peptide polymerizes to form oligomers (thought currently to be the primary neurotoxic agents in the disease process) and later to polymers which clump together to form several types of amyloid inclusions.

Neurofibrillary tangles (NFTs) are intracellular, insoluble filamentous deposits which are composed of an abnormal form of a microtubule-associated protein called *tau*, which plays a role in the assembly and stabilization of the neuronal cytoskeleton. This function is compromised if *tau* becomes hyperphosphorylated, resulting in paired helical filaments which reduce the flow of materials along axons and often in neuronal death. It is felt that this process is the common final pathway of altered signaling mechanisms in degenerating neurons (Gong *et al.*, 2010).

Of the many neurotransmitters within the brain most attention has focused on the role of acetylcholine in understanding cognitive changes in AD. Cortical pathways utilizing acetylcholine are widely distributed throughout the central nervous system. Efferent projections from the nucleus basalis of Meynert to the olfactory bulbs, amygdala, hippocampus and the entire cerebral cortex are pathways affected in AD. The synthesis of acetylcholine from choline and acetyl coenzyme A in presynaptic neurons is catalyzed by cholineacetyltransferase. When released, acetylcholines' effects are mediated via pre- and post-synaptic muscarinic and nicotinic receptors with either excitatory or inhibitory results. Acetylcholine is broken down in the synaptic cleft by the enzyme acetylcholinesterase (AChE). The cholinergic hypothesis is widely accepted to be based on many different demonstrated abnormalities within the cholinergic system including a loss of cholineacetyltransferase in the cerebral cortex and hippocampus of patients with AD, photon emission tomography (PET) scans demonstrating reduced activity of AChE in AD, and a significant loss of neurons in the nucleus basalis of patients with the disease compared with age-matched controls. Consistent with this is the cognitive dysfunction and confusion in otherwise healthy individuals produced by anti cholinergic drugs. It is worth noting that antipsychotics and antidepressants, used in treating the behavioral and psychological symptoms of AD, often have strong anticholinergic effects which can inevitably exacerbate the cognitive dysfunction evident in AD.

Current options for pharmacotherapy

This section will describe the medications currently available to treat Alzheimer's disease and critically review the available evidence for their use. This is followed by a suggested management strategy, with an added focus on the management of BPSD.

Medications currently available

Four agents are licensed for the treatment of Alzheimer's disease in both Europe and the USA: these are donepezil (Aricept©), rivastigmine (Exelon©), galantamine (Reminyl©) and memantine (Ebixa©). A fifth, tacrine (Cognex©), has a similar licence in the USA but is rarely used due to an established and significant risk of hepatotoxicity. Donepezil functions purely as an acetycholinesterase inhibitor (ACHEI), rivastigmine as a dual acetyl-cholinesterase and butyrylcholinesterase inhibitor, and galantamine acts as an acetyl-cholinesterase inhibitor and an allosteric nicotinic agonist. The pharmacological premise underlying the development of these drugs is derived from the cholinergic hypothesis of AD suggesting that enhancement of levels of acetylcholine, through inhibition of degradation of the existing neurotransmitter, should provide symptomatic relief. It remains to be proven whether there is cognitive benefit derived from the nicotinic modulation demonstrated by galantamine.

Memantine is a non-competitive NMDA receptor antagonist with moderate affinity

The action of glutamate on the N-methyl-D-aspartate (NMDA) receptor is known to be important in the process of learning and memory via the mechanism of long-term potenti-ation. In addition persistent high levels of glutamate result in excitotoxicity, a state in which there is increased neuronal apoptosis. This state has been shown to be induced by $A\beta$ plaques in Alzheimer's disease (Harkany et al., 2000). Thus modulation of this pathway is an attractive option for disease modification in the illness.

In other types of dementia, rivastigmine is licensed for the treatment of neuropsychiatric symptoms in Lewy body dementia and mild to moderate dementia associated with Parkin-son's disease. Other cholinesterase inhibitors may be equally effective (Josif & Graham, 2008), however, there is a noticeable absence of sufficient randomized, placebo-controlled trials in this area.

Current evidence to support efficacy

The evidence base to support an effect on cognition

Evidence for the benefits of cholinesterase inhibitors in the treatment of Alzheimer's disease has been subject to extensive and regular review (Burns et al., 2006; Raina et al., 2008; Ritchie et al., 2004), including a Cochrane review (Birks, 2006) which accesses all available evidence, both published and unpublished. While almost all studies have revealed a reduced rate of cognitive decline or even some improvement in cognitive function, effect sizes have been consistently small, averaging an approximate 3-point difference in the ADAS-COG after 3–6 months of therapy. It has been argued that the widespread acceptance that this difference represents a significant response does not translate into a clinically meaningful outcome. The FDA has suggested a minimum 4-point difference should represent a clinical response, and a separate meta-analysis by Lanctot et al. (2003) using these criteria found that only 10% more patients responded to a cholinesterase inhibitor than placebo. An opposing debate argues that the ADAS-COG is over-dependent on language skills and relatively light in assessing visuospatial memory, apathy, depression, and executive dysfunction. Additionally, the scale loses sensitivity when applied to patients with severe dementia, where a more appropriate tool may be the Severe Impairment Battery (SIB) which has been validated for use in this cohort (Albert & Cohen, 1992). Another clear concern is that the subjects used in trials on these agents do not represent the patients seen in clinical practice. Two separate studies revealed that 50–90% of patients in two separate sites in the USA and Canada (Gill *et al.*, 2004; Schneider *et al.*, 1997) would have been ineligible for inclusion in all relevant trials due to a combination of comorbid illness, concomitant medication, or the presence of neuropsychiatric symptoms.

A review of the research methodology

The majority of randomized controlled trials that enabled the cognitive enhancers to gain their licence lasted on average between 3–6 months. With a median survival time of 6–8 years from point of diagnosis, and the recognition that cognitive ability can fluctuate markedly in response to both individual and environmental influences, it is debated that these trials are not long enough to provide clinically meaningful data. However it is also recognized that longer trials are subject to high rates of attrition. Birks *et al.* (2006) reported that after 6 months of treatment 29% of patients in the cholinesterase inhibitor arms had withdrawn, compared with 18% receiving placebo ($p < 0.00001$). It can also be argued that the use of the standard "last observation carried forward (LOCF) – intention to treat (ITT)" method of inclusive analysis may create bias towards treatment arms. AD is a progressive illness therefore an early discontinuation (for side-effects, as an example) would contribute data recording a reduced rate of decline using this method, particularly if this event occurred early in treatment (Molnar *et al.*, 2009). This would clearly create bias towards the treatment arm. The National Institute of Clinical Excellence (NICE) assessment group, in their recently released draft guidance on the management of Alzheimer's Disease (October 7, 2010), described the quality of the placebo-controlled studies on cognitive enhancers since its initial review in 2004 as "disappointing" for precisely these reasons. They also highlighted the lack of long-term data, the lack of research on the impact of technological interventions on patients and carers, and the heterogeneity of outcome measures utilized as particular concerns.

Evidence for cost-effectiveness

NICE in its revised guidance (TA111 2007 and 2009) concluded that the use of medication beyond the moderate stage of the illness was not cost-effective within the current framework of care in the National Health Service in the UK. This decision provoked significant distress but resulted in a necessary focus on the statistical models used in economic analyses on an older cohort, in particular the appropriateness of using Quality Adjusted Life Years (QALYs), the equations used for calculating the predicted cost of full-time care, the use of various scores not validated for use in an older population, and a lack of consideration to caregiver burden (Burns *et al.*, 2006). More recently the NICE assessment group (October 2010) reviewed 23 subsequent economic analyses, most using the model originally used by NICE to determine its revised guidance, and concluded that cholinesterase inhibitors and memantine are cost-effective at all stages of the illness. They did however also raise significant concerns regarding the validity of their own model. Equally, the impact of generic forms of cholinesterase inhibitors becoming available over the next 2 years has not been determined.

Evidence for non-cognitive measures of improvement

The overemphasis on cognitive improvement together with the impact of cost concerns has seen attention shift away from cognitive measures such as the ADAS-COG and the SIB onto non-cognitive measures of efficacy. This move has also been aided by the requirement of some regulatory bodies (such as the European Medicines Evaluation Agency – January 1997) that evidence of efficacy requires assessment in two of the domains of cognition, global assessment and function. More than 40 different instruments have been used to capture benefits that are deemed important to the caregiver and/or the clinician. In the early stages these have focused on measures of improved cognition and disease delay. The mid stages have been characterized by efforts to capture improved functionality and delay movement into full-time care, and the later stages by measures of the impact on the behavioral and psychological manifestations of the illness. The Clinician-Based Impression of Change scale (with caregiver input) (CIBIC-plus), the Alzheimer's Disease Cooperative Study subscale for Activities of Daily Living (ADCS-ADL), time to institutional care, and the Neuropsychiatric Inventory (NPI) have been the most widely utilized. Clearly the use of such a wide variety of measures has hampered effective statistical comparisons and prevented meaningful quantitative meta-analysis. In general, non-cognitive measures have demonstrated similar levels of improvement to cognitive measures, with equally small effect sizes.

Management strategies for clinicians

In the face of such debate there are significant challenges posed to clinicians faced with the management of such an emotive and debilitating illness.

Assessment and diagnosis

The diagnosis of AD has traditionally been a clinical one, made following the collation of a detailed history from the patient and carer, the exclusion of organic causes of cognitive impairment, the use of an appropriate cognitive screening tool – most commonly the Mini-Mental State Examination (MMSE) (Folstein et al., 1975) – and the judicious use of either CT or MRI scanning. This task is becoming increasingly complex. Over the last 10 years particularly, the notion that many patients would present with a "pure" form of AD has been challenged. Neuropathological studies have suggested that AD and particularly vascular dementia frequently coexist (Abraham et al., 2000) and additional evidence has emerged that they share risk factors such as smoking (Anstey et al., 2007), hypertension (Skoog et al., 1996), as well as dietary factors and obesity (Beydoun et al., 2008). It has been estimated that even with the most careful diagnostic evaluation a clinical diagnosis of AD made during a patient's lifetime correlates with histopathological findings only in about 70–90% of cases (Rabins et al., 2007). New scanning techniques such as SPECT (single photon emission computed tomography) and PET (positron emission tomography) are becoming more accessible and can enhance diagnostic sensitivity. Although there is no evidence that vascular dementia can be treated with cognitive enhancers, if there is evidence of coexisting AD then a trial of an ACHEI would be appropriate for that component of the presentation.

Cognitive assessment tools used in research trials are not amenable to clinical practice. Thus the MMSE still remains the most practically useful tool to enable the clinician to explore deficits and then categorize their patient into levels of severity in a practical and timely manner, once a diagnosis of AD has been made. There are valid concerns over its ability to capture the true extent of cognitive deficit, the influence of premorbid intellectual functioning, and also its ability to capture changes in cognitive status accurately. However, as a screening tool it has been widely validated and all guidelines rely on its result to categorize the severity of dementia. Three categories can be generated: mild dementia (21–26 points); moderate dementia (10–20 points); and severe (or advanced) dementia (< 10 points). A fourth category describing moderate to severe dementia is sometimes used (10–14 points). On average, untreated patients lose 2 MMSE points per year, although significant fluctuation can occur (Birks, 2006). A score of 27–30 points may suggest a mild cognitive impairment (MCI) – a subjective and objective cognitive impairment with minimal impact on functional ability, such that the patient would not meet the criteria for a dementia. Although the concept of MCI has been much debated, it is becoming increasingly accepted as a separate entity which may be prodromal to the development of a neurodegenerative condition. The most widely used categorical system separates MCI into the following forms: amnestic – single domain (objective impairment in memory only); amnestic – multiple domain (i.e. memory with another cognitive domain); non-amnestic – single domain (non-memory cognitive impairment only); and non-amnestic – multiple domain (two cognitive domains not involving memory) (Petersen, 2004; Winblad et al., 2004).

Treatment strategies

Treatment strategies will focus here on pharmacological management, as an appraisal of the various environmental, social, and psychological interventions that may be beneficial to patients and their carers is beyond the scope of this review. Readers are directed elsewhere (Burns et al., 2002; Clare et al., 2003; Logsdon et al., 2007; Rabins et al., 2007) for further information.

Mild cognitive impairment

There is evidence suggesting a 10–15% transition rate from MCI to dementia per year (Grundman et al., 2002) and that a third of patients with MCI, in particular the "amnestic subtype," will progress cumulatively to developing AD (Mitchell & Shiri-Feshki, 2008; Petersen, 2004).

A number of risk factors have been identified that place individuals at increased risk of transition including biomarker variables, characteristics on functional imaging, increased age, and low education (Mariani et al., 2007). It is clear, however, that for a significant proportion of sufferers any cognitive deficits will remain stable. There are currently no approved drugs for the treatment of MCI. Trials on all cholinesterase inhibitors, memantine and indeed other agents such as rofecoxib, vitamin E, folic acid, piracetam or statins (Farlow, 2009; Jelic et al., 2006; Petersen, 2005) have demonstrated no significant influence over the progression to dementia, or the development of AD. Evidence from two unpublished trials have even suggested an increased mortality associated with galantamine, which remains unexplained (Burns et al., 2006). As the cholinesterase inhibitors and memantine have only offered symptomatic relief it should come as no surprise that they are unable to influence the pathogenesis of the illness. Despite this it is clear that "off-label" prescription of medication does occur supported by the finding that 28–35% of MCI patients received cholinesterase inhibitors and roughly 11% received memantine in two separate sites (Weinstein et al., 2009). Thus all that can be advocated with certainty for this heterogeneous group of patients is a period of "watchful waiting" and the modification of dietary and lifestyle factors known to increase risk

(Middleton & Yaffe, 2009). Cognitive deficits can be more thoroughly unmasked and monitored through cognitive examinations such as the Montreal Cognitive Assessment tool (MOCA) (Nasreddine *et al.*, 2005) or the Addenbrookes Cognitive Examination (ACE) (Mathuranath *et al.*, 2000) both of which can be administered in a time-efficient manner in an outpatient setting and may be more descriptive than the MMSE in this cohort.

Mild to moderate dementia

The American Psychiatric Association (APA) guidelines (October 2007) advise that cholinesterase inhibitors should be offered to patients with both mild (MMSE 21–26) and moderate (MMSE 10–20) AD. In the UK the current NICE guidance only supports use of an ACHEI at moderate stages, though on legal challenge it was accepted that there was a need to exercise clinical judgment in individual patients. The most recent draft guidelines issued by NICE have recommended bringing UK guidance in line with the current APA recommendations. There is no clear evidence of efficacy of one cholinesterase inhibitor over the others, or of any preparation over another, although relatively few trials have performed adequate comparisons (Bullock *et al.*, 2005; Jones *et al.*, 2004; Wilcock *et al.*, 2003; Wilkinson *et al.*, 2002). It is difficult to predict who will respond to these agents and choice is generally guided by tolerability issues, side-effect profiles, and clinician experience. Donepezil is more widely prescribed and this is likely to be due to a lower incidence of gastrointestinal adverse effects (Birks, 2006; Lockhart *et al.*, 2009).This may change as clinicians become more familiar with the rivastigmine transdermal preparation. Rates of between 18–48% improvement have been reported (Lanctot *et al.*, 2003) and this improvement may come in different forms. It may be in memory domains but may also be in areas such as attention and initiative, more commonly related to frontal lobe function (Rockwood *et al.*, 2004).There is increasing evidence that a developing understanding of the influence of genetic variation in ApoE ε4 status, butyryl-cholinesterase and cytochrome P450 2D6 (CYP2D6) –a vital member of the hepatic mixed-function oxidase system – may enable a better prediction of who is likely both to respond to medication, as well as develop side–effects (Lam *et al.*, 2009). Memantine has only demonstrated significant benefit at this stage in one trial (Peskind *et al.*, 2006) which has not been replicated.

Severe dementia

It is estimated that between 21% and 43% of patients with AD fall in the moderately severe to severe range (Hebert *et al.*, 2003; Helmer *et al.*, 2006). There is relatively less evidence supporting the use of pharmacotherapy in this cohort, however, similar effect sizes to those found in mild to moderate disease have been found for donepezil (Black *et al.*, 2007; Feldman *et al.*, 2005; Winblad *et al.*, 2009), memantine (McShane *et al.*, 2006) and galantamine (Burns *et al.*, 2009). Only memantine and donepezil are licensed for use in severe AD and therefore a therapeutic trial (supported by the APA but not current NICE guidance) with these agents in therapy-naive patients could be supported. However, it is likely that the majority of patients will migrate into this category having been already initiated on an ACHEI. It is hoped that the results of the DOMINO-AD trial (Jones *et al.*, 2009) will provide some much-needed clarity regarding the optimum treatment for this subgroup. In their recent draft guidance (2010) the NICE assessment group suggest an approach broadly similar to that of the APA, suggesting the use of memantine in resistance to, or intolerance of, cholinesterase inhibitors in the moderate stages, and as a first-line agent in severe illness. This is despite concluding that an appraisal of all new evidence on trials using memantine did not support "evidence of benefit for memantine monotherapy compared with placebo on any measure."

Duration of treatment

There is no certainty regarding the optimum duration of treatment. Relatively few trials have examined treatment effect for longer than 1 year, primarily due to high attrition rates and ethical concerns. The AD2000 study (Courtney et al., 2004) remains the longest placebo-controlled randomized trial to date; however, while proving continued benefit, it was hampered by dropout rates of 66–70% at 2 years. Due to the paucity of such placebo-controlled trials, one looks to open-label studies for guidance despite obvious concerns regarding cohort effects, survivor bias, and extrapolation of data. The majority of these have demonstrated a significant difference in both cognitive and non-cognitive measures for periods of up to 4–5 years (Bullock & Dengiz, 2005; Burns et al., 2007; Feldman et al., 2009; Lyketsos et al., 2004; Rockwood et al., 2008; Winblad & Jelic, 2004) and have demonstrated acceptable tolerability (Burns et al., 2007; Rockwood et al., 2008). The level of improvement in cognitive function may not be as noticeable to clinicians or carers (McLendon & Doraiswamy, 1999) as that of non-cognitive measures, particularly the emergence of specific behavioral symptoms and the preservation of daily living skills.

Most guidelines support a therapeutic trial of a cognitive enhancer for a period of 3 months. Patient-specific objective and targeted measures of cognitive and functional ability should be detailed and examined at the end of that period. Improvement in or preservation of a deficit would count as a response and the pattern could be continued, extending the interval of follow-up to 6-monthly after 6 months. The decision on when to stop treatment may be more challenging. Most clinicians would agree that using an objective measure (i.e. an MMSE score as advocated by NICE) as the point at which to cease prescribing is clinically and ethically unjustifiable. If there is a suspicion that the effect of the medication may be wearing off, a short (3–6 week) "treatment holiday" may be attempted through a gradual withdrawal of medication and close observation of objective measures. The clinician must be cogniscent of the fact that patients become less likely to regain their previous level of functioning the longer the trial period continues (Burns et al., 2007; Doody et al., 2001). Generally such an approach results in re-institution of therapy in 30–40% of cases (Loveman et al., 2006) and thus is a decision best taken with wide consultation with carers and professionals.

Treatment resistance/non-response

In the event of treatment non-response an alternative ACHEI could be tried. No studies to date have studied a switch to donepezil, however, there is sufficient evidence to suggest a switch from donepezil to another oral formulation may show clinical benefit (Auriacombe et al., 2002; Bartorelli et al., 2005; Bullock & Connolly, 2002; Gauthier et al., 2003). A direct switch with no washout period has proven to be safe and well tolerated. There is developing evidence to support a similar strategy when switching from an ACHEI to the rivastigmine transdermal formulation (Sadowsky et al., 2010). In the moderate-severe to severe stage a switch to memantine may also be attempted safely, either directly or in a stepwise fashion (Waldemar et al., 2008). There is evidence to support further improvement if memantine is added to an ACHEI (Klinger et al., 2005; Tariot et al., 2004), however, these findings need to be replicated. One of the treatment arms of the DOMINO-AD trial (Jones et al., 2009) includes this strategy and thus may contribute some necessary clarification.

Management of behavioral and psychological symptoms of dementia (BPSD)

BPSD constitute a spectrum of non-cognitive symptoms found in Alzheimer's disease, and include agitation and aggression, psychotic symptoms, mood disorders, disrupted sleep patterns, and behavioral disturbances. Managing these symptoms can be a significant challenge, and is clearly important as they have significant prognostic implications. The presence of BPSD has been associated with accelerated morbidity and increased mortality (Holtzer *et al.*, 2003; Lopez *et al.*, 1999), earlier institutionalization (Yaffe *et al.*, 2002), increased carer stress (Clyburn *et al.*, 2000), and increased care costs (Herrmann *et al.*, 2006). More than 90% of patients will exhibit at least one BPSD at some point during their illness (Lyketsos *et al.*, 2000) with psychosis (40%) and agitation (80%) being highly prevalent during the course of the illness. There have been relatively fewer studies examining BPSD as a primary outcome. Results from earlier trials examining BPSD as a secondary outcome are difficult to draw conclusions from, mainly because measures of BPSD were low at baseline. More recently meta-analyses focusing on the role of cholinesterase inhibitors in more relevant trials have revealed on average a modest 2–4 point reduction in overall scores on the Neuropsychiatric Inventory(NPI) (Ames *et al.*, 2008; Beier, 2007; Birks, 2006; Campbell *et al.*, 2008; Cummings, 1997; Cummings *et al.*, 1994).

Increasing attention has focused on the specific pharmacological management of agitation, aggression, and psychosis in AD which cause the most distress to carers and cost to health services. Only risperidone has a licence for the short-term (up to 6 weeks) treatment of aggression in Alzheimer's disease (since 2008) although both typical and atypical antipsychotics have been subject to critical appraisal and have been found to have modest benefits (Kindermann *et al.*, 2002; Lanctot *et al.*, 1998; Schneider *et al.*, 2006). A recent Cochrane review (Ballard & Waite, 2006) suggested that risperidone and olanzapine can be effective in reducing aggression, and risperidone in treating psychosis. This was supported by the CATIE-AD trial (Schneider *et al.*, 2006) with superiority of both agents evident over both quetiapine and placebo, however, there were high discontinuation rates in both arms and effect sizes were modest. The use of antipsychotics has however been associated with a 65% increase in all-cause mortality (Schneider *et al.*, 2005) with risperidone in particular associated with a three-times increased mortality (Herrmann & Lanctot, 2005). The use of atypical antipsychotics in dementia carries a "black box" warning from the US Food and Drug Administration (FDA) (in 2005) and a similar caution from the UK Medicines and Healthcare products Regulatory Agency (MHRA) (in 2008). Typical antipsychotics do not provide a suitable alternative, due to an associated excess mortality of 40% over and above that of atypicals (Wang *et al.*, 2005). There is uncertainty regarding the precise mechanism through which this risk is generated although concerns have been raised regarding increased cardiac QTc intervals, and the impact of metabolic side-effects. Attempts to demonstrate an effect of ACHEIs (Gauthier *et al.*, 2002; Howard *et al.*, 2007), mood stabilizers, antidepressants, benzodiazepines, and beta-blockers (Herrmann, 2007) on reducing aggression and agitation in AD have been inconclusive. There is some suggestion that carbamazepine may be effective (Tariot *et al.*, 1998) but its use is unpopular, primarily due to the high potential for drug–drug interactions. There is early evidence suggesting memantine may provide an alternative strategy (Gauthier *et al.*, 2008; Grossberg *et al.*, 2009), however, further evidence is required. Thus a sensible management strategy would suggest an initial focus on optimizing environmental and psychosocial strategies. If these fail, then the use of either risperidone or olanzapine following wide consultation and a detailed risk–benefit analysis could be trialed with ongoing review every 6 weeks. Memantine may be an alternative if antipsychotics are contraindicated. The NPI is the most practical and valid tool for measuring the baseline and change in BPSD in individual cases. It can be used to identify target symptoms, guide management, and measure response. A clinically relevant change has been suggested as a 50% reduction in baseline score (Kaufer et al., 1998) in relevant domains.

The management of other BPSDs has less theoretical support. In depression associated with AD there is some evidence to support the use of SSRIs (Thompson et al., 2007), however, a recent study has suggested any benefit from SSRIs may be outweighed by side-effects (Rosenberg et al., 2010). Alternative emergent psychiatric symptoms would by necessity need to be approached according to existing guidelines for non-cognitively impaired individuals.

Future therapeutic options

The use of gene therapy is still some way distant and therefore current strategies are targeting symptomatic relief and disease modification as primary strategies for both the inherited and sporadic forms of the illness. Most approaches are either aiming to reduce amyloid burden, through reducing production or enhancing clearance of Aβ peptides, or to modify alternative pathogenetic mechanisms. Amongst the latter, mitochondrial dysfunction (Mancuso et al., 2010), oxidative stress (Lee et al., 2010), the influence of heavy metals (Bush & Tanzi, 2008), specific infectious agents (Holmes & Cotterell, 2009), hormonal deficiencies (Hogervorst & Bandelow, 2010) and periodontal disease (Kamer et al., 2008) have all been widely debated as contributory mechanisms, but consistent evidence of a defining role remains elusive at present. No supplements, vitamins, or herbal remedies have demonstrated any significant effect currently (Sano et al., 2008).

Significant attention is currently focused on the amyloid pathway. There are currently three γ-secretase inhibitors in development, all of which are at separate phases of pharmaceutical trials, and an agent which reduces the aggregation of Aβ oligomers, scyllo-inositol, is currently in Phase II development. Approaches harnessing the immune system to clear centrally deposited amyloid include the agent bapineuzumab (Phase III), which consists of monoclonal antibodies against Aβ peptides, as well as the passive immunization of preformed antibodies against Aβ peptides (also currently in Phase III).

Interest in the role of neuroinflammation in dementia was initially stimulated by early findings that the risk of developing AD was reduced by two-fold in those taking regular non-steroidal anti-inflammatory drugs (NSAIDS) (odds ratio (OR) = 0.5; $p = 0.0002$) (McGeer et al., 1996). The largest case–control study to date (49 349 cases and 196 850 matched controls) (Vlad et al., 2008) showed a significant effect of NSAIDS after 5 years of regular use, with a combined OR of 0.76 (0.68–0.85). Interestingly, NSAIDS have not been shown to alter the course of the illness or reduce the rate of cognitive decline (de Craen et al., 2005). However, individual components of the inflammatory pathway are currently being targeted and include etanercept, a tumor necrosis factor–alpha antagonist, which is currently in Phase II trials.

Latrepirdine (Dimebon), an antihistamine widely used in Russia, is in a Phase III trial in the USA after significant improvement in cognitive and functional measures were confirmed in a recent placebo-controlled trial (Doody et al., 2008). Although the precise mechanism causing improvement is unclear, it is felt this may be due to NMDA antagonistic properties and the enhancement of mitochondrial function.

Strategies aimed at reducing the formation of neurofibrillary tangles include the investigation of methylene blue, which recently passed a Phase II trial. Methylene blue is felt to act by reducing the aggregation of tau, and also by possibly enhancing mitochondrial function (Oz *et al.*, 2009). A Phase III trial is planned.

An exhaustive list of agents currently in development can be found on the website www.alzforum.org. It is likely that future approaches will look to combine a variety of agents in a focused strategy aimed at addressing individual vulnerabilities, in what is clearly a heterogeneous disease process.

Conclusion

Alzheimer's disease is increasingly being recognized as a huge worldwide challenge for health and social care organizations, particularly associated with demographic changes in population. The advent of the ACHEIs and memantine as symptomatic treatments for AD in the late 1990s has already had a significant effect on the practice of dementia care and assessment. This availability of treatments has contributed to a significantly raised profile for dementia with the general public and has contributed to dramatically shortened periods before patients with possible cognitive changes are referred for specialist assessment. This important raising of the profile of dementia awareness can never be captured in any financial modeling for the cost-effectiveness of these drugs. Whilst there has been widespread variation in the use of these drugs, most clinicians would see them as an important part of their therapeutic armory. Possible easing of the criteria for access to symptomatic treatments for dementia allied to the end of existing patents for these drugs offers the opportunity to ensure that even greater numbers of patients may derive benefit in the future. However, these factors arise at a time of unprecedented international financial pressures and clinicians will have to demonstrate optimum practice to justify their continuing prescription.

References

Abraham I, Harkany T, Horvath KM *et al* (2000). Chronic corticosterone administration dose-dependently modulates Abeta(1–42)- and NMDA-induced neurodegeneration in rat magnocellular nucleus basalis. *Journal of Neuroendocrinology* 12, 486–494.

Albert M, Cohen C (1992). The Test for Severe Impairment: an instrument for the assessment of patients with severe cognitive dysfunction. *Journal of the American Geriatric Society* 40, 449–453.

Ames D, Kaduszkiewicz H, van den Bussche H *et al.* (2008). For debate: is the evidence for the efficacy of cholinesterase inhibitors in the symptomatic treatment of Alzheimer's disease convincing or not? *International Psychogeriatrics* 20, 259–292.

Anstey KJ, von Sanden C, Salim A, O'Kearney R (2007). Smoking as a risk factor for dementia and cognitive decline: a meta-analysis of prospective studies. *American Journal of Epidemiology* 166, 367–378.

Auriacombe S, Pere JJ, Loria-Kanza Y, Vellas B (2002). Efficacy and safety of rivastigmine in patients with Alzheimer's disease who failed to benefit from treatment with donepezil. *Current Medical Research and Opinion* 18, 129–138.

Ballard C, Waite J (2006). The effectiveness of atypical antipsychotics for the treatment of aggression and psychosis in Alzheimer's disease. *Cochrane Database of Systematic Reviews* 1, CD003476.

Bartorelli L, Giraldi C, Saccardo M *et al.* (2005). Effects of switching from an AChE inhibitor to a dual AChE-BuChE inhibitor in patients with Alzheimer's disease. *Current Medical Research and Opinion* 21, 1809–1818.

Beier MT (2007). Treatment strategies for the behavioral symptoms of Alzheimer's disease:

focus on early pharmacologic intervention. *Pharmacotherapy* 27, 399–411.

Beydoun MA, Beydoun HA, Wang Y (2008). Obesity and central obesity as risk factors for incident dementia and its subtypes: a systematic review and meta-analysis. *Obesity Review* 9, 204–218.

Birks J (2006). Cholinesterase inhibitors for Alzheimer's disease. *Cochrane Database of Systematic Reviews* 1, CD005593.

Black SE, Doody R, Li H et al. (2007). Donepezil preserves cognition and global function in patients with severe Alzheimer disease. *Neurology* 69, 459–469.

Bullock R, Connolly C (2002). Switching cholinesterase inhibitor therapy in Alzheimer's disease – donepezil to rivastigmine, is it worth it? *International Journal of Geriatric Psychiatry* 17, 288–289.

Bullock R, Dengiz A (2005). Cognitive performance in patients with Alzheimer's disease receiving cholinesterase inhibitors for up to 5 years. *International Journal of Clinical Practice* 59, 817–822.

Bullock R, Touchon J, Bergman H et al. (2005). Rivastigmine and donepezil treatment in moderate to moderately-severe Alzheimer's disease over a 2-year period. *Current Medical Research and Opinion* 21, 1317–1327.

Burns A, Bernabei R, Bullock R et al. (2009). Safety and efficacy of galantamine (Reminyl) in severe Alzheimer's disease (the SERAD study): a randomised, placebo-controlled, double-blind trial. *Lancet Neurology* 8(1), 39–47.

Burns A, Byrne J, Ballard C, Holmes C (2002). Sensory stimulation in dementia. *British Medical Journal* 325(7376), 1312–1313.

Burns A, Gauthier S, Perdomo C (2007). Efficacy and safety of donepezil over 3 years: an open-label, multicentre study in patients with Alzheimer's disease. *International Journal of Geriatric Psychiatry* 22, 806–812.

Burns A, O'Brien J, Auriacombe S et al. (2006). Clinical practice with anti-dementia drugs: a consensus statement from the British Association for Psychopharmacology. *Journal of Psychopharmacology* 20, 732–755.

Bush AI, Tanzi RE (2008). Therapeutics for Alzheimer's disease based on the metal hypothesis. *Neurotherapeutics* 5, 421–432.

Campbell N, Ayub A, Boustani MA et al. (2008). Impact of cholinesterase inhibitors on behavioral and psychological symptoms of Alzheimer's disease: a meta-analysis. *Journal of Clinical Interventions in Aging* 3(4), 719–728.

Campion D, Dumanchin C, Hannequin D et al. (1999). Early-onset autosomal dominant Alzheimer disease: prevalence, genetic heterogeneity, and mutation spectrum. *American Journal of Human Genetics* 65(3), 664–670.

Clare L, Woods RT, Moniz Cook ED et al. (2003). Cognitive rehabilitation and cognitive training for early-stage Alzheimer's disease and vascular dementia. *Cochrane Database of Systematic Reviews* 4, CD003260.

Clyburn LD, Stones MJ, Hadjistavropoulos T, Tuokko H (2000). Predicting caregiver burden and depression in Alzheimer's disease. *Journals of Gerontology Series B: Psychological Sciences and Social Sciences*, 55(1), S2–S13.

Corder EH, Saunders AM, Strittmatter WJ et al. (1993). Gene dose of apolipoprotein E type 4 allele and the risk of Alzheimer's disease in late onset families. *Science* 261(5123), 921–923.

Courtney C, Farrell D, Gray R et al. (2004). Long-term donepezil treatment in 565 patients with Alzheimer's disease (AD2000): randomised double-blind trial. *Lancet* 363(9427), 2105–2115.

Cummings JL (1997). The Neuropsychiatric Inventory: assessing psychopathology in dementia patients. *Neurology* 48(5 Suppl. 6), S10–S16.

Cummings JL, Mega M, Gray K et al. (1994). The Neuropsychiatric Inventory: comprehensive assessment of psychopathology in dementia. *Neurology* 44, 2308–2314.

de Craen AJ, Gussekloo J, Vrijsen B, Westendorp RG (2005). Meta-analysis of nonsteroidal antiinflammatory drug use and risk of dementia. *American Journal of Epidemiology* 161, 114–120.

Dementia UK (2007). Details available at: http://alzheimers.org.uk/site/scripts/documents_info.php?documentID=342

Doody RS, Gavrilova SI, Sano M et al. (2008). Effect of dimebon on cognition, activities of daily living, behaviour, and global function in patients with mild-to-moderate Alzheimer's disease: a randomised, double-blind, placebo-controlled study. *Lancet* 372(9634), 207–215.

Doody RS, Massman P, Dunn JK (2001). A method for estimating progression rates in Alzheimer disease. *Archives of Neurology* 58, 449–454.

Farlow MR (2009). Treatment of mild cognitive impairment (MCI). *Current Alzheimer Research* 6, 362–367.

Feldman H, Gauthier S, Hecker J et al. (2005). Efficacy and safety of donepezil in patients with more severe Alzheimer's disease: a subgroup analysis from a randomized, placebo-controlled trial. *International Journal of Geriatric Psychiatry* 20, 559–569.

Feldman HH, Pirttila T, Dartigues JF et al. (2009). Treatment with galantamine and time to nursing home placement in Alzheimer's disease patients with and without cerebrovascular disease. *International Journal of Geriatric Psychiatry* 24, 479–488.

Folstein MF, Folstein SE, McHugh PR (1975). "Mini-mental state". A practical method for grading the cognitive state of patients for the clinician. *Journal of Psychiatric Research* 12(3), 189–198.

Gauthier S, Emre M, Farlow MR, Bullock R et al. (2003). Strategies for continued successful treatment of Alzheimer's disease: switching cholinesterase inhibitors. *Current Medical Research and Opinion* 19(8): 707–714.

Gauthier S, Feldman H, Hecker J et al. (2002). Efficacy of donepezil on behavioral symptoms in patients with moderate to severe Alzheimer's disease. *International Psychogeriatrics* 14, 389–404.

Gauthier S, Loft H, Cummings J (2008). Improvement in behavioural symptoms in patients with moderate to severe Alzheimer's disease by memantine: a pooled data analysis. *International Journal of Geriatric Psychiatry* 23, 537–545.

Gill SS, Bronskill SE, Mamdani M et al. (2004). Representation of patients with dementia in clinical trials of donepezil. *Canadian Journal of Clinical Pharmacology* 11(2), e274–e285.

Gong CX, Grundke-Iqbal I, Iqbal K (2010). Targeting tau protein in Alzheimer's disease. *Drugs and Aging* 27(5), 351–365.

Grossberg GT, Pejovic V, Miller ML, Graham SM (2009). Memantine therapy of behavioral symptoms in community-dwelling patients with moderate to severe Alzheimer's disease.

Dementia and Geriatric Cognitive Disorders 27, 164–172.

Grundman M, Sencakova D, Jack CR Jr et al. (2002). Brain MRI hippocampal volume and prediction of clinical status in a mild cognitive impairment trial. *Journal of Molecular Neuroscience* 19(1–2), 23–27.

Harkany T, Abraham I, Timmerman W et al. (2000). Beta-amyloid neurotoxicity is mediated by a glutamate-triggered excitotoxic cascade in rat nucleus basalis. *European Journal of Neuroscience* 12(8), 2735–2745.

Hebert LE, Scherr PA, Bienias JL et al. (2003). Alzheimer disease in the US population: prevalence estimates using the 2000 census. *Archives of Neurology* 60, 1119–1122.

Helmer C, Peres K, Letenneur L et al. (2006). Dementia in subjects aged 75 years or over within the PAQUID cohort: prevalence and burden by severity. *Dementia and Geriatric Cognitive Disorders* 22, 87–94.

Herrmann N (2007). Treatment of moderate to severe Alzheimer's disease: rationale and trial design. *Canadian Journal of Neurological Science* 34 (Suppl. 1), S103–S108.

Herrmann N, Lanctot KL (2005). Do atypical antipsychotics cause stroke? *CNS Drugs* 19, 91–103.

Herrmann N, Lanctot KL, Sambrook R et al. (2006). The contribution of neuropsychiatric symptoms to the cost of dementia care. *International Journal of Geriatric Psychiatry* 21, 972–976.

Hogervorst E, Bandelow S (2010). Sex steroids to maintain cognitive function in women after the menopause: a meta-analyses of treatment trials. *Maturitas* 66(1), 56–71.

Holmes C, Cotterell D (2009). Role of infection in the pathogenesis of Alzheimer's disease: implications for treatment. *CNS Drugs* 23, 993–1002.

Holtzer R, Tang MX, Devanand DP et al. (2003). Psychopathological features in Alzheimer's disease: course and relationship with cognitive status. *Journal of the American Geriatric Society* 51, 953–960.

Howard RJ, Juszczak E, Ballard CG et al. (2007). Donepezil for the treatment of agitation in Alzheimer's disease. *New England Journal of Medicine* 357(14), 1382–1392.

Jelic V, Kivipelto M, Winblad B (2006). Clinical trials in mild cognitive impairment: lessons for the future. *Journal of Neurology, Neurosurgery and Psychiatry* **77**, 429–438.

Jones R, Sheehan B, Phillips P *et al.* (2009). DOMINO-AD protocol: donepezil and memantine in moderate to severe Alzheimer's disease – a multicentre RCT. *Trials* **10**, 57.

Jones RW, Soininen H, Hager K *et al.* (2004). A multinational, randomised, 12-week study comparing the effects of donepezil and galantamine in patients with mild to moderate Alzheimer's disease. *International Journal of Geriatric Psychiatry* **19**, 58–67.

Josif S, Graham K (2008). Diagnosis and treatment of dementia with Lewy bodies. *Journal of the American Academy of Physician Assistants* **21**(5), 22–26.

Kamer AR, Craig RG, Dasanayake AP *et al.* (2008). Inflammation and Alzheimer's disease: possible role of periodontal diseases. *Alzheimer's and Dementia* **4**(4), 242–250.

Kaufer DI, Cummings JL, Christine D *et al.* (1998). Assessing the impact of neuropsychiatric symptoms in Alzheimer's disease: the Neuropsychiatric Inventory Caregiver Distress Scale. *Journal of the American Geriatric Society* **46**(2), 210–215.

Kindermann SS, Dolder CR, Bailey A *et al.* (2002). Pharmacological treatment of psychosis and agitation in elderly patients with dementia: four decades of experience. *Drugs and Aging* **19**, 257–276.

Klinger T, Ibach B, Schoenknecht P *et al.* (2005). Effect of donepezil in patients with Alzheimer's disease previously untreated or treated with memantine or nootropic agents in Germany: an observational study. *Current Medical Research and Opinion* **21**, 723–732.

Lam B, Hollingdrake E, Kennedy JL *et al.* (2009). Cholinesterase inhibitors in Alzheimer's disease and Lewy body spectrum disorders: the emerging pharmacogenetic story. *Human Genomics* **4**(2), 91–106.

Lanctot KL, Best TS, Mittmann N *et al.* (1998). Efficacy and safety of neuroleptics in behavioral disorders associated with dementia. *Journal of Clinical Psychiatry* **59**, 550–561; quiz 562–553.

Lanctot KL, Herrmann N, Yau KK *et al.* (2003). Efficacy and safety of cholinesterase inhibitors in Alzheimer's disease: a meta-analysis. *Canadian Medical Association Journal* **169**, 557–564.

Lee HP, Zhu X, Casadesus G *et al.* (2010). Antioxidant approaches for the treatment of Alzheimer's disease. *Expert Reviews in Neurotherapeutics* **10**(7), 1201–1208.

Lockhart IA, Mitchell SA, Kelly S (2009). Safety and tolerability of donepezil, rivastigmine and galantamine for patients with Alzheimer's disease: systematic review of the 'real-world' evidence. *Dementia and Geriatric Cognitive Disorders* **28**(5), 389–403.

Logsdon RG, McCurry SM, Teri L (2007). Evidence-based interventions to improve quality of life for individuals with dementia. *Alzheimer's Care Today*, **8**(4), 309–318.

Lopez OL, Wisniewski SR, Becker JT *et al.* (1999). Psychiatric medication and abnormal behavior as predictors of progression in probable Alzheimer disease. *Archives of Neurology* **56**, 1266–1272.

Loveman E, Green C, Kirby J *et al.* (2006). The clinical and cost-effectiveness of donepezil, rivastigmine, galantamine and memantine for Alzheimer's disease. *Health Technology Assessment* **10**(1), iii–iv, ix–xi, 1–160.

Lyketsos CG, Reichman WE, Kershaw P, Zhu Y (2004). Long-term outcomes of galantamine treatment in patients with Alzheimer disease. *American Journal of Geriatric Psychiatry* **12**, 473–482.

Lyketsos CG, Steinberg M, Tschanz JT *et al.* (2000). Mental and behavioral disturbances in dementia: findings from the Cache County Study on Memory in Aging. *American Journal of Psychiatry* **157**, 708–714.

Mancuso M, Orsucci D, LoGerfo A *et al.* (2010). Clinical features and pathogenesis of Alzheimer's disease: involvement of mitochondria and mitochondrial DNA. *Advances in Experimental and MedicalBiology* **685**, 34–44.

Mariani E, Monastero R, Mecocci P (2007). Mild cognitive impairment: a systematic review. *Journal of Alzheimer's Disease* **12**, 23–35.

Mathuranath PS, Nestor PJ, Berrios GE *et al.* (2000). A brief cognitive test battery to differentiate Alzheimer's disease and frontotemporal dementia. *Neurology* **55**, 1613–1620.

McGeer PL, Schulzer M, McGeer EG (1996). Arthritis and anti-inflammatory agents as possible protective factors for Alzheimer's disease: a review of 17 epidemiologic studies. *Neurology* **47**, 425–432.

McLendon BM, Doraiswamy PM (1999).
Defining meaningful change in Alzheimer's
disease trials: the donepezil experience.
Journal of Geriatric Psychiatry and Neurology
12, 39–48.

McShane R, Areosa Sastre A, Minakaran N
(2006). Memantine for dementia. *Cochrane
Database of Systematic Reviews* **2**, CD003154.

Middleton LE, Yaffe K (2009). Promising
strategies for the prevention of dementia.
Archives of Neurology **66**, 1210–1215.

Mitchell AJ, Shiri-Feshki M (2008). Temporal
trends in the long term risk of progression of
mild cognitive impairment: a pooled
analysis. *Journal of Neurology, Neurosurgery
and Psychiatry* **79**, 1386–1391.

Molnar FJ, Man-Son-Hing M, Hutton B,
Fergusson DA (2009). Have last-observation-
carried-forward analyses caused us to favour
more toxic dementia therapies over less toxic
alternatives? A systematic review. *Open
Medicine* **3**(2), e31–e50.

Nasreddine ZS, Phillips NA, Bedirian V *et al.*
(2005). The Montreal Cognitive Assessment,
MoCA: a brief screening tool for mild
cognitive impairment. *Journal of the
American Geriatric Society* **53**, 695–699.

Oz M, Lorke DE, Petroianu GA. (2009).
Methylene blue and Alzheimer's disease.
Biochemical Pharmacology **78**, 927–932.

Peskind ER, Potkin SG, Pomara N *et al.* (2006).
Memantine treatment in mild to moderate
Alzheimer disease: a 24-week randomized,
controlled trial. *American Journal of
Geriatric Psychiatry* **14**, 704–715.

Petersen RC (2004). Mild cognitive impairment
as a diagnostic entity. *Journal of Internal
Medicine* **256**(3), 183–194.

Petersen RC (2005). Mild cognitive impairment:
where are we? *Alzheimer's Disease and
Associated Disorders* **19**(3), 166–169.

Rabins PV, Blacker D, Rovner BW *et al.* (2007).
American Psychiatric Association practice
guideline for the treatment of patients with
Alzheimer's disease and other dementias.
Second edition. *American Journal of
Psychiatry* **164**(12 Suppl.), 5–56.

Raina P, Santaguida P, Ismaila A *et al.* (2008).
Effectiveness of cholinesterase inhibitors and
memantine for treating dementia: evidence
review for a clinical practice guideline.
Annals of Internal Medicine **148**(5),
379–397.

Ritchie CW, Ames D, Clayton T, Lai R (2004).
Metaanalysis of randomized trials of the
efficacy and safety of donepezil, galantamine,
and rivastigmine for the treatment of
Alzheimer disease. *American Journal of
Geriatric Psychiatry* **12**(4), 358–369.

Rockwood K, Black SE, Robillard A, Lussier I
(2004). Potential treatment effects of
donepezil not detected in Alzheimer's
disease clinical trials: a physician survey.
International Journal of Geriatric Psychiatry
19(10), 954–960.

Rockwood K, Dai D, Mitnitski A (2008).
Patterns of decline and evidence of
subgroups in patients with Alzheimer's
disease taking galantamine for up to 48
months. *International Journal of Geriatric
Psychiatry* **23**(2), 207–214.

Rosenberg PB, Drye LT, Martin BK *et al.* (2010).
Sertraline for the treatment of depression in
Alzheimer disease. *American Journal of
Geriatric Psychiatry* **18**, 136–145.

Rovelet-Lecrux A, Hannequin D, Raux G *et al.*
(2006). APP locus duplication causes
autosomal dominant early-onset Alzheimer
disease with cerebral amyloid angiopathy.
Nature Genetics **38**(1), 24–26.

Sadowsky C, Perez JA, Bouchard RW *et al.*
(2010). Switching from oral cholinesterase
inhibitors to the rivastigmine transdermal
patch. *CNS Neuroscience and Therapeutics*
16(1), 51–60.

Sano M, Grossman H, Van Dyk K (2008).
Preventing Alzheimer's disease: separating
fact from fiction. *CNS Drugs* **22**(11),
887–902.

Schneider LS, Dagerman KS, Insel P (2005).
Risk of death with atypical antipsychotic
drug treatment for dementia: meta-analysis
of randomized placebo-controlled trials.
Journal of the American Medical Association
294(15), 1934–1943.

Schneider LS, Olin JT, Lyness SA, Chui HC
(1997). Eligibility of Alzheimer's disease
clinic patients for clinical trials. *Journal of the
American Geriatrics Society* **45**(8): 923–928.

Schneider LS, Tariot PN, Dagerman KS *et al.*
(2006). Effectiveness of atypical antipsychotic
drugs in patients with Alzheimer's disease.
New England Journal of Medicine **355**(15),
1525–1538.

Skoog I, Lernfelt B, Landahl S *et al.* (1996).
15-year longitudinal study of blood pressure

and dementia. *Lancet* **347**(9009), 1141–1145.

Tariot PN, Erb R, Podgorski CA *et al.* (1998). Efficacy and tolerability of carbamazepine for agitation and aggression in dementia. *American Journal of Psychiatry* **155**, 54–61.

Tariot PN, Farlow MR, Grossberg GT *et al.* (2004). Memantine treatment in patients with moderate to severe Alzheimer disease already receiving donepezil: a randomized controlled trial. *Journal of the American Medical Association* **291**, 317–324.

Thompson S, Herrmann N, Rapoport MJ, Lanctot KL (2007). Efficacy and safety of antidepressants for treatment of depression in Alzheimer's disease: a metaanalysis. *Canadian Journal of Psychiatry* **52**(4), 248–255.

Vlad SC, Miller DR, Kowall NW, Felson DT (2008). Protective effects of NSAIDs on the development of Alzheimer disease. *Neurology* **70**(19), 1672–1677.

Waldemar G, Hyvarinen M, Josiassen MK *et al.* (2008). Tolerability of switching from donepezil to memantine treatment in patients with moderate to severe Alzheimer's disease. *International Journal of Geriatric Psychiatry* **23**, 979–981.

Wang PS, Schneeweiss S, Avorn J *et al.* (2005). Risk of death in elderly users of conventional vs. atypical antipsychotic medications. *New England Journal of Medicine* **353**(22), 2335–2341.

Weinstein AM, Barton C, Ross L *et al.* (2009). Treatment practices of mild cognitive impairment in California Alzheimer's Disease Centers. *Journal of the American Geriatrics Society* **57**, 686–690.

Wilcock G, Howe I, Coles H *et al.* (2003). A long-term comparison of galantamine and donepezil in the treatment of Alzheimer's disease. *Drugs and Aging* **20**(10), 777–789.

Wilkinson DG, Passmore AP, Bullock R *et al.* (2002). A multinational, randomised, 12-week, comparative study of donepezil and rivastigmine in patients with mild to moderate Alzheimer's disease. *International Journal of Clinical Practice* **56**(6), 441–446.

Winblad B, Black SE, Homma A *et al.* (2009). Donepezil treatment in severe Alzheimer's disease: a pooled analysis of three clinical trials. *Current Medical Research and Opinion* **25**(11), 2577–2587.

Winblad B, Jelic V (2004). Long-term treatment of Alzheimer disease: efficacy and safety of acetylcholinesterase inhibitors. *Alzheimer's Disease and Associated Disorders* **18** (Suppl. 1), S2–S8.

Winblad B, Palmer K, Kivipelto M *et al.* (2004). Mild cognitive impairment – beyond controversies, towards a consensus: report of the International Working Group on Mild Cognitive Impairment. *Journal of Internal Medicine* **256**, 240–246.

Yaffe K, Fox P, Newcomer R *et al.* (2002). Patient and caregiver characteristics and nursing home placement in patients with dementia. *Journal of the American Medical Association* **287**(16), 2090–2097.

Evidence-based pharmacotherapy of personality disorders

Luis H. Ripoll, Joseph Triebwasser, and Larry J. Siever

Introduction

Personality disorders are defined by an "enduring pattern of inner experience and behavior that…is inflexible and pervasive across a broad range of personal and social situations," with symptomatic disturbances in cognition, affect, impulsivity, and interpersonal functioning leading to distress (APA, 1994). Until recently, guidelines recommended sparing use of pharmacotherapy, and expectations remained guarded regarding expected benefits from medications. Since then, distinctions between Axis I disorders, considered "genetic…biological…brain disorders" treated with medications; and Axis II disorders, alternatively considered "psychological" and therefore treated with psychotherapy, have undergone a paradigm shift (Siever & Davis, 1991). In this atmosphere, clinicians must rely on the most up-to-date, evidence-based practices for pharmacotherapy to be effective.

Component dimensions of personality, such as impulsivity or aggressiveness, have demonstrable neurobiological correlates, as shown via a variety of endocrine, electrophysiological, and neuroimaging measures (Brambilla et al., 2004; Goodman et al., 2004; Houston et al., 2004; Juengling et al., 2003; Levitt et al., 2004; Minzenberg et al., 2006; New et al., 1997, 2004; Ogiso et al., 1993; Oquendo et al., 2005; Prossin et al., 2010; Rusch et al., 2003; Russ et al., 1991; Simeon et al., 1992; Soderstrom & Foresman, 2004). Identifying neurobiological substrates of personality has allowed for increasingly specific pharmacotherapy. Nevertheless, improvement from effective pharmacotherapeutic interventions is often transient and/or restricted to several symptom domains. In the USA, there are no FDA-approved medications for treating personality disorders. Thus, pharmacotherapy for personality disorders remains off-label, and psychopharmacological strategies for evidence-based practices remain lacking.

The majority of psychopharmacological research on personality disorders has focused on borderline personality disorder (BPD). In the most recent treatment guidelines for BPD, the American Psychiatric Association (APA, 2001), acknowledges that "pharmacotherapy has an important adjunctive role," along with "extended psychotherapy to attain and maintain lasting improvement in…personality, interpersonal problems, and overall functioning." Similarly, others have described psychopharmacological treatment of BPD as resulting only in "a mild degree of symptom relief" (Paris, 2005). Moreover, there remains a dearth of evidence-based medication treatments for other personality disorders.

Often, pharmacotherapy for severe personality disorders is used to stabilize patients' symptoms sufficiently in order to facilitate psychosocial interventions and foster reflective

Essential Evidence-Based Psychopharmacology, Second Edition, ed. Dan J. Stein, Bernard Lerer, and Stephen M. Stahl. Published by Cambridge University Press. © Cambridge University Press.

functioning. Close communication between psychotherapists and psychopharmacologists remains crucial. Although functional gains can be expected from medications, the magnitude and time-course vary. There is little evidence regarding distinctions between acute and maintenance pharmacotherapy, or how long to continue patients on a medication. Empirical data on recurrence or relapse are similarly scarce. Therefore, evidence-based practices must be judged case-by-case, weighing clinical risks and benefits.

Clinicians can refer to the accompanying tables for the best available evidence regarding pharmacotherapy for personality disorders (see Tables 14.1–14.4). These data were compiled by searching the MEDLINE database with the main combinations pharmacotherapy and each of the various DSM–IV personality disorder diagnoses. In addition, we paid particularly close attention to randomized, placebo-controlled trials (along with some lower-level evidence if this type of evidence was severely limited). We focused on studies published in the past 3 years, since the publication of the last World Federation of Societies of Biological Psychiatry guidelines for the biological treatment of personality disorders (Herpertz et al., 2007). Additional research regarding medications for treating impulsive aggression was found via a similar MEDLINE search on impulsivity, aggression, and pharmacotherapy.

Unfortunately, only a few novel trials of pharmacotherapy for personality disorders have been published during this recent period. Several recent meta-analyses have been published in this time, which we utilized to establish areas of consensus for evidence-based practice, and identify gaps that need to be addressed with future research. Many prior reviews cover only BPD, but we expanded our scope to include all personality disorders. Thus, we include a comprehensive summary of the best, current evidence, with commentary on recent consensus and recommendations for evidence-based practices, and future directions regarding pharmacotherapeutic strategies that have been insufficiently tested, but appear promising for further research. This situates this review as a nexus, compiling evidence-based practices for treating personality disorders for interested clinicians, as well as providing avenues for future psychopharmacological research.

Schizotypal personality disorder (SPD)

Schizotypal personality disorder (SPD) is characterized by interpersonal deficits and psychotic-like symptoms. Like schizophrenia patients, SPD patients often demonstrate cognitive deficits in working memory, particularly sustained attention and executive functioning (Bergida & Lenzenweger, 2006; McClure et al., 2007a; Pare & McTigue, 1997), as well as significant abnormalities in empathic understanding (Langdon & Coltheart, 2004; Pickup, 2006; Ripoll et al., unpublished data). Unlike schizophrenic patients, there is greater preservation of frontal volume in SPD (Siever & Davis, 2004).

Overall, clinical trials for SPD have been complicated by comorbidity, particularly with other personality disorders. Most early RCTs on BPD also included SPD patients (Goldberg et al., 1986; Serban & Siegel, 1984; Soloff et al., 1986c), because both SPD and BPD were considered rooted in "borderline" schizophrenia; but psychotic symptoms in SPD and BPD are clinically distinguishable.

The conceptualization of SPD within the schizophrenia spectrum supports treatment with antipsychotic medications. Antipsychotics appear to be useful in the treatment of SPD, particularly in terms of psychotic-like symptoms (Goldberg et al., 1986; Koenigsberg et al., 2003). Open-label studies have suggested a role for antidepressants in treating self-injury, psychotic-like, and depressive symptomatology (Jensen & Andersen, 1989;

Table 14.1. Schizotypal personality disorder (SPD).

Study	Diagnosis	N	Medication(s)	Dosage(s)	Design, duration	Results in active drug group(s)
Koenigsberg et al. (2003)	SPD	25 males and females	Risperidone	Started at 0.25 mg/day, titrated up to 2 mg/day	Parallel design, 9 weeks	Significantly lower scores on PANSS negative and general symptom scales by week 3 and positive symptoms by week 7
McClure et al. (2007b)	SPD	29 males and females	Guanfacine	Titrated up to 2 mg/day within first 2 weeks	Parallel design, 4 weeks	After 4 weeks, greater improvements from baseline in neuropsychological measures of working memory (Modified AX-Continuous Performance Task) compared with placebo
McClure et al. (2010)	SPD	25 males and females	Pergolide	0.025 mg/day for first 3 days, then 0.05 mg/day for 4 days, then 0.1 mg/day for 1 week, then 0.2 mg/day for 1 week, then 0.3 mg/day	Parallel design, 4 weeks	Greater improvement from baseline in tasks measuring executive function (Trail-Making Test Part B), verbal memory (Word List Learning-immediate and delayed recall), verbal working memory (Letter Number Span), long-term visuospatial memory (Wechsler Memory Scale Visual Reproduction Test), and visuospatial working memory (Dot Test), compared to placebo. Dot findings were largely driven by worsening in placebo group

PANSS, Positive and Negative Symptom Scale.

Markovitz *et al.*, 1991), but the evidence is weaker. Recent RCTs targeting cognitive deficits in SPD compared performance on neuropsychological tasks before and after treatment with medication or placebo. Both pergolide, a dopaminergic agonist active at both the D1 and D2 receptor (McClure *et al.*, 2010), and the noradrenergic a_{2A} agonist guanfacine (McClure *et al.*, 2007*b*) improved SPD patients' cognitive performance, on distinct neuropsychological measures. Whether this improvement extends to overall clinical functioning in SPD remains subject to future investigation.

In sum, SPD patients respond to low-dose, atypical antipsychotics, targeting psychotic-like symptoms and general functioning. First-generation antipsychotic medication and antidepressants may also play a role, although the evidence is not as reliable. Evidence-based practice requires weighing risk of extrapyramidal side-effects or tardive dyskinesia against potential benefits. Cognitive enhancement via noradrenergic a_{2A} or dopaminergic agonism may be future avenues of research, given that, by analogy with schizophrenia, the cognitive impairment in SPD may be responsible for the overall dysfunction observed in the disorder. Research efforts to understand neurobiological substrates of social cognitive dysfunction have heretofore mainly focused on BPD and schizophrenia. Because SPD involves social isolation, relational paranoia, and empathic deficits, research on pharmacotherapeutic effects on social cognition may also be fruitful.

Antisocial personality disorder (AsPD)

Peer-reviewed trials of antisocial personality disorder (AsPD) include studies on groups of individuals likely to have been antisocial based on histories of repeated violence and criminality and an absence of other stated causes for these behaviors. Lithium has been associated with decreases in serious rule infractions in incarcerated males (Sheard, 1971; Sheard *et al.*, 1976). Prisoners treated with phenytoin committed fewer aggressive acts and evidenced decreased tension-anxiety and depression-dejection (although not anger-hostility), and improvements in aggression appeared to be limited to impulsive (not pre-meditated) aggression (Barratt *et al.*, 1991, 1997). At present, evidence-based pharmacotherapy for AsPD is restricted to treatment of impulsive aggression. Future neurobiological research in AsPD and psychopathy will probably increase our understanding of the dysfunctional emotional empathy often seen in this disorder (Blair, 2005) and whether this may be susceptible to psychopharmacological intervention.

Borderline personality disorder

Most RCTs on personality disorders focused on BPD, which consists of several domains of dysfunction: affective instability, impulsivity and anger, transient psychotic or dissociative symptoms, and intense, unstable relationships (Lieb *et al.*, 2004; Zanarini *et al.*, 1990). BPD patients often demonstrate high comorbidity (Zanarini *et al.*, 2004*a, c*) and make numerous suicide attempts and parasuicidal gestures, conferring significantly higher risk for completed suicide (Welch & Linehan, 2002).

Early studies employed a distinct nosology in characterizing subjects, some of whom actually had what might be called BPD today (Rifkin *et al.*, 1972). In studies on suicidal or parasuicidal subjects, the majority often have BPD (Battaglia *et al.*, 1999; Montgomery & Montgomery, 1982; Montgomery *et al.*, 1983; Verkes *et al.*, 1998). Early studies often included combinations of BPD and SPD subjects (Goldberg *et al.*, 1986; Serban & Siegel, 1984; Soloff

Table 14.2. Antisocial personality disorder.

Study	Diagnosis	N	Medication(s)	Dosage(s)	Design, duration	Results in active drug group(s)
Sheard (1971)	Inmates of maximum security prison with verbal and physical aggression while in prison	12 males	Lithium carbonate	Lithium levels of 0.6–1.5 meq/1, mean dose 1200 mg/day	Cross-over/single-blind, three 4-week phases	Decrease in serious incidents of verbal or physical aggression. Improvements in self-rated anger and tension. Single-blind. Aggressive incidents scored on basis of prison guards' issuing of punitive tickets, not by psychiatrists' ratings
Sheard et al. (1976)	Prisoners convicted of "serious aggressive crimes"	80 males	Lithium carbonate	Lithium levels of 0.6–1.0 meq/1, mean lithium level during last week of medication phase 0.89 meq/1	Parallel design, 5 months with first and last months medication-free and 3 months lithium vs. placebo	Decrease in violent infractions of prison rules in lithium group
Lion (1979)	"All patients had past histories of temper outbursts, belligerence, assaultive behavior and impulsiveness, had experienced legal difficulties and some had committed criminal acts"	65 males and females	Chlordiazepoxide, oxazepam	Chlordiazepoxide: 100 mg/day for 2 weeks, then 200 mg/day for 2 weeks. Oxazepam: 120 mg/day for 2 weeks, then 240 mg/day for 2 weeks	Parallel design, 4 weeks	Oxazepam superior to chlordiazepoxide and placebo for indirect hostility (Buss–Durkee Hostility Scale), anxiety
Barratt et al. (1991)	Maximum security prison inmates with impulsive aggression while in prison	19 males	Phenytoin	100 mg/day or 300 mg/day	Cross-over design, three 4-week phases	Significant reduction in aggressive acts at 300 mg/day but not 100 mg/day. Improvements in tension-anxiety and depression-dejection at 300 mg/day, but not anger-hostility
Barratt et al. (1997)	Prison inmates with aggression while in prison	150 total, but only 30 males with primarily impulsive aggression and 30 males with primarily pre-meditated aggression included in analysis (other 66 had mixture of both types)	Phenytoin	300 mg/day	Cross-over design, two 6-week phases	Significant reduction in frequency and intensity of aggressive acts in impulsive aggressive group but not pre-meditated aggressive group

et al., 1986*c*), and studies recruiting a range of all personality disorders ultimately include BPD as the most frequent diagnosis (Coccaro & Kavoussi, 1997; Hollander *et al.*, 2003).

Clinicians should exercise caution in attempting to apply research findings to severely ill BPD patients, as many RCTs recruited only outpatients, who further were excluded if they expressed acute suicidality (Frankenburg & Zanarini, 2002; Tritt *et al.*, 2005; Zanarini & Frankenburg, 2003; Zanarini *et al.*, 2004*b*) or had made a recent suicide attempt (Bogenschutz & Nurnberg, 2004). In addition, small sample sizes predominated, and most studies lasted ≤ 3 months. The few trials lasting ≥ 6 months suffered from high dropout rates (Frankenburg & Zanarini, 2002; Zanarini & Frankenburg, 2001) or concomitant recruitment of subjects without BPD (Battaglia *et al.*, 1999; Montgomery *et al.*, 1983; Verkes *et al.*, 1998). Moreover, RCTs with BPD subjects appear to be prone to high placebo response rates (Lieb *et al.*, 2004; Salzman *et al.*, 1995), meaning that open-label trial data should be interpreted with caution.

APA practice guidelines (APA, 2001) recommended a symptom-targeted approach in pharmacotherapy of BPD. This leaves open the possibility for patients to improve in some but not all symptom dimensions. Some clinicians have based their decision to implement polypharmacy on this, but there is actually little evidence as to the effectiveness of this strategy. The only study on combined pharmacotherapy in BPD (Zanarini *et al.*, 2004*b*) found no superior efficacy for combination treatment compared with one medication alone. Using as few medications as possible to target central areas of clinical dysfunction, together with evidence-based psychotherapy, is usually the optimal treatment strategy. In light of this, although the 2001 guidelines suggest a prominent role for serotonergic pharmacotherapy, recent reviews have questioned this and instead emphasized anticonvulsants and antipsychotics (Abraham & Calabrese, 2008; Mercer *et al.*, 2009).

Tricyclic antidepressants (TCAs)

Disturbances of serotonin have been associated with BPD, impulsive aggression, self-harm, and suicidality (Coccaro *et al.*, 1995; Evenden, 1999; Malone *et al.*, 1996; Pitchot *et al.*, 2005). Low cerebrospinal fluid (CSF) levels of serotonin metabolites have been associated with suicide attempts and completion (Samuelsson *et al.*, 2006; Traskman *et al.*, 1981), impulsivity, aggression (Mehlman *et al.*, 1994; Virkkunen *et al.*, 1994), lifetime aggressiveness, and suicidal lethality (Placidi *et al.*, 2001). Impulsive aggression with suicidality has been linked to blunted prolactin responses to the serotonergic probe fenfluramine (Coccaro *et al.*, 1989). PET scans of personality-disordered subjects high in impulsive aggression have demonstrated reduced response to fenfluramine in orbitofrontal, ventromedial, and cingulate regions (Siever *et al.*, 1999).

Nevertheless, early research on TCAs for BPD proved disappointing (Montgomery *et al.*, 1983; Soloff *et al.*, 1989). Amitriptyline has been associated with paradoxical increases in suicidality, paranoia, and behavioral dysregulation, attributed to "generalized disinhibition of cognitive and affective controls" (Soloff *et al.*, 1986*a*, 1987). Indeed, borderline patients have difficulty cognitively resolving conflict among stimulus dimensions (Posner *et al.*, 2002), and prefrontal hypofunction can be seen after a serotonergic stimulus in subjects with prominent impulsive aggression (New *et al.*, 2002). Thus, medications with adverse cognitive sequelae, including anticholinergic side-effects, may contribute to worsening impulsivity. As mentioned in prior reviews, the use of TCAs in treating BPD is discouraged (Abraham &

Calabrese, 2008; Mercer *et al.*, 2009). Their use is also associated with potentially significant risk of overdose.

Monoamine oxidase inhibitors (MAOIs)

Despite hesitancy in prescribing monoamine oxidase inhibitors (MAOIs) to patients with prominent impulsivity or self-injurious behavior, some recommend these medications for BPD patients who can take them safely and reliably. Interest in MAOIs for BPD is rooted in their differential efficacy for conditions such as hysteroid dysphoria or atypical depression, viewed as being related to one other and BPD (Kayser *et al.*, 1985; Liebowitz & Klein, 1981). In a cross-over trial with multiple medication phases, only tranylcypromine was associated with higher patient-rated improvement scores and completion rates (Cowdry & Gardner, 1988).

Similarly, relative prominence of BPD symptoms predicted superiority of phenelzine (Parsons *et al.*, 1989). Phenelzine is beneficial in the treatment of hostility, anxiety, and borderline symptoms (Soloff *et al.*, 1993). In some patients, it could cause uncomfortable excitement and emotional reactivity (Cornelius *et al.*, 1993). Thus, although there is evidence for their efficacy, many patients may not tolerate these medications. Other associated risks of MAOIs include toxicity in overdose and potentially fatal hypertensive crises or serotonin syndrome.

Selective serotonin reuptake inhibitors (SSRIs)

Selective serotonin reuptake inhibitors (SSRIs) are thought to potentiate serotonergic neuromodulation but demonstrate more favorable side-effect profiles. Fluoxetine reduced anger in BPD independent of any antidepressant effect (Salzman *et al.*, 1995). It also improved verbal and impulsive aggression, irritability, and overall functioning (Coccaro & Kavoussi, 1997). Similarly, a RCT with paroxetine demonstrated efficacy in preventing recurrent suicidal behavior but no significant effect on depression, hopelessness, or anger (Verkes *et al.*, 1998). By contrast, there was little added benefit from fluoxetine when added to dialectical behavioral therapy (DBT) (Simpson *et al.*, 2004).

On the other hand, fluvoxamine decreased affective lability, but not scores of impulsivity or aggression (Rinne *et al.*, 2002). Although SSRIs decrease impulsivity and aggression in BPD patients with comorbid intermittent explosive disorder (IED; Coccaro & Kavoussi, 1997; New *et al.*, 2004), data from BPD subjects without comorbid IED are inconsistent (Rinne *et al.*, 2002). Previous reviews have emphasized that effect sizes for antidepressant pharmacotherapy vary widely between classes and trials (Ingenhoven *et al.*, 2010; Lieb *et al.*, 2010; Mercer *et al.*, 2009). Nevertheless, current evidence-based practice recommends use of SSRIs, due to potential benefits on impulsive aggression that may outweigh associated risks. There has been no evidence that antidepressants alleviate the chronic emptiness, shameful self-concept, and intra-psychic pain in BPD.

First-generation antipsychotics

An early interest in antipsychotic medications for treating BPD probably arose from a conception of BPD as a variant of schizophrenia (e.g. Deutsch, 1942). Antipsychotics have demonstrated partial efficacy, reflecting underlying abnormalities in dopaminergic signaling. Borderline subjects demonstrate high levels of the dopamine metabolite, homovallinic

Study	Diagnosis	N	Medication(s)	Dosage(s)	Design, duration	Results in active drug group(s)
Rifkin et al. (1972)	EUCD (emotionally unstable character disorder, characterized by "chronic maladaptive behavior patterns…poor acceptance of reasonable authority, truancy, poor work history, manipulativeness…with a core psychopathological disturbance of depressive and hypomanic mood swings lasting hours to days")	21 (sex distribution not specified)	Lithium carbonate	Dosed to levels between 0.6–1.5 meq/1	Cross-over design, two 6-week phases	Mood swings and overall clinical status judged better on lithium
Leone (1982)	BPD	80 males and females	Loxapine succinate, chlorpromazine	Mean doses, loxapine: 14.5 mg/day, chlorpromazine: 110 mg/day	Parallel design but not placebo-controlled, 6 weeks	Both groups with significant improvements. Loxapine group improved more, especially in depression and anger-hostility
Montgomery & Montgomery (1982)	BPD, DPD, and/or HPD, all hospitalized after a suicidal act with history of at least two prior suicidal acts	Not specified. 30 males and females completed the study, 23 with BPD, 15 with HPD, and two with DPD	Depot flupenthixol	20 mg IM every 4 weeks	Parallel design, 6 months	Flupenthixol group showed reduction in number of suicidal acts
Montgomery et al. (1983)	BPD and/or HPD, all hospitalized after a suicidal act with history of at least two prior suicidal acts	Not specified. 38 male and female subjects completed, 30 with BPD and 12 with HPD	Mianserin	30 mg q.h.s.	Parallel design, 6 months	Mianserin group showed fewer suicidal acts but this did not reach trend levels
Serban & Siegel (1984)	BPD, SPD	52 males and females	Thiothixene, haloperidol	Thiothixene: began at 2 mg/day, then adjusted up or down, mean dose 9.4 mg/day. Haloperidol: began at 0.8 mg b.i.d., then adjusted dose up or down, mean dose 3 mg/day	Parallel design but not placebo-controlled, 3 months	Final drop-out rate unspecified, but 19% dropped out during the first month. 84% of all subjects moderately to markedly improved (mainly in cognitive disturbance, derealization, ideas of reference, anxiety, depression. Thiothixene superior to haloperidol. BPD vs. SPD diagnoses did not predict outcome

(cont.)

Table 14.3. (cont.)

Study	Diagnosis	N	Medication(s)	Dosage(s)	Design, duration	Results in active drug group(s)
Goldberg et al. (1986)	BPD and/or SPD, all subjects with at least one psychotic symptom	50 males and females	Thiothixene	Started at 5 mg/day, then increased gradually to maximum of 35 mg/day	Parallel design, 12 weeks	48% dropout rate. Significant improvement in ideas of reference, illusions, phobic anxiety, psychoticism, and obsessive-compulsive symptoms but not depression (SCL-90). Predictors of response from pre-treatment MMPI, discussed in Goldberg et al. (1986)
Soloff et al. (1986b)	BPD and/or SPD, 64 total, with 28 BPD only, four SPD only, and 32 comorbid BPD and SPD		Haloperidol, amitriptyline	Amitriptyline: began at 25 mg/day, then titrated upward to mean final dose of 147.62 mg/day. Haloperidol: began at 2 mg/day, then titrated upward to mean final dose of 7.24 mg/day	Parallel design, 5 weeks	Observer-rated measures did not demonstrate significant medication effects. Haloperidol superior to amitriptyline in self-report measures of hostility, paranoia, anxiety, and depression. Little benefit from amitriptyline even on depression. Results presented again in Soloff et al. (1989) but outpatients deleted from analyses (n = 13)
Soloff et al. (1986c)	See above	See above	See above	See above	See above	Haloperidol better than both amitriptyline and placebo for overall symptom severity. Improvements described as "modest," more apparent in self-rated than observer-rated measures. No differences between amitriptyline and placebo
Soloff et al. (1986a, 1987)	See above	Papers analyze paradoxical response to amitriptyline during study first described in Soloff et al. (1986b). Compared 15 amitriptyline non-responders, 14 placebo non-responders, 13 amitriptyline responders, and 10 placebo responders	Amitriptyline	See above. Mean final amitriptyline + nortriptyline blood levels were 246 ng/ml for responders and 245.9 ng/ml for non-responders	See above	Amitriptyline associated with paradoxical increases in hostility, irritability, impulsivity, paranoia, suicide threats, and demanding and assaultive behavior in non-responders

Study	Diagnosis	Sample	Drugs	Dosing	Design	Results
Cowdry & Gardner (1988)	BPD with "prominent behavioral dyscontrol"	16 females	Alprazolam, carbamazepine, trifluoperazine hydrochloride, tranylcypromine sulfate	Mean doses of alprazolam: 4.7 mg/day, carbamazepine: 820 mg/day, trifluoperazine: 7.8 mg/day, and tranylcypromine: 40 mg/day	Cross-over design, each phase lasting 6 weeks	Tranylcypromine and carbamazepine had lowest drop-out rates (25% and 33%, respectively, compared with average 45%) and were associated with physician-rated improvements. Tranylcypromine also associated with patient-rated improvements. Trifluoperazine completers showed some improvements. Carbamazepine group showed improvement especially in behavioral dyscontrol (Gardner & Cowdry, 1986b). Alprazolam group showed worsening behavioral dyscontrol (Cowdry & Gardner, 1988). Three subjects on carbamazepine developed worsening melancholia that remitted on discontinuation (Gardner & Cowdry, 1986a)
Parsons et al. (1989)	BPD and atypical depression	First sample of subjects were required to meet five BPD criteria (n = 40), second sample met four BPD criteria (n = 19)	Phenelzine, imipramine	Phenelzine: titration to 60 mg/day with option to increase to 90 mg/day if no response by week 5. Imipramine: titration to 200 mg/day with option to increase to 300 mg/day if no response by week 5	Cross-over design, two 6-week phases	Greater proportion of subjects responded to phenelzine than imipramine. Presence of BPD symptoms was negative predictor of response to imipramine: in subjects with four or more BPD symptoms, higher number of symptoms predicted superiority of phenelzine
Soloff et al. (1989)	Same as Soloff et al. (1986b)	90 total, with 35 "unstable" BPD, four SPD, and 51 "mixed" BPD and SPD	Same as Soloff et al. (1986b)	Same procedure as Soloff et al. (1985b). Mean dose of haloperidol was 4.8 mg/day and mean dose of amitriptyline was 149.1 mg/day on day 35	Parallel design, 5 weeks	Significant differences between haloperidol and placebo in global functioning, depression, hostility, schizotypy, and impulsivity. Differences between amitriptyline and placebo limited to depressive symptoms. Final results of 4-year study only analyzed data from inpatients, deleting data from outpatients in prior reports

(cont.)

Table 14.3. (cont.)

Study	Diagnosis	N	Medication(s)	Dosage(s)	Design, duration	Results in active drug group(s)
Links et al. (1990)	BPD	17 males and females	Lithium carbonate, desipramine	Not specified	Cross-over design, two 6-week phases	No statistically significant effects on depression. Trend towards decrease in anger and suicidality in lithium group, relative to desipramine. Therapists' perceptions favored lithium over placebo. Trend towards favoring lithium over desipramine. Therapists did not find desipramine superior to placebo
Soloff et al. (1993)	BPD	108 males and females	Haloperidol, phenelzine	Haloperidol: began at 1 mg/day, then titrated up to mean dose of 4 mg/day. Phenelzine: began at 15 mg/day, then titrated up to mean dose of 60 mg/day	Parallel design, 5 weeks	Improvements observed with haloperidol in Soloff et al. (1986a–c, 1987, 1989) were not replicated. Phenelzine associated with improvements in depression, borderline symptoms, anxiety, anger, and hostility, but not atypical depression/hysteroid dysphoria
Cornelius et al. (1993)	BPD	54 males and females	Haloperidol, phenelzine	Haloperidol: up to 6 mg/day, phenelzine: up to 90 mg/day. Doses generally did not change from final dose of prior 5-week acute phase (Soloff et al., 1993)	Parallel design, 16 weeks following 5-week acute phase (Soloff et al., 1993)	Drop-out rate during entire 22-week study, acute phase (Soloff et al., 1993) and continuation, was 73% (79/108). Only benefit in haloperidol group was decreased irritability. Haloperidol contributed to worsening depression, leaden paralysis, and hypersomnia. Phenelzine showed modest efficacy on depression and irritability, but unpleasant activation
de la Fuente & Lotstra (1994)	BPD	20 males and females	Carbamazepine	Dosed to obtain therapeutic blood levels	Parallel design, 32 days	No significant benefit
Salzman et al. (1995)	BPD	27 males and females	Fluoxetine	Started at 20 mg/day, titrated up to a maximum of 60 mg/day, with mean dose of 40 mg/day	Parallel design, 12 weeks	Decrease in anger with fluoxetine, but high placebo response rate. Subjects from outpatient sample without Axis I comorbidity, limiting generalizability

Study	Subjects	Drug	Dosing	Design	Results
Coccaro & Kavoussi (1997)	All subjects had at least one PD, as well as current problems with impulsive aggression and irritability. Most frequent PD was BPD	Fluoxetine	Started at 20 mg/day, and after end of week 4, could be increased to 40 mg/day, with further increase to 60 mg/day poss ble after end of week 8	Parallel design, 12 weeks	Reduction in irritability and aggression subscales of OAS-M. Higher proportion of CGI responders in fluoxetine group relative to placebo. D-fenfluramine challenge of subset of 15 subjects showed positive correlation in fluoxetine-treated but not placebo-treated subjects between improvement in OAS-M subscales and pre-treatment prolactin response (Coccaro & Kavoussi, 1997)
Verkes et al. (1998)	Non-depressed subjects who had recently attempted suicide for at least the second time. 81% met criteria for a Cluster B PD	Paroxetine	Started at 20 mg/day, increased to 40 mg/day after 1 week	Parallel design, 52 week	79% (72/91) dropped out prematurely. Significant efficacy in preventing suicidal behavior after controlling for number of prior suicide attempts. Paroxetine more effective in patients who met fewer than 15 Cluster BPD criteria. Paroxetine group did not differ from placebo in depressed mood, hopelessness, or anger
Battaglia et al. (1999)	Multiple suicide attempters. 85% had BPD	Fluphenazine decanoate	12.5 mg IM monthly or 1.5 mg IM monthly	Parallel design but not placebo-controlled, 6 months	60% (35/58) dropped out prematurely. Marked reduction in self-harm behaviors, but 12.5 mg dose did not significantly differ from 1.5 mg dose. According to authors, "The 'ultra-low' 1.5 mg dose was chosen to represent the extreme low end of possible pharmacological effect for fluphenazine treatment. The investigators believed that the ethics review board would not approve a study with the use of a placebo in such a critically ill group of patients"

(cont.)

Table 14.3. (cont.)

Study	Diagnosis	N	Medication(s)	Dosage(s)	Design, duration	Results in active drug group(s)
Hollander et al. (2001)	BPD	16 males and females	Divalproex sodium	Started at 250 mg q.h.s., increased gradually to maintain valproate levels of 80 (µg/ml or highest tolerable dose. Mean end-point valproate level 64.57 µg/ml	Parallel design, 10 week	50% (6/12) of medication group and 100% (6/12) of placebo group dropped out. No statistically significant benefits in ITT analyses. Among completers, significant improvements from baseline in CGI and GAS. ITT data showed changes in expected directions in BDI and AQ
Zanarini & Frankenburg (2001)	BPD	28 females	Olanzapine	Started with 1.25 mg/day, then titrated up to mean dose of 5.33 mg/day at end-point	Parallel design, 6 months	68% (19/28) dropped out prematurely. Improvements in olanzapine group in anxiety, paranoia, anger/hostility, and interpersonal sensitivity subscales but not depression subscale of SCL-90
Frankenburg & Zanarini (2002)	BPD and bipolar disorder type II	30 females	Divalproex sodium	Started at 250 mg bid, then titrated to target serum levels of 50–100 mg/1	Parallel design, 6 months	63% (19/30) dropped out prematurely. Improvements in medication group in interpersonal sensitivity, anger/hostility, and overall aggression
Rinne et al. (2002)	BPD	38 females	Fluvoxamine	Began with 150 mg/day, then titrated up to a maximum of 250 mg/day after week 10 if insufficient response	6-week double-blind placebo-controlled phase followed by 6-week single-blind half-cross-over phase in which all subjects received fluvoxamine. This was followed by 12-week open-label study of fluvoxamine	Significant reduction in BPD Severity Index rapid mood shift subscale, but not in impulsivity or aggression

Study	Diagnosis	Sample	Medication	Dosing	Design	Results
Hollander et al. (2003)	Cluster BPD, IED, or PTSD with OAS-M Aggression score > 15	Males and females. Cluster BPD: 96, with 55% BPD, 13% NPD, 10% AsPD, 1% HPD, PD NOS 21%); IED: 116; PTSD: 34	Divalproex sodium	Began with 250 mg b.i.d., then increased by 250 mg/day every 3–7 days during first 3 weeks. Recommended valproate levels were 80–120 µg/ml by third week. Maximum dose 30 mg/kg/day	Parallel design, 12 weeks	44% (54/124) divalproex group and 39% (47/122) placebo group dropped out. No differences in ITT data sets when all subjects included. In Cluster BPD subjects, significant decreases in CGI scores, OAS-M irritability scores, and verbal assault and assault against objects items of OAS-M aggression scale in medication group. Secondary analysis (Hollander et al., 2005) revealed improvements in impulsive aggression in a subset of BPD subjects, and that high BIS scores and high OAS-M aggression scores predicted better responses
Zanarini & Frankenburg (2003)	BPD	30 females	Ethyl-eicosapentaenoic acid (E-EPA)	500 mg b.i.d.	Parallel design, 8 weeks	Better than placebo in reducing aggression and severity of depressive symptoms
Bogenschutz & Nurnberg (2004)	BPD	40 males and females	Olanzapine	Started at 2.5 mg/day, then increased by 2.5–5 mg/day/week up to 10 mg/day. After week 8, dose could be further increased to maximum of 20 mg/day. Most patients received less than 10 mg/day	Parallel design, 12 week	Superior to placebo on CGI and CGI-BPD
Nickel et al. (2004)	BPD	31 females	Topiramate	Began with 50 mg/day, then increased to 250 mg/day by last 3 weeks	Parallel design, 8 weeks	Significant improvements in State-Anger, Trait-Anger, Anger-Out, and Anger-Control subscales of STAXI

(cont.)

Table 14.3. (cont.)

Study	Diagnosis	N	Medication(s)	Dosage(s)	Design, duration	Results in active drug group(s)
Philipsen et al. (2004a)	BPD	22 females	Clonidine	75 μg or 150 μg	Cross-over design in which each subject received one 75 μg dose and one 150 μg dose in randomized cross-over fashion during separate episodes of "strong aversive inner tension and urge to commit self-injurious behavior," no placebo-control, single-blind	Significant decreases in aversive inner tension, dissociative symptoms, suicidal ideation, and urges to commit self-injurious behavior 30–60 min after clonidine, for both doses. Dose did not affect response; no placebo-control
Philipsen et al. (2004b)	BPD	9 females	Naloxone hydrochloride	0.4 mg IV administered over 30 s	Cross-over design in which each subject received one dose of naloxone and one dose of placebo in randomized cross-over fashion during separate acute dissociative episodes	Dissociative symptoms decreased after both naloxone and placebo, but no difference between groups
Simpson et al. (2004)	BPD	25 females	Fluoxetine plus concurrent DBT	Started at 20 mg/day, increased to 40 mg/day at week 3	Parallel design, 12 week	No significant group differences from pre-treatment to post-treatment
Zanarini et al. (2004b)	BPD	45 females	Fluoxetine, olanzapine, and olanzapine-fluoxetine combination (OFC)	Fluoxetine: started at 10 mg/day, with end-point mean dose of 15 mg/day. Olanzapine: started at 2.5 mg/day, with end-point mean dose of 3.3 mg/day. OFC: started at olanzapine 2.5 mg/day and fluoxetine 10 mg/day, with end-point mean doses of 3.2 mg/day and 12.7 mg/day respectively	Parallel design but not placebo-controlled, 8 week	Olanzapine and OFC superior to fluoxetine for depression and impulsive aggression, although patients on fluoxetine improved in both as well. Weight gain greater in olanzapine group than fluoxetine or OFC groups

Nickel et al. (2005)	BPD	44 males	Topiramate	Began with 50 mg/day, then increased to 250 mg/day by last 3 weeks	Parallel design, 8 weeks	Significant improvements for medication group in State-Anger, Trait-Anger, Anger-Out, and Anger-Control subscales of STAXI. Subsequent open-label follow-up (Nickel & Loew, 2008) demonstrated continued benefits in topiramate group in ITT analysis
Soler et al. (2005)	BPD	60 males and females	Olanzapine with concurrent DBT	Flexible dosing from 5–20 mg/day, with mean dose 8.83 mg/day	Parallel design, 12 week	Olanzapine superior to placebo for depression, anxiety, and impulsive aggression
Tritt et al. (2005)	BPD	27 females	Lamotrigine	Started at 50 mg/day, then increased to 100 mg/day during week 3, 150 mg/day during weeks 4 and 5, and 200 mg/day during weeks 6–8	Parallel design, 8 weeks	Significant improvement on State-Anger, Trait-Anger, Anger-Out, and Anger-Control subscales of STAXI in medication group
Nickel et al. (2006)	BPD	52 males and females	Aripiprazole	15 mg/day	Parallel design, 8 weeks	Aripiprazole group evidenced greater improvements in SCL-90 subscales of obsessive-compulsive symptoms, insecurity in social contacts, depression, anxiety, hostility, phobic anxiety, paranoia, and psychoticism, as well as global psychological stress. Medication group also improved on HAMD and HAMA as well as all subscales of the STAXI. Less self-injurious behavior observed in medication group

(cont.)

Table 14.3. (cont.)

Study	Diagnosis	N	Medication(s)	Dosage(s)	Design, duration	Results in active drug group(s)
Loew et al. (2006)	BPD	59 females	Topiramate	Began with 25 mg/day, increasing to a target dose of 200 mg/day by week 6	Parallel design, 10 week	Significant improvements in medication group in SCL-90 subscales of somatization symptoms, interpersonal sensitivity, anxiety, hostility, phobic anxiety, and global stress, but not in obsessive–compulsive, depression, paranoia, or psychoticism subscales. Medication group significantly improved relative to placebo in measures of health-related quality of life (SF-36) and subscales relating to dominance, competitiveness, social avoidance, and importunateness in Inventory of Interpersonal Problems. Weight loss observed, but no subjects dropped out due to side-effects. Subsequent open-label follow-up demonstrated continued improvements in topiramate group in ITT analysis (Loew & Nickel, 2008)
Schulz et al. (2008)	BPD	314 males and females	Olanzapine	Flexible dosing, starting with 2.5–5 mg/day and increasing after 1 week by 2.5–5 mg/day to a maximum of 20 mg/day. Dose could also be lowered at investigator's judgment. After 4 weeks, if subjects did not demonstrate sufficient improvement, 2.5–5 mg dose increases were prescribed	Parallel design, 12 week. 52 sites included in nine different countries	ZAN-BPD scores decreased in both groups, but no significant differences between medication and placebo. Olanzapine group associated with greater weight gain, worse fasting lipid profiles, and higher elevations in prolactin compared to placebo group. Authors suggest that patients on olanzapine may have been under-dosed

Study	Diagnosis	Sample	Medication	Dosing	Design	Results
Pascual et al. (2008)	BPD	60 males and females	Ziprasidone	Flexible dosing starting at 40 mg/day up to a maximum of 200 mg/day, with mean dose 84.1 mg/day	Parallel design, 12 week after 2-week baseline evaluation	No significant improvements in CGI-BPD or measures of anxiety, psychotic symptoms, or impulsivity
Reich et al. (2009)	BPD, with all subjects also scoring "serious" on affective instability in Zanarini Rating Scale for Borderline Personality Disorder (ZAN-BPD) and > 14 on anger items of Affective Lability Scale (ALS), but did not meet criteria for bipolar disorder	28 males and females	Lamotrigine	Began with 25 mg/day for first 2 weeks, after which flexible dosing followed with possible increases of 25 mg/day/week and mean final dose of 106.7 mg/day	Parallel design, 12 week	Significant improvements in affective lability (ALS and ZAN-BPD subscale) and scores of general impulsivity (not associated with self-injury or suicidality) in ZAN-BPD. 20% (3/15) of lamotrigine group experienced rash requiring discontinuation
Ziegenhorn et al. (2009)	BPD patients with prominent hyperarousal, Clinician-Administered PTSD Scale-part D (CAPS-D) scores > 20 (sleep problems, anger, concentration problems, hypervigilance, exaggerated startle reflex)	17 females and 1 male. 67% (12/18) had comorbid PTSD	Clonidine	Slow-dose escalation over first week to target dose of 0.15 mg cam and 0.3 mg qhs	Double-blind cross-over design, each phase lasted 2 weeks	Statistically significant improvements in hyperarousal (CAPS-D), subjective sleep latency and restorative qualities of sleep, and anxiety, but not borderline-specific symptoms for the total sample. Improvements in hyperarousal and sleep did not reach significance in non-PTSD subsample
Shafti & Shahveisi (2010)	BPD	28 females, recruited shortly after inpatient psychiatric admission and subsequent 7-day washout	Olanzapine, haloperidol	Both medications began at 2.5 mg/day and increased weekly by 2.5 mg/day as needed or tolerated to a maximum of 10 mg/day by week 4. Doses at week 4 were maintained for remainder of study	Parallel design but no placebo-control, 8 weeks	Olanzapine group trended towards greater improvement in Buss–Durkee Hostility scores. Haloperidol trended towards greater improvement in CGI scores. No significant between-group differences. Olanzapine group associated with worsening metabolic profile. Higher rates of extra-pyramidal symptoms in haloperidol group

AQ, Aggression Questionnaire; AsPD, antisocial personality disorder; AvPD, avoidant personality disorder; BDI, Beck Depression Inventory; BPD, borderline personality disorder; CGI, Clinical Global Impression; CGI-BPD, Clinical Global Impression for Borderline Personality Disorder; DPD, dependent personality disorder; GAS, Global Assessment Scale; HAMA, Hamilton Anxiety Scale; HAMD, Hamilton Depression Scale; HPD, histrionic personality disorder; MMPI, Minnesota Multiphasic Personality Inventory; OAS-M, Modified Overt Aggression Scale; PANSS, Positive and Negative Symptom Scale; PD, personality disorder; PTSD, posttraumatic stress disorder; SCL-90, Symptom Checklist-90; STAXI, State-Trait Anger Expression Inventory; ZAN-PBD, Zanarini Rating Scale for Borderline Personality Disorder.

Table 14.4. Avoidant personality disorder (AvPD).

Study	Diagnosis	N	Medication(s)	Dosage(s)	Design, duration	Results in active drug group(s)
Versiani et al. (1992)	Social phobia	78 males and females (percent AvPD or generalized type not reported)	Moclobemide, phenelzine	Moclobemide: started with 100 mg b.i.d., with flexible dose increases after 4 days, again after 4 weeks and 5 weeks. Mean dose 580 mg/day. Phenelzine: started with 15 mg b.i.d., with flexible dose increases after 4 days, again after 4 weeks, 5 weeks Mean dose 67.5 mg/day	Parallel design, 16 weeks (with 8 additional weeks follow-up in which half of each medication group gradually switched to placebo, others continued on last dosage)	Both agents better than placebo in reducing social anxiety and improving social function. 82% response rate for moclobemide group; 91% for phenelzine group. Moclobemide better tolerated than phenelzine
Van Vliet et al. (1994)	Social phobia	30 males and females (53% generalized subtype)	Fluvoxamine	150 mg/day	Parallel design, 12 weeks	Reduction of social and general anxiety, but not phobic avoidance
Fahlen (1995)	Social phobia	63 males and females (34 with comorbid AvPD, 1 with comorbid DPD)	Brofaromine	Started at 50 mg/day, then increased to 100 mg/day in week 2 and 150 mg/day in week 3	Parallel design, 12 weeks	Improvement in social anxiety. More marked improvements in maladaptive personality traits. 2/3 of subjects in medication group with comorbid AvPD and 1 DPD comorbid subject no longer met criteria
Katzelnick et al. (1995)	Social phobia	12 males and females (percent AvPD or generalized type not reported)	Sertraline	Began with 50 mg/day, with flexible increases by 50 mg every 2 weeks if no clinical response, to maximum of 200 mg. Mean dose 133.5 mg/day at end-point	Parallel design, 10 weeks	Reduction of social anxiety, bodily pain and improvement in social functioning. 50% of sertraline group rated moderately or markedly improved vs. 9% of placebo group
IMCTGMSP & Katschnig (1997)	Social phobia	578 males and females (78% generalized type; 49% comorbid AvPD)	Moclobemide	300 mg/day vs. 600 mg/day (after 4 days of 300 mg initial dose)	Parallel design, 12 weeks	Reduction of social anxiety and improved social functioning in 600 mg group (47% responders vs. 34% in placebo group). No differences between groups with/without AvPD in response, but comorbid AvPD patients responded less to placebo

Study	Diagnosis	Sample	Drug	Dosing	Design	Results
Lott et al. (1997)	Social phobia	102 males and females (percent AvPD or generalized type not reported)	Brofaromine	After 1–8 weeks washout, started on 50 mg/day with flexible dosing to maximum of 150 mg/day	Parallel design, 10 weeks	Reduction of social anxiety but no significant effect in social functioning. 50% response rate vs. 19% in placebo group
Noyes et al. (1997)	Social phobia	583 males and females (62.5% generalized type; 47.8% comorbid AvPD)	Moclobemide	Fixed dose comparison of 75 mg/day vs. 150 mg/day vs. 300 mg/day vs. 900 mg/day. 600 mg/day vs. 900 mg/day. 75–150 mg/day began with full dose, other groups began with 150 mg/day and increased by 150 mg q.i.d. to target dosage	Parallel design, 12 weeks	No improvement independent of dose at 12 weeks, only at 8 weeks. 35% much improved but high placebo response rate. As above, no difference between groups with/without AvPD, but less drug/placebo difference in comorbid AvPD patients
Heimberg et al. (1998)	Social phobia	133 males and females (70.7% generalized type)	Phenelzine	Began with 15 mg/day, with increases to 30 mg after 4 days, then 45 mg after 8 days, then 60 mg after 15 days. Further flexible dose increases possible after 4 weeks to 75 mg/day and after 5 weeks to 90 mg/day	Parallel design but non-randomized, comparing medication to group cognitive–behavioral therapy (CBT) or supportive/educational therapy or placebo; 12 weeks	Phenelzine and CBT better than both comparison conditions. Phenelzine effect earlier and on more subscales. 77% response rate to phenelzine and 75% to CBT. Phenelzine group showed trend towards greater relapse in subsequent treatment-free follow-up (Liebowitz et al., 1999)
Schneier et al. (1998)	Social phobia	77 males and females (85% generalized type; 38% comorbid AvPD)	Moclobemide	Began with 100 mg b.i.d., flexibly dosed to a maximum of 400 mg b.i.d. Mean dose: 728 mg/day at end-point	Parallel design, 8 weeks	Reduction of 2 of 10 subscores of social anxiety (total fear, avoidance). 17.5% response rate vs. 13.5% in placebo group
Stein et al. (1998)	Social phobia	183 males and females (100% generalized subtype)	Paroxetine	Began with 20 mg/day, with possible 10 mg increases every 2 weeks to a maximum of 50 mg/day. Mean dose 35.6 mg/day at end-point	Parallel design, 12 weeks	Reduction of social anxiety and improvement in social functioning

(cont.)

Table 14.4. (cont.)

Study	Diagnosis	N	Medication(s)	Dosage(s)	Design, duration	Results in active drug group(s)
Allgulander (1999)	Social phobia	99 males and females (percent with comorbid AvPD or generalized type not reported)	Paroxetine	Began with 20 mg/day, with possible 10 mg increases every week to maximum of 50 mg/day	Parallel design, 12 weeks	Reduction of social anxiety and improvement in social functioning. 70.5% response rate *vs.* 8.3% in placebo group. Rate of response lower amongst those with comorbid dysthymia
Baldwin et al. (1999)	Social phobia	290 males and females (percent with comorbid AvPD or generalized type not reported)	Paroxetine	Began with 20 mg/day, with possible 10 mg increases every week to maximum of 50 mg/day. Mean dose 34.7 mg/day at end-point	Parallel design, 12 weeks	Reduction of social anxiety and improvement in social functioning. 65.7% response rate *vs.* 32.4% in placebo group
Stein et al. (1999)	Social phobia	92 males and females (91.3% generalized type)	Fluvoxamine	Began with 50 mg/day with further weekly 50 mg/day increases possible after week 1, to maximum of 300 mg/day. Mean dose 202 mg/day at end-point	Parallel design, 12 weeks	Reduction of social anxiety and improvement in social functioning. 65.7% response rate *vs.* 32.4% in placebo group
Blomhoff et al. (2001)	Social phobia	387 males and females (100% generalized type)	Sertraline	Began with 50 mg/day, increased to 100 mg/day after 4 weeks if insufficient improvement noted. Further dose escalation to 150 mg/day allowed after 8 or 12 weeks	Parallel design comparing sertraline + general medical care, sertraline + prolonged exposure therapy (PE), placebo + PE, and placebo + general medical care; 24 weeks	Sertraline and combined sertraline/PE groups superior to placebo groups in reduction of social anxiety. Greatest improvement in combination group, though not significantly different than sertraline alone
van Ameringen et al. (2001)	Social phobia	204 males and females (100% generalized type; 61% comorbid AvPD)	Sertraline	Began with 50 mg/day, with option to increase after 4 weeks by 50 mg every 3 weeks to maximum of 200 mg/day. Mean dose 146.7 mg/day at end-point	Parallel design, 20 weeks	Reduction of social anxiety and improvement in social functioning. 53% response rate *vs.* 29% in placebo group

Reference	Diagnosis	Sample	Drug	Dosing	Design	Results
et al. (2002)	(100% generalized type)			of 20 mg/day vs. 40 mg/day vs. 60 mg/day. All groups began with 20 mg/day, increasing to 40 mg/day after 1 week, and to 60 mg/day after 2 weeks in each respective group		social anxiety in 20 mg group. Highest response rate (based on CGI) in 40 mg group
Stein et al. (2002)	Social phobia	257 males and females (100% generalized type)	Paroxetine	Began with 20 mg/day, flexibly increased by 10 mg at 2, 3, 4, and 8 weeks, to maximum of 50 mg/day	Parallel design, single-blind 12-week acute phase with those whose CGI decreased by at least 2 points entering 24-week double-blind continuation phase	Relapse in paroxetine group 14% compared with 39% in placebo group
Davidson et al. (2004b)	Social phobia	279 males and females (100% generalized type)	Fluvoxamine CR	Began with 100 mg/day and flexibly increased by 50 mg every week to maximum of 300 mg/day. Mean dose 174 mg/day	Parallel design, 12 week	Reduction of social anxiety and improvement in social functioning
Davidson et al. (2004a)	Social phobia	295 (100% generalized type)	Fluoxetine	Began with 10 mg/day, increasing to 20 mg/day on day 8, to 30 mg/day on day 15, and to 40 mg/day on day 29 Dose could be further increased to 50–60 mg/day on days 43 and 57, if insufficient improvement	Parallel design comparing fluoxetine, group CBT, fluoxetine + group CBT, placebo, placebo + group CBT; 14 weeks	All treatments superior to placebo. No differences between treatments at 14 weeks. Combined treatment without further advantage
Lepola et al. (2004)	Social phobia	372 males and females (percent with comorbid AvPD or generalized type not reported)	Paroxetine CR	Began with 12.5 mg/day for 2 weeks, with flexible increases by 12.5 mg every week to maximum of 37.5 mg/day. Mean dose 32.3 mg/day at end-point	Parallel design, 12 weeks	Reduction of social anxiety and improvement in social functioning. 57% response rate vs. 30.4% in placebo group

(cont.)

Table 14.4. (cont.)

Study	Diagnosis	N	Medication(s)	Dosage(s)	Design, duration	Results in active drug group(s)
Rickels et al. (2004)	Social phobia	272 males and females (100% generalized type)	Venlafaxine ER	Began with 75 mg/day, with increase to 150 mg after 1 week and possible further increase to maximum of 225 mg/day after at least one more week	Parallel design, 12 weeks	Reduction of social anxiety and improvement in social functioning
Lader et al. (2004)	Social phobia	839 males and females (100% generalized type)	Escitalopram, paroxetine	Escitalopram: fixed dose comparison of 5 mg/day vs. 10 mg/day vs. 20 mg/day. Paroxetine: 20 mg/day	Parallel design, 12 weeks with 24 weeks continuation and follow-up	Reduction of social anxiety and improvement in social functioning for all doses of escitalopram and paroxetine. Escitalopram 20 mg/day superior to paroxetine 20 mg/day
Allgulander et al. (2004)	Social phobia	434 males and females (100% generalized type)	Venlafaxine ER, paroxetine	Venlafaxine ER: Began with 75 mg/day, with flexible increases by 75 mg after 1 week and after 3 weeks to maximum of 225 mg/day. Mean dose 192.4 mg/day at end-point. Paroxetine: Began with 20 mg/day, with flexible increases by 10 mg every week to maximum of 50 mg/day. Mean dose 44.2 mg/day at end-point	Parallel design, 12 weeks	Both venlafaxine and paroxetine groups similarly efficacious in reducing social anxiety and improvement in social functioning. Possibly more rapid effect of venlafaxine
Kasper et al. (2005)	Social phobia	358 males and females (100% generalized type)	Escitalopram	Began with 10 mg/day, with possible increase to 20 mg/day after 4, 6, or 8 weeks for unsatisfactory response. Mean dose 17.6 mg/day at end-point	Parallel design, 12 weeks	Reduction of social anxiety and improvement in social functioning. 54% response rate vs. 39% in placebo group

Study	Disorder	Sample	Drug	Dosing	Design	Results
Liebowitz et al. (2005b)	Social phobia	271 males and females (100% generalized type)	Venlafaxine ER	Began with 75 mg/day for week 1, with increase to 150mg in week 2 and to maximum of 225 mg in week 3, if clinically indicated		Reduction of social anxiety and improvement in social functioning. 44% response rate vs. 30% in placebo group
Liebowitz et al. (2005a)	Social phobia	413 males and females (100% generalized type)	Venlafaxine ER, paroxetine	Venlafaxine ER: Began with 75 mg/day up to 225 mg/day, with flexible 75 mg increases each week to maximum of 225 mg/day. Mean dose 201.7 mg/day at end-point. Paroxetine: Began with 20 mg/day, with flexible 10 mg increases to maximum of 50 mg/day. Mean dose 46 mg/day at end-point		Reduction of social anxiety and improvement in social functioning compared with placebo, for both medication groups. Both medications equally efficacious. 56.6% response rate for venlafaxine; 62.5% for paroxetine; and 36.1% for placebo group
Stein et al. (2005)	Social phobia	386 males and females (100% generalized type)	Venlafaxine	Comparison of low-dose (fixed) to higher-dose (flexible). All began with 75 mg/day and, if randomized to higher-dose, increased to 150 mg/day after week 1, with further flexible increase to 225 mg/day after week 2	Parallel design, 24 weeks	Reduction in social phobia and improvement in social functioning in both dosage groups. 31% remission rate for both venlafaxine groups combined vs. 16% in placebo group. Relapse rate 22% vs. 50% in placebo group. Median time to relapse was 407d vs. 144 days for placebo group. No direct comparison made between doses
Montgomery et al. (2005)	Social phobia	517 males and females (100% generalized type)	Escitalopram	During open-label phase, began with 10 mg-day with possible increase to 20 mg/day at weeks 2, 4, or 8. CGI responders entered relapse prevention phase with last dose continued for remainder	12-week open-label phase, followed by 24-week fixed-dose relapse prevention (parallel design, double-blind RCT)	Relapse rate 22% vs. 50% in placebo group. Median time to relapse was 407 days vs. 144 days for placebo group. No direct comparison made between doses

For abbreviations in table see notes to Table 14.3.

acid, in both plasma and cerebrospinal fluid (Siever *et al.* unpublished data). Prior to more widespread use of SSRIs, antipsychotics demonstrated efficacy in decreasing psychotic-like symptoms (Goldberg *et al.*, 1986; Soloff *et al.*, 1986*b*), depression (Soloff *et al.*, 1986*b*), irritability (Cornelius *et al.*, 1993), and general symptom severity (Cowdry & Gardner, 1988; Soloff *et al.*, 1986*b*).

A recent Cochrane review suggests haloperidol is efficacious in reducing anger in BPD, and treatment with flupenthixol decanoate reduced suicidal behavior (Lieb *et al.*, 2010). By contrast, evidence for efficacy of neuroleptics on affective symptoms, psychosis, and anxiety remains inconsistent. The dosage of antipsychotic medication for evidence-based treatment of BPD is usually lower than schizophrenia. High dropout rates are noted, and risk of extrapyramidal symptoms may further limit the utility of neuroleptics.

Second-generation antipsychotics

Classical neuroleptics have largely been superseded by atypical antipsychotics, whose broader therapeutic benefits may be explained by activity beyond the D2 receptor. As mentioned in prior reviews, olanzapine has proven beneficial in treatment of BPD patients' anxiety, anger, interpersonal sensitivity, and paranoia, but not depression (Zanarini & Frankenburg, 2001), as well as improving general clinical functioning and BPD symptomatology (Bogenschutz & Nurnberg, 2004). A recent, large RCT demonstrated no effect of olanzapine on BPD symptoms (Schulz *et al.*, 2008), although the authors suggested that patients may have been underdosed. A study comparing olanzapine with haloperidol showed no between-group differences except with respect to side-effects, with more weight gain associated with olanzapine and more extrapyramidal side-effects with haloperidol (Shafti & Shahveisi, 2010).

Adding fluoxetine to olanzapine did not elicit further benefit, except that subjects receiving both medications gained less weight than those receiving only olanzapine (Zanarini *et al.*, 2004*b*). The addition of olanzapine to DBT reduced depression, anxiety, and impulsive aggression, but the magnitude and timing of these benefits relative to DBT was difficult to interpret (Soler *et al.*, 2005).

Aripiprazole has a novel mechanism of action (partial agonist at the dopamine D2 receptor and serotonin 5-HT$_{1A}$ receptor, antagonist at the 5-HT$_{2A}$ receptor). It may be more favorable than other atypicals with respect to metabolic side-effects. A longer half-life may be more effective for patients susceptible to non-adherence. In non-suicidal BPD patients, aripiprazole was effective in reducing aggression, anxiety, depression, psychosis, interpersonal symptoms, self-injurious behavior, and subjective distress. There were no significant differences between groups in weight gain (Nickel *et al.*, 2006). An 18-month, open-label follow-up showed sustained improvements and continued tolerability (Nickel *et al.*, 2007).

Previously, open-label trials suggested possible efficacy of ziprasidone in BPD patients during acute exacerbations (Pascual *et al.*, 2004, 2006). The side-effect and psychopharmacological profiles of ziprasidone indicated lesser metabolic risks and antidepressant and anxiolytic effects thought to be independent of antidopaminergic activity (Keck *et al.*, 1998; Tandon, 2000; Wilner *et al.*, 2002). Despite such promise, a recent RCT with ziprasidone was negative (Pascual *et al.*, 2008). Thus, evidence-based practice supports use of aripiprazole but not ziprasidone in treating BPD.

In meta-analyses, the class of antipsychotics had moderate effect in treating aggression, but no significant effect on depression, although aripiprazole and olanzapine may be exceptions (Lieb *et al.*, 2010; Mercer *et al.*, 2009). For atypicals, metabolic side-effects may limit clinical utility. Because 29–53% of borderline patients fulfil criteria for an eating disorder at some point in their lives (Lieb et al., 2004), and a significant number suffer from obesity (Frankenburg & Zanarini, 2006), iatrogenic metabolic risks must be regarded as serious. Although evidence-based practices have advanced in treating aggression associated with BPD, chronic emptiness, affective lability, and interpersonal dysfunction lack effective, evidence-based medication treatments.

Mood stabilizers and anticonvulsants

Due to BPD patients' affective dysregulation and comorbidity with bipolar disorder, some have classified BPD within the bipolar spectrum (Akiskal, 2004; Smith et al., 2004), although most continue to distinguish between the two, particularly with regard to interpersonal dysfunction (Bolton & Gunderson, 1996; Henry et al., 2001; Paris, 2004). Mood stabilizers are indeed becoming a more integral component of evidence-based treatment practices for BPD.

Lithium is beneficial in treating BPD, particularly in terms of quieting affective instability (Links et al., 1990; Rifkin et al., 1972). Lithium toxicity and/or non-compliance may be problematic, due to BPD patients' characteristic impulsive, self-destructive behavior.

However, anticonvulsants are more often recommended for treatment of rapid-cycling bipolar disorder, the variant most closely resembling BPD. Carbamazepine demonstrated "dramatic" reductions in behavioral dyscontrol and improvements in global functioning, anxiety, anger, euphoria, impulsivity, and suicidality, but it was associated with worsening melancholic depression (Gardner & Cowdry, 1986a, 1986b), and therapeutic benefits could not be replicated in inpatients (de la Fuente & Lotstra, 1994).

Although high dropout rates were reported with divalproex (Hollander et al., 2001), it subsequently demonstrated benefits on interpersonal sensitivity, anger, and aggression in euthymic borderline women with bipolar II (Frankenburg & Zanarini, 2002). Divalproex reduced aggression, irritability, and overall disease severity in patients with Cluster B personality disorders and prominent impulsive aggression (Hollander et al., 2003). Differential treatment response in Cluster B subjects was enhanced by baseline trait impulsivity and state aggression, although not affective instability (Hollander et al., 2005).

Lamotrigine extends periods of euthymia in bipolar patients (e.g. Goodwin et al., 2004). Potential benefits also include pro-cognitive activity, as previously demonstrated in normal volunteers (Aldenkamp et al., 2002). Lamotrigine effectively reduced BPD patients' anger (Tritt et al., 2005), and an 18-month follow-up demonstrated maintenance of this anti-aggressive effect (Leiberich et al., 2008). More recently, BPD patients without comorbid bipolar disorder but with prominent affective instability demonstrated reduced affective lability and impulsivity, but no change in other BPD symptoms, when treated with lamotrigine (Reich et al., 2009). Documented effects on impulsivity, anger, and affective lability in BPD thus make lamotrigine an attractive pharmacotherapeutic option. Nevertheless, the latter study reported higher rates of skin rash than reported elsewhere. Due to this life-threatening risk, clinicians should monitor patients closely and titrate the dose slowly.

Although topiramate's utility in bipolar disorder is controversial, it is efficacious for BPD. Topiramate reduced anger in female BPD subjects (Nickel et al., 2004), and a similar RCT reported this effect in males with BPD (Nickel et al., 2005). A separate RCT conducted with female BPD patients taking topiramate also demonstrated improvements in somatization, anxiety, health-related quality of life, overall stress, interpersonal sensitivity, hostility, and other facets of interpersonal functioning (Loew et al., 2006). Although no dropouts were due to side-effects, cognitive impairment, reduced appetite, and weight loss were commonly reported.

Open-label follow-up studies to these initial RCTs demonstrated maintenance of therapeutic gains and additional weight loss associated with topiramate, and the authors therefore encouraged longer-term use (Loew & Nickel, 2008; Nickel & Loew, 2008). The authors admit that the patients studied were not the most severe. Because cognitive side-effects of topiramate may more adversely affect severely impulsive or suicidal BPD patients, a careful risk–benefit analysis should be undertaken before prescribing.

Overall, mood stabilizers and anticonvulsants are effective in treating BPD, particularly symptoms of impulsivity and aggression. As a class, they also demonstrate a moderate effect in treating depression in BPD (Ingenhoven et al., 2010; Mercer et al., 2009). Although they are an important component of evidence-based practice, patients should be closely monitored, because some may not tolerate these medications. The relatively slow titration schedules and the necessity of drawing plasma levels to reach an optimal dose may limit clinical effectiveness, particularly in a population often characterized by impulsive non-compliance. Although impulsivity and aggression appear to respond to treatment, there is little evidence of any effect from mood stabilizers in improving interpersonal dysfunction or disturbances of identity. Future research should focus more closely on these domains.

Other medications

Although there have been case reports of improvement in BPD patients treated with alprazolam (Faltus, 1984), the class of benzodiazepines has been associated with disinhibition, worsening impulsivity, suicidal ideation, and behavioral dyscontrol in BPD (Cowdry & Gardner, 1988). Benzodiazepines are vehemently discouraged, due to these risks, as well as elevated risks of dependence. Patients may abuse benzodiazepines to self-medicate intrapsychic pain, interfering with progress in psychotherapy and adversely affecting cognition.

The omega-3 fatty acid, ethyl-eicosapentaenoic acid (E-EPA) decreased aggression and depression in women with moderate to severe BPD (Zanarini & Frankenburg, 2003). A similar anti-aggressive effect was observed in two other RCTs with healthy subjects (Hamazaki et al., 1996, 2002). Omega-3 fatty acids may act by inhibiting protein kinase C, a mechanism thought to be involved in lithium and valproic acid pharmacotherapy (Peet & Stokes, 2005).

Clonidine, a presynaptic a$_2$ noradrenergic agonist, has been studied in a trial comparing two doses given to BPD patients amidst states of "acute aversive inner tension." Although tension, dissociative symptoms, self-injurious urges, and suicidal ideation decreased for both doses, there was no difference between the two doses (Philipsen et al., 2004a). Ziegenhorn et al. (2009) conducted an RCT of clonidine with BPD subjects with prominent symptoms of hyperarousal. Most of them therefore also met criteria for comorbid PTSD, which limited generalizability of findings. In the total sample, clonidine treatment improved hyperarousal, subjective quality of sleep, and anxiety, but not borderline-specific symptoms, and these benefits were not seen in the minuscule non-PTSD subsample. Although clonidine and similar agents have been efficacious in the treatment of PTSD (e.g. Southwick et al., 1999; Strawn & Geracioti, 2008), their role in treating BPD remains unclear.

A subset of borderline patients engage in self-injurious behavior or more indirect forms of self-destructiveness (e.g. bulimia, substance abuse), which may reflect disturbances in endogenous opioids. Some BPD patients become disinhibited and aggressive after receiving opiate medications (Saper, 2000), and morphine administration increased self-injurious behavior in one patient with BPD (Thurauf & Washeim, 2000). Naloxone used during acute states of aversive tension and dissociation in BPD demonstrated no significant benefit (Philipsen *et al.*, 2004*b*). Naltrexone has been used successfully in open-label trials to treat self-harm (Griengl *et al.*, 2001; McGee, 1997; Roth *et al.*, 1996) and dissociation (Bohus *et al.*, 1999). Therefore, evidence for treatment of BPD with medications acting upon opioid receptors remains inconsistent. Treatment with full agonists or antagonists may be complicated by differences between chronic effects on post-synaptic receptor density on the one hand, and distinct, acute effects of receptor agonism or antagonism on the other (Prossin *et al.*, 2010; Stanley & Siever, 2010). The potential for abuse of full opioid agonists may pose too great a risk for an effective treatment. For both these reasons, future trials with partial opioid agonists may be more effective in reducing self-injury, interpersonal dysfunction, and intrapsychic pain.

Avoidant personality disorder (AvPD)

AvPD is a common personality disorder (Loranger *et al.*, 1994), existing as a comorbid condition in up to one-third of all patients with anxiety disorders (Alden *et al.*, 2002). Up to 56% of AvPD patients continue to meet criteria after 2 years (Skodol *et al.*, 2005). Nevertheless, distinguishing between this and generalized social phobia has been difficult, due to similarities in diagnostic criteria as well as frequently reported comorbidity. No neurobiological evidence indicates how the etiology and psychopathology of AvPD differs from social phobia.

At present, clinicians should "extrapolate from data which are primarily related to anxiety disorders … to apply treatment strategies … that have primarily been developed for social phobia" (Herpertz *et al.*, 2007). Evidence-based treatment for AvPD would thereby include venlafaxine and SSRIs as first-line agents. A potential caveat is mentioned for sertraline if symptoms began in childhood or adolescence, in which case lesser efficacy was reported (van Ameringen *et al.*, 2004). Gabapentin (Pande *et al.*, 1999) and pregabalin (Pande *et al.*, 2004) have also demonstrated efficacy in social phobia. Second-line agents would include reversible MAOIs brofaromine and moclobemide, for which there is presently less robust evidence, and the irreversible MAOI phenelzine, which entails risk of serious side-effects.

Other personality disorders and maladaptive traits

Pharmacological research is strikingly absent from other personality disorders. In these cases, medication is particularly indicated in the treatment of comorbid Axis I disorders, particularly mood and anxiety disorders that frequently co-occur with narcissistic, histrionic, and dependent personality disorders. SSRIs may be of particular clinical benefit relative to TCAs, given their more favorable side-effect profile and the possibility of an independent effect on personality factors (Ekselius & von Knorring, 1998; Reich, 2002). With the advent of the next DSM, a greater emphasis on a dimensional diagnostic approach to personality disorders will probably cast greater importance upon pharmacotherapeutic interventions targeting dimensions common to a variety of current Axis II diagnoses.

One such dimension of personality dysfunction is impulsive aggression. Recent trials with levetiracetam and oxcarbazepine for impulsive aggression recruited individuals with IED without significant comorbidity (e.g. Mattes, 2005, 2008), while other trials recruited subjects with personality disorders and a history of impulsive aggression (e.g. Coccaro *et al.*,

2009; Hollander *et al.*, 2003). Coccaro *et al.* (2009) found an anti-aggressive effect of fluoxetine in patients with IED and personality disorders. Several anticonvulsants (most notably divalproex, oxcarbazepine, and phenytoin) have also demonstrated evidence in treating impulsive aggression across diagnoses (Huband *et al.*, 2010).

Future directions

Although the past two decades of research have ushered a paradigm shift in personality disorders, most research has been limited to BPD and SPD. Future research should be directed towards the treatment of other Axis II diagnoses and dimensions of dysfunction across diagnoses. Although research has made great strides towards understanding impulsivity and aggression, similar neurobiological substrates should be sought for other dimensions of personality. Only by clarifying these gaps in the evidence base can clinicians anticipate more effective evidence-based psychopharmacological practices for the treatment of personality disorders.

Further efforts to understand to what extent AvPD differs from generalized social phobia are warranted. This may require understanding distinctions between these diagnoses in neurobiology of fear and social inhibition, and in the developmental trajectory of each disorder. For SPD, the effects of pro-cognitive interventions should be evaluated with respect to social isolation and overall functioning. More comprehensive efforts are needed to understand the underlying neurobiology of SPD to improve evidence-based practices. Further characterization of the interpersonal dysfunction and cognitive, sensory-gating abnormalities seen in SPD will probably improve the effect of treatment on general functioning. Efforts at understanding the neurobiology of schizophrenia and its prodrome will also assist in defining targets for pharmacotherapy. Clarifying the respective roles of genes and environment in shaping the course of the schizophrenia spectrum will also uncover future pharmacotherapeutic targets.

Within BPD, research has detailed more extensive evidence-based practices for treating impulsive aggression. Anticonvulsants and atypical antipsychotics are acquiring more prominent roles in the treatment of BPD, relative to SSRIs. Nevertheless, greater serotonergic specificity will probably improve the efficacy of treatments. For example, selective 5-HT_{2A} antagonism, but not 5-HT_{2C} antagonism, has been shown to decrease impulsivity (Higgins *et al.*, 2003; Winstanley *et al.*, 2004).

Future research will also focus on treating affective instability, intrapsychic pain, dissociation, and interpersonal dysfunction associated with BPD. BPD has been conceptualized as related to disturbed attachment (Fonagy & Luyten, 2009) and dysfunctional representations of self and other (Bender & Skodol, 2007), with other symptoms seen as sequelae to this core feature. Oxytocin, vasopressin, and opioids may therefore be of particular relevance for treating BPD (Stanley & Siever, 2010), given the developmental role of these neuropeptides in attachment and the relationship between attachment security and stable social cognitive representations of self and other (Fonagy & Luyten, 2009). Although these domains have been exclusively treated with psychotherapy, research in the neurobiology of affiliative behavior (e.g. Depue & Morrone-Strupinsky, 2005) as well as self-injury and dissociation (Mauchnik & Schmahl, 2010) may eventually provide novel pharmacotherapeutic targets.

For all personality disorders, integrating psychopharmacology with neurobiological effects of psychotherapy may produce synergistic and long-lasting benefits. Evidence-based practice continues to recommend an approach that includes both psychotherapy and pharmacotherapy. Although experienced therapists' contributions to personality theory and empirical research often continue to be at odds with one another, future research should attempt to connect theory with empirically validated psychopharmacological targets. By understanding the neurobiology underlying increasingly complex behavior, pharmacotherapy can be optimized and targeted to personality dimensions previously considered susceptible only to psychotherapy.

References

Abraham PF, Calabrese JR (2008). Evidence-based pharmacologic treatment of borderline personality disorder: a shift from SSRIs to anticonvulsants and atypical antipsychotics? *Journal of Affective Disorders* **111**, 21–30.

Akiskal HS (2004). Demystifying borderline personality: critique of the concept and unorthodox reflections on its natural kinship with the bipolar spectrum. *Acta Psychiatrica Scandinavica* **110**, 401–407.

Alden LE, Paosa JM, Taylor CT, Ryder AG (2002). Avoidant personality disorder: current status and future directions. *Journal of Personality Disorders* **16**, 1–29.

Aldenkamp AP, Arends J, Boorsma HPR *et al.* (2002). Randomized double-blind parallel-group study comparing cognitive effects of a low-dose lamotrigine with valproate and placebo in healthy volunteers. *Epilepsia* **43**, 19–26.

Allgulander C (1999). Paroxetine in social anxiety disorder: a randomized placebo-controlled study. *Acta Psychiatrica Scandinavica* **100**, 193–198.

Allgulander C, Mangano R, Zhang J *et al.* (2004). Efficacy of venlafaxine ER in patients with social anxiety disorder: a double-blind, placebo-controlled, parallel-group comparison with paroxetine. *Human Psychopharmacology* **19**, 387–396.

American Psychiatric Association (APA) (1994). *Diagnostic and Statistical Manual of Mental Disorders*, 4th edn. Washington, DC: American Psychiatric Association.

American Psychiatric Association (APA) (2001). Practice guideline for the treatment of patients with borderline personality disorder. *American Journal of Psychiatry* **158** (October suppl.), 1–52.

Baldwin D, Bobes J, Stein DJ *et al.* (1999). Paroxetine in social phobia/social anxiety disorder. Randomised double-blind, placebo-controlled study. Paroxetine Study. *British Journal of Psychiatry* **175**, 120–126.

Barratt ES, Kent TA, Bryant SG, Felthous AR (1991). A controlled trial of phenytoin in impulsive aggression. *Journal of Clinical Psychopharmacology* **11**, 388–389.

Barratt ES, Stanford MS, Felthous AR, Kent TA (1997). The effects of phenytoin on impulsive and pre-meditated aggression: a controlled study. *Journal of Clinical Psychopharmacology* **17**, 341–349.

Battaglia J, Wolff TK, Wagner Johnson DS *et al.* (1999). Structured diagnostic assessment and depot fluphenazine treatment of multiple suicide attempters in the emergency department. *International Clinical Psychopharmacology* **14**, 361–372.

Bender DS, Skodol AE (2007). Borderline personality as a self-other representational disturbance. *Journal of Personality Disorders* **21**, 500–517.

Bergida H, Lenzenweger MF (2006). Schizotypy and sustained attention: confirming evidence from an adult community sample. *Journal of Abnormal Psychology* **115**, 545–551.

Blair RJR (2005). Responding to the emotions of others: dissociating forms of empathy through the study of typical and psychiatric populations. *Consciousness and Cognition* **14**, 698–718.

Blomhoff S, Haug TT, Hellstrom K *et al.* (2001). Randomised controlled general practice trial of sertraline, exposure therapy and combined treatment in generalised social phobia. *British Journal of Psychiatry* **179**, 23–30.

Bogenschutz MP, Nurnberg PH (2004). Olanzapine *vs.* placebo in the treatment of borderline personality disorder. *Journal of Clinical Psychiatry* **65**, 104–109.

Bohus MJ, Landwehrmeyer GB, Stiglmayr CE *et al.* (1999). Naltrexone in the treatment of dissociative symptoms in patients with borderline personality disorder: an open-label trial. *Journal of Clinical Psychiatry* **60**, 598–603.

Bolton S, Gunderson JG (1996). Distinguishing borderline personality disorder from bipolar disorder: differential diagnosis and implications. *American Journal of Psychiatry* **153**, 1202–1207.

Brambilla P, Soloff PH, Sala M *et al.* (2004). Anatomical MRI study of borderline personality disorder patients. *Psychiatry Research* **131**, 125–133.

Coccaro EF, Kavoussi RJ (1997). Fluoxetine and impulsive aggressive behavior in personality-disordered subjects. *Archives of General Psychiatry* **54**, 1081–1088.

Coccaro EF, Kavoussi RJ, Hauger RL (1995). Physiological responses to d-fenfluramine and ipsapirone challenge correlate with indices of aggression in males with personality disorder. *International Clinical Psychopharmacology* **10**, 177–179.

Coccaro EF, Lee RJ, Kavoussi RJ (2009). A double-blind, randomized, placebo-controlled trial of fluoxetine in patients with intermittent explosive disorder. *Journal of Clinical Psychiatry* **70**, 653–662.

Coccaro EF, Siever LJ, Klar HM *et al.* (1989). Serotonergic studies in patients with affective and personality disorders: correlates with suicidal and impulsive aggressive behavior. *Archives of General Psychiatry* **46**, 587–599.

Cornelius JR, Soloff PH, Perel JM, Ulrich RF (1993). Continuation pharmacotherapy of borderline personality disorder with haloperidol and phenelzine. *American Journal of Psychiatry* **150**, 1843–1848.

Cowdry RW, Gardner DL (1988). Pharmacotherapy of borderline personality disorder: alprazolam, carbamazepine, trifluoperazine, and tranylcypromine. *Archives of General Psychiatry* **45**, 111–119.

Davidson J, Yaryura-Tobias J, DuPont R *et al.* (2004*b*). Fluvoxamine-controlled release formulation for the treatment of generalized social anxiety disorder. *Journal of Clinical Psychopharmacology* **24**, 118–125.

Davidson JR, Foa EB, Huppert JD *et al.* (2004*a*). Fluoxetine, comprehensive cognitive behavioral therapy, and placebo in generalized social phobia. *Archives of General Psychiatry* **61**, 1005–1013.

de la Fuente JM, Lotstra F (1994). A trial of carbamazepine in borderline personality disorder. *European Neuropsychopharmacology* **4**, 479–486.

Depue RA, Morrone-Strupinsky JV (2005). A neurobehavioral model of affiliative bonding: implications for conceptualizing a human trait of affiliation. *Behavioral and Brain Sciences* **28**, 313–395.

Deutsch H (1942). Some forms of emotional disturbance and their relationship to schizophrenia. *Psychoanalytic Quarterly* **11**, 301–321.

Ekselius L, von Knorring L (1998). Personality disorder comorbidity with major depression and response to treatment with sertraline or citalopram. *International Clinical Psychopharmacology* **13**, 205–211.

Evenden J (1999). Impulsivity: a discussion of clinical and experimental findings. *Journal of Psychopharmacology* **13**, 180–192.

Fahlen T (1995). Personality traits in social phobia, II: changes during drug treatment. *Journal of Clinical Psychiatry* **56**, 569–573.

Faltus FJ (1984). The positive effect of alprazolam in the treatment of three patients with borderline personality disorder. *American Journal of Psychiatry* **141**, 802–803.

Fonagy P, Luyten P (2009). A developmental, mentalization-based approach to the understanding and treatment of borderline personality disorder. *Development and Psychopathology* **21**, 1355–1381.

Frankenburg FR, Zanarini MC (2002). Divalproex sodium treatment of women with borderline personality disorder and bipolar II disorder: a double-blind placebo-controlled pilot study. *Journal of Clinical Psychiatry* **63**, 442–446.

Frankenburg FR, Zanarini MC (2006). Obesity and obesity-related illnesses in borderline patients. *Journal of Personality Disorders* **20**, 71–80.

Gardner DL, Cowdry RW (1986*a*). Development of melancholia during carbamazepine treatment in borderline personality disorder. *Journal of Clinical Psychopharmacology* **6**, 236–239.

Gardner DL, Cowdry RW (1986*b*). Positive effects of carbamazepine on behavioral dyscontrol in borderline personality disorder. *American Journal of Psychiatry* **143**, 519–522.

Goldberg SC, Schulz SC, Schulz PM *et al.* (1986). Borderline and schizotypal personality disorders treated with low-dose thiothixene *vs.* placebo. *Archives of General Psychiatry* **43**, 680–686.

Goodman M, New A, Siever L (2004). Trauma, genes, and the neurobiology of personality disorders. *Annals of the New York Academy of Sciences* **1032**, 104–116.

Goodwin GM, Bowden CL, Calabrese JR *et al.* (2004). A pooled analysis of 2 placebo-controlled 18-month trials of lamotrigine and lithium maintenance in bipolar I disorder. *Journal of Clinical Psychiatry* **65**, 432–441.

Griengl H, Sendera A, Dantendorfer K (2001). Naltrexone as a treatment of self-injurious behavior – a case report. *Acta Psychiatrica Scandinavica* **103**, 234–236.

Hamazaki T, Sawazaki S, Itomura M *et al.* (1996). The effect of docosahexaenoic acid on aggression in young adults. A placebo-controlled double-blind study. *Journal of Clinical Investigation* **97**, 1129–1133.

Hamazaki T, Thienprasert A, Kheovichai K *et al.* (2002). The effect of docosahexaenoic acid on aggression in elderly Thai subjects – a placebo-controlled double-blind study. *Nutritional Neuroscience* **5**, 37–41.

Heimberg RG, Liebowitz MR, Hope DA *et al.* (1998). Cognitive behavioral group therapy *vs.* phenelzine therapy for social phobia: 12-week outcome. *Archives of General Psychiatry* **55**, 1133–1141.

Henry C, Mitropoulou V, New AS *et al.* (2001). Affective instability and impulsivity in borderline personality and bipolar II disorders: similarities and differences. *Journal of Psychiatric Research* **35**, 307–312.

Herpertz SC, Zanarini M, Schulz CS *et al.* (2007). World Federation of Societies of Biological Psychiatry (WFSBP) guidelines for biological treatment of personality disorders. *World Journal of Biological Psychiatry* **8**, 212–244.

Higgins GA, Enderlin M, Haman M, Fletcher PJ (2003). The 5-HT2A receptor antagonist M100,907 attenuates motor and 'impulsive-type' behaviours produced by NMDA receptor antagonism. *Psychopharmacology* (Berlin) **170**, 309–319.

Hollander E, Allen A, Lopez RP *et al.* (2001). A preliminary double-blind, placebo-controlled trial of divalproex sodium in borderline personality disorder. *Journal of Clinical Psychiatry* **62**, 199–203.

Hollander E, Swann AC, Coccaro EF *et al.* (2005). Impact of trait impulsivity and state aggression on divalproex *vs.* placebo response in borderline personality disorder. *American Journal of Psychiatry* **162**, 621–624.

Hollander E, Tracy KA, Swann AC *et al.* (2003). Divalproex in the treatment of impulsive aggression: efficacy in cluster B personality disorders. *Neuropsychopharmacology* **28**, 1185–1197.

Houston RJ, Bauer LO, Hesselbrock VM (2004). Effects of borderline personality disorder features and a family history of alcohol or drug dependence on P300 in adolescents. *International Journal of Psychophysiology* **53**, 57–70.

Huband N, Ferriter M, Nathan R, Jones H (2010). Antiepileptics for aggression and associated impulsivity. *Cochrane Database for Systematic Reviews* **2**, CD003499.

IMCTGMSP, Katschnig H (1997). The International Multicenter Clinical Trial Group on Moclobemide in Social Phobia. Moclobemide in social phobia: a double-blind, placebo-controlled clinical study. *European Archives of Psychiatry and Clinical Neuroscience* **247**, 71–80.

Ingenhoven T, Lafay P, Rinne T *et al.* (2010). Effectiveness of pharmacotherapy for severe personality disorders: meta-analyses of randomized controlled trials. *Journal of Clinical Psychiatry* **71**, 14–25.

Jensen HV, Andersen J (1989). An open, noncomparative study of amoxapine in borderline disorders. *Acta Psychiatrica Scandinavica* **79**, 89–93.

Juengling FD, Schmahl C, Hesslinger B *et al.* (2003). Positron emission tomography in female patients with borderline personality disorder. *Journal of Psychiatric Research* **37**, 109–115.

Kasper S, Stein DJ, Loft H, Nil R (2005). Escitalopram in the treatment of social anxiety disorder: randomised, placebo-controlled, flexible-dosage study. *British Journal of Psychiatry* **186**, 222–226.

Katzelnick DJ, Kobak KA, Greist JH *et al.* (1995). Sertraline for social phobia: a double-blind, placebo-controlled crossover study. *American Journal of Psychiatry* **152**, 1368–1371.

Kayser A, Robinson DS, Nies A, Howard D (1985). Response to phenelzine among depressed patients with features of hysteroid dysphoria. *American Journal of Psychiatry* **142**, 486–488.

Keck P, Buffenstein A, Ferguson J et al. (1998). Ziprasidone 40 and 120 mg/day in the acute exacerbation of schizophrenia and schizoaffective disorder: a 4-week placebo-controlled trial. *Psychopharmacology* **140**, 173–184.

Koenigsberg HW, Reynolds D, Goodman M et al. (2003). Risperidone in the treatment of schizotypal personality disorder. *Journal of Clinical Psychiatry* **64**, 628–634.

Lader M, Stender K, Burger V, Nil R (2004). Efficacy and tolerability of escitalopram in 12- and 24-week treatment of social anxiety disorder: randomised, double-blind, placebo-controlled, fixed-dose study. *Depression and Anxiety* **19**, 241–248.

Langdon R, Coltheart M (2004). Recognition of metaphor and irony in young adults: the impact of schizotypal personality traits. *Psychiatry Research* **125**, 9–20.

Leiberich P, Nickel MK, Tritt K, Pedrosa Gil F (2008). Lamotrigine treatment of aggression in female borderline patients, part II: an 18-month follow-up. *Journal of Psychopharmacology* **22**, 805–808.

Leone NF (1982). Response of borderline patients to loxapine and chlorpromazine. *Journal of Clinical Psychiatry* **43**, 148–150.

Lepola U, Bergtholdt B, St Lambert J et al. (2004). Controlled-release paroxetine in the treatment of patients with social anxiety disorder. *Journal of Clinical Psychiatry* **65**, 222–229.

Levitt JJ, Westin CF, Nestor PG et al. (2004). Shape of caudate nucleus and its cognitive correlates in neuroleptic-naïve schizotypal personality disorder. *Biological Psychiatry* **55**, 177–184.

Lieb K, Vollm B, Rucker G et al. (2010). Pharmacotherapy for borderline personality disorder: Cochrane systematic review of randomized trials. *British Journal of Psychiatry* **196**, 4–12.

Lieb K, Zanarini MC, Schmahl C et al. (2004). Borderline personality disorder. *Lancet* **364**, 453–461.

Liebowitz MR, Klein DF (1981). Interrelationship of hysteroid dysphoria and borderline personality disorder. *Psychiatric Clinics of North America* **4**, 67–87.

Liebowitz MR, Gelenberg AJ, Munjack D (2005a). Venlafaxine extended release *vs.* placebo and paroxetine in social anxiety disorder. *Archives of General Psychiatry* **62**, 190–198.

Liebowitz MR, Heimberg RG, Schneier FR et al. (1999). Cognitive-behavioral group therapy versus phenelzine in social phobia: long-term outcome. *Depression and Anxiety* **10**, 89–98.

Liebowitz MR, Mangano RM, Bradwejn J et al. (2005b). A randomized controlled trial of venlafaxine extended release in generalized social anxiety disorder. *Journal of Clinical Psychiatry* **66**, 238–247.

Liebowitz MR, Stein MB, Tancer M et al. (2002). A randomized, double-blind, fixed-dose comparison of paroxetine and placebo in the treatment of generalized social anxiety disorder. *Journal of Clinical Psychiatry* **63**, 66–74.

Links PS, Steiner M, Boiago I, Irwin D (1990). Lithium therapy for borderline patients: preliminary findings. *Journal of Personality Disorders* **4**, 173–181.

Lion JR (1979). Benzodiazepines in the treatment of aggressive patients. *Journal of Clinical Psychiatry* **40**, 70–71.

Loew TH, Nickel MK (2008). Topiramate treatment of women with borderline personality disorder, part II: an open 18-month follow-up. *Journal of Clinical Psychopharmacology* **28**, 355–357.

Loew TH, Nickel MK, Muehlbacher M et al. (2006). Topiramate treatment of women with borderline personality disorder: a double-blind, placebo-controlled study. *Journal of Clinical Psychopharmacology* **26**, 61–66.

Loranger AW, Sartorius N, Andreoli A et al. (1994). The international personality disorders examination. The World Health Organization/alcohol, drug abuse, and mental health administration international pilot study of personality disorders. *Archives of General Psychiatry* **51**, 215–224.

Lott M, Greist JH, Jefferson JW et al. (1997). Brofaromine for social phobia: a multicenter, placebo-controlled, double-blind study. *Journal of Clinical Psychopharmacology* **17**, 255–260.

Malone KM, Corbitt EM, Li S, Mann JJ (1996). Prolactin response to fenfluramine and suicide attempt lethality in major depression. *British Journal of Psychiatry* **168**, 324–329.

Markovitz PJ, Calabrese JR, Schulz SC, Meltzer HY (1991). Fluoxetine in the treatment of borderline and schizotypal personality disorders. *American Journal of Psychiatry* **148**, 1064–1067.

Mattes JA (2005). Oxcarbazepine in patients with impulsive aggression: a double-blind, placebo-controlled trial. *Journal of Clinical Psychopharmacology* **25**, 575–579.

Mattes JA (2008). Levetiracetam in patients with impulsive aggression: a double-blind, placebo-controlled trial. *Journal of Clinical Psychiatry* **69**, 310–315.

Mauchnik J, Schmahl C (2010). The latest neuroimaging findings in borderline personality disorder. *Current Psychiatry Reports* **12**, 46–55.

McClure MM, Barch DM, Romero MJ et al. (2007b). The effects of guanfacine on context-processing abnormalities in schizotypal personality disorder. *Biological Psychiatry* **61**, 1157–1160.

McClure MM, Harvey PD, Goodman M et al. (2010). Pergolide treatment of cognitive deficits associated with schizotypal personality disorder: continued evidence of the importance of the dopamine system in the schizophrenia spectrum. *Neuropsychopharmacology* **35**, 1356–1362.

McClure MM, Romero MJ, Bowie CR et al. (2007a). Visual-spatial learning and memory in schizotypal personality disorder: continued evidence for the importance of working memory in the schizophrenia spectrum. *Archives of Clinical Neuropsychology* **22**, 109–116.

McGee MD (1997). Cessation of self-mutilation in a patient with borderline personality disorder treated with naltrexone. *Journal of Clinical Psychiatry* **58**, 32–33.

Mehlman PT, Higley JD, Faucher I et al. (1994). Low CSF 5-HIAA concentrations and severe aggression and impaired impulse control in nonhuman primates. *American Journal of Psychiatry* **151**, 1485–1491.

Mercer D, Douglass AB, Links PS (2009). Meta-analyses of mood stabilizers, antidepressants and antipsychotics in the treatment of borderline personality disorder:

effectiveness for depression and anger symptoms. *Journal of Personality Disorders* **23**, 156–174.

Minzenberg MJ, Grossman R, New AS et al. (2006). Blunted hormone responses to ipsapirone are associated with trait impulsivity in personality disorder patients. *Neuropsychopharmacology* **31**, 197–203.

Montgomery SA, Montgomery D (1982). Pharmacological prevention of suicidal behavior. *Journal of Affective Disorders* **4**, 291–298.

Montgomery SA, Nil R, Durr-Pal N et al. (2005). A 24-week randomized, double-blind, placebo-controlled study of escitalopram for the prevention of generalized social anxiety disorder. *Journal of Clinical Psychiatry* **66**, 1270–1278.

Montgomery SA, Roy D, Montgomery DB (1983). The prevention of recurrent suicidal acts. *British Journal of Clinical Pharmacology* **15**, 183S–188S.

New AS, Hazlett EA, Buchsbaum MS et al. (2002). Blunted prefrontal cortical 18 fluorodeoxyglucose positron emission tomography response to meta-chlorophenylpiperazine in impulsive aggression. *Archives of General Psychiatry* **59**, 621–629.

New AS, Trestman R, Mitropoulou V et al. (1997). Serotonergic function and self-injurious behavior in personality disorder patients. *Psychiatry Research* **69**, 17–26.

New AS, Trestman R, Mitropoulou V et al. (2004). Low prolactin response to fenfluramine in impulsive aggression. *Journal of Psychiatric Research* **38**, 223–230.

Nickel MK, Loew TH (2008). Treatment of aggression with topiramate in male borderline patients, part II: 18-month follow-up. *European Psychiatry* **23**, 115–117.

Nickel MK, Loew TH, Pedrosa Gil F (2007). Aripiprazole in treatment of borderline patients, part II: an 18-month follow-up. *Psychopharmacology* **191**, 1023–1026.

Nickel MK, Muehlbacher M, Nickel C et al. (2006). Aripiprazole in the treatment of patients with borderline personality disorder: a double-blind, placebo-controlled study. *American Journal of Psychiatry* **163**, 833–838.

Nickel MK, Nickel C, Kaplan P et al. (2005). Treatment of aggression with topiramate in male borderline patients: a double-blind, placebo-controlled study. *Biological Psychiatry* **57**, 495–499.

Nickel MK, Nickel C, Mitterlehner FO *et al.* (2004). Topiramate treatment of aggression in female borderline personality disorder patients: a double-blind, placebo-controlled study. *Journal of Clinical Psychiatry* **65**, 1515–1519.

Noyes R, Moroz G, Davidson JR *et al.* (1997). Moclobemide in social phobia: a controlled dose-response trial. *Journal of Clinical Psychopharmacology* **17**, 247–254.

Ogiso Y, Moriya N, Ikuta N *et al.* (1993). Relationship between clinical symptoms and EEG findings in borderline personality disorder. *Japanese Journal of Psychiatry and Neurology* **47**, 37–46.

Oquendo MA, Krunic A, Parsey RV *et al.* (2005). Positron emission tomography of regional brain metabolic responses to a serotonergic challenge in major depressive disorder with and without borderline personality disorder. *Neuropsychopharmacology* **30**, 1163–1172.

Pande AC, Davidson JR, Jefferson JW *et al.* (1999). Treatment of social phobia with gabapentin: a placebo-controlled study. *Journal of Clinical Psychopharmacology* **19**, 341–348.

Pande AC, Feltner DE, Jefferson JW *et al.* (2004). Efficacy of the novel anxiolytic pregabalin in social anxiety disorder. *Journal of Clinical Psychopharmacology* **24**, 141–149.

Pare S, McTigue K (1997). Working memory and the syndromes of schizotypal personality. *Schizophrenia Research* **29**, 213–220.

Paris J (2004). Borderline or bipolar? Distinguishing borderline personality disorder from bipolar spectrum disorders. *Harvard Review of Psychiatry* **12**, 140–145.

Paris J (2005). Borderline personality disorder. *Canadian Medical Association Journal* **172**, 1579–1583.

Parsons B, Quitkin FM, McGrath PJ *et al.* (1989). Phenelzine, imipramine, and placebo in borderline patients meeting criteria for atypical depression. *Psychopharmacological Bulletin* **25**, 524–534.

Pascual JC, Madre M, Soler J *et al.* (2006). Injectable atypical antipsychotics for agitation in borderline personality disorder. *Pharmacopsychiatry* **39**, 117–118.

Pascual JC, Oller S, Soler J *et al.* (2004). Ziprasidone in the acute treatment of borderline personality disorder in psychiatric emergency services. *Journal of Clinical Psychiatry* **65**, 1281–1283.

Pascual JC, Soler J, Puigdemont D *et al.* (2008). Ziprasidone in the treatment of borderline personality disorder: a double-blind, placebo-controlled, randomized study. *Journal of Clinical Psychiatry* **69**, 603–608.

Peet M, Stokes C (2005). Omega-3 fatty acids in the treatment of psychiatric disorders. *Drugs* **65**, 1051–1059.

Philipsen A, Richter H, Schmahl C *et al.* (2004*a*). Clonidine in acute aversive inner tension and self-injurious behavior in female patients with borderline personality disorder. *Journal of Clinical Psychiatry* **65**, 1414–1419.

Philipsen A, Schmahl C, Lieb K (2004*b*). Naloxone in the treatment of acute dissociative states in female patients with borderline personality disorder. *Pharmacopsychiatry* **37**, 196–199.

Pickup GJ (2006). Theory of mind and its relation to schizotypy. *Cognitive Neuropsychiatry* **11**, 177–192.

Pitchot W, Hansenne M, Pinto E *et al.* (2005). 5-Hydroxytryptamine 1A receptors, major depression, and suicidal behavior. *Biological Psychiatry* **58**, 854–858.

Placidi GP, Oquendo MA, Malone KM *et al.* (2001). Aggressivity, suicide attempts, and depression: relationship to cerebrospinal fluid monoamine metabolite levels. *Biological Psychiatry* **50**, 783–791.

Posner MI, Rothbart MK, Vizueta N *et al.* (2002). Attentional mechanisms of borderline personality disorder. *Proceedings of the National Academy of Sciences USA* **99**, 16366–16370.

Prossin AR, Love TM, Koeppe RA *et al.* (2010). Dysregulation of regional endogenous opioid function in borderline personality disorder. *American Journal of Psychiatry* **167**, 925–933.

Reich DB, Zanarini MC, Bieri KA (2009). A preliminary study of lamotrigine in the treatment of affective instability in borderline personality disorder. *International Clinical Psychopharmacology* **24**, 270–275.

Reich J (2002). Drug treatment of personality disorder traits. *Psychiatric Annals* **32**, 590–596.

Rickels K, Mangano R, Khan A (2004). A double-blind, placebo-controlled study of a flexible dose of venlafaxine ER in adult outpatients with generalized social anxiety disorder. *Journal of Clinical Psychopharmacology* 24, 488–496.

Rifkin A, Quitkin F, Carrillo C et al. (1972). Lithium carbonate in emotionally unstable character disorder. *Archives of General Psychiatry* 27, 519–523.

Rinne T, van den Brink W, Wouters L, van Dyck R (2002). SSRI treatment of borderline personality disorder: a randomized, placebo-controlled clinical trial for female patients with borderline personality disorder. *American Journal of Psychiatry* 159, 2048–2054.

Roth AS, Rostroff RB, Hoffman RE (1996). Naltrexone as a treatment for repetitive self-injurious behavior: an open-label trial. *Journal of Clinical Psychiatry* 57, 233–237.

Rusch N, van Elst LT, Ludaescher P et al. (2003). A voxel-based morphometric MRI study in female patients with borderline personality disorder. *Neuroimage* 20, 385–392.

Russ MJ, Campbell SS, Kakuma T et al. (1991). EEG theta activity and pain insensitivity in self-injurious borderline patients. *Psychiatry Research* 89, 201–214.

Salzman C, Wolfson AN, Schatzberg A et al. (1995). Effects of fluoxetine on anger in symptomatic volunteers with borderline personality disorder. *Journal of Clinical Psychopharmacology* 15, 23–29.

Samuelsson M, Jokinen J, Nordstrom AL, Nordstrom P (2006). CSF 5-HIAA, suicide intent and hopelessness in the prediction of early suicide in male high-risk suicide attempters. *Acta Psychiatrica Scandinavica* 113, 44–47.

Saper JR (2000). Borderline personality, opioids, and naltrexone. *Headache* 40, 765–766.

Schneier FR, Gortz D, Campeas R et al. (1998). Placebo-controlled trial of moclobemide in social phobia. *British Journal of Psychiatry* 172, 70–77.

Schulz SC, Zanarini MC, Bateman A et al. (2008). Olanzapine for the treatment of borderline personality disorder: variable-dose 12-week randomized double-blind placebo-controlled study. *British Journal of Psychiatry* 193, 485–492.

Serban G, Siegel S (1984). Response of borderline and schizotypal patients to small doses of thiothixene and haloperidol. *American Journal of Psychiatry* 141, 1455–1458.

Shafti SS, Shahveisi B (2010). Olanzapine *vs.* haloperidol in the management of borderline personality disorder: a randomized double-blind trial. *Journal of Clinical Psychopharmacology* 30, 44–47.

Sheard MH (1971). Effect of lithium on human aggression. *Nature* 230, 113–114.

Sheard MH, Marini JL, Bridges CI, Wagner E (1976). The effect of lithium on impulsive aggressive behavior in man. *American Journal of Psychiatry* 133, 1409–1413.

Siever LJ, Buchsbaum MS, New AS et al. (1999). D,L-fenfluramine response in impulsive personality disorder assessed with [18F]fluorodeoxyglucose positron emission tomography. *Neuropsychopharmacology* 20, 413–423.

Siever LJ, Davis KL (1991). A psychobiological perspective on the personality disorders. *American Journal of Psychiatry* 148, 1647–1658.

Siever LJ, Davis KL (2004). The pathophysiology of schizophrenia disorders: perspectives from the spectrum. *American Journal of Psychiatry* 161, 398–413.

Simeon D, Stanley B, Frances A et al. (1992). Self-mutilation in personality disorders: psychological and biological correlates. *American Journal of Psychiatry* 149, 221–226.

Simpson EB, Yen S, Costello E et al. (2004). Combined dialectical behavior therapy and fluoxetine in the treatment of borderline personality disorder. *Journal of Clinical Psychiatry* 65, 379–385.

Skodol AE, Gunderson JG, Shea MT et al. (2005). The collaborative longitudinal personality disorders study (CLPS): overview and implications. *Journal of Personality Disorders* 19, 487–504.

Smith DJ, Muir WJ, Blackwood DH (2004). Is borderline personality disorder part of the bipolar spectrum? *Harvard Review of Psychiatry* 12, 133–139.

Soderstrom H, Foresman A (2004). Elevated triiodothyronine in psychopathy – possible physiological mechanisms. *Journal of Neural Transmission* 111, 739–744.

Soler J, Pascual JC, Campins J et al. (2005). Double-blind, placebo-controlled study of dialectical behavior therapy plus olanzapine for borderline personality disorder. American Journal of Psychiatry 162, 1221–1224.

Soloff PH, Cornelius J, George A et al. (1993). Efficacy of phenelzine and haloperidol in borderline personality disorder. Archives of General Psychiatry 50, 377–385.

Soloff PH, George A, Nathan RS et al. (1986a). Paradoxical effects of amitryptiline on borderline patients. American Journal of Psychiatry 143, 1603–1605.

Soloff PH, George A, Nathan RS et al. (1986b). Amitryptiline and haloperidol in unstable and schizotypal borderline disorders. Psychopharmacology Bulletin 22, 177–182.

Soloff PH, George A, Nathan RS et al. (1986c). Progress in pharmacotherapy of borderline disorders. Archives of General Psychiatry 43, 691–697.

Soloff PH, George A, Nathan RS et al. (1987). Behavioral dyscontrol in borderline patients treated with amitryptiline. Psychopharmacology Bulletin 23, 177–181.

Soloff PH, George A, Nathan RS et al. (1989). Amitryptiline vs. haloperidol in borderlines: final outcomes and predictors of response. Journal of Clinical Psychopharmacology 9, 238–246.

Southwick SM, Bremner JD, Rasmusson A et al. (1999). Role of norepinephrine in the pathophysiology and treatment of posttraumatic stress disorder. Biological Psychiatry 46, 1192–1204.

Stanley B, Siever LJ (2010). The interpersonal dimension of borderline personality disorder: toward a neuropeptide model. American Journal of Psychiatry 167, 24–39.

Stein DJ, Versiani M, Hair T, Kumar R (2002). Efficacy of paroxetine for relapse prevention in social anxiety disorder. Archives of General Psychiatry 59, 1111–1118.

Stein MB, Fyer AJ, Davidson JR et al. (1999). Fluvoxamine treatment of social phobia (social anxiety disorder): a double-blind, placebo-controlled study. American Journal of Psychiatry 156, 756–760.

Stein MB, Liebowitz MR, Lydiard RB et al. (1998). Paroxetine treatment of gereralized social phobia (social anxiety disorder): a randomized controlled trial. Journal of the American Medical Association 280, 708–713.

Stein MB, Pollack MH, Bystritsky A et al. (2005). Efficacy of low and higher dose extended-release venlafaxine in generalized social anxiety disorder: a 6-month randomized controlled trial. Psychopharmalogy 177, 280–288.

Strawn JR, Geracioti TD (2008). Noradrenergic dysfunction and the psychopharmacology of posttraumatic stress disorder. Depression and Anxiety 25, 260–271.

Tandon R (2000). Introduction: ziprasidone appears to offer important therapeutic and tolerability advantages over conventional, and some novel, antipsychotics. British Journal of Clinical Pharmacology 49(Suppl. 1), 1S–3S.

Thurauf NJ, Washeim HA (2000). The effects of exogenous analgesia in a patient with borderline personality disorder (BPD) and severe self-injurious behavior. European Journal of Pain 4, 107–109.

Traskman L, Asberg M, Bertilsson L, Sjostrand L (1981). Monoamine metabolites in CSF and suicidal behavior. Archives of General Psychiatry 38, 631–636.

Tritt K, Nickel C, Lahmann C et al. (2005). Lamotrigine treatment of aggression in female borderline patients: a randomized, double-blind, placebo-controlled study. Journal of Psychopharmacology 19, 287–291.

van Ameringen M, Oakman J, Mancini C et al. (2004). Predictors of response in generalized social phobia: effect of age of onset. Journal of Clinical Psychopharmacology 24, 42–48.

van Ameringen MA, Lane RM, Walker JR et al. (2001). Sertraline treatment of generalized social phobia: a 20-week, doubleblind, placebo-controlled study. American Journal of Psychiatry 158, 275–281.

van Vliet IM, den Boer JA, Westenberg HG (1994). Psychopharmacological treatment of social phobia; a double blind placebo controlled study with fluvoxamine. Psychopharmacology (Berlin) 115, 128–134.

Verkes RJ, van der Mast RC, Hengeveld MW et al. (1998). Reduction by paroxetine of suicidal behavior in patients with repeated suicide attempts but not major depression. American Journal of Psychiatry 155, 543–547.

Versiani M, Nardi AE, Mundim FD et al. (1992). Pharmacotherapy of social phobia. A controlled study with moclobemide and phenelzine. *British Journal of Psychiatry* **161**, 353–360.

Virkkunen M, Rawlings R, Tokola R *et al.* (1994). CSF biochemistries, glucose metabolism, and diurnal activity rhythms in alcoholic, violent offenders, fire setters, and healthy volunteers. *Archives of General Psychiatry* **51**, 20–27.

Welch SS, Linehan MM (2002). High-risk situations associated with parasuicide and drug use in borderline personality disorder. *Journal of Personality Disorders* **16**, 561–569.

Wilner KD, Anziano RJ, Johnson AC *et al.* (2002). The anxiolytic effect of the novel antipsychotic ziprasidone compared with diazepam in subjects anxious before dental surgery. *Journal of Clinical Psychopharmacology* **22**, 206–210.

Winstanley CA, Theobald DE, Dalley JW *et al.* (2004). 5-HT2A and 5-HT2C receptor antagonists have opposing effects on a measure of impulsivity. Interactions with global 5-HT depletion. *Psychopharmacology (Berlin)* **176**, 376–385.

Zanarini MC, Frankenburg FR (2001). Olanzapine treatment of female borderline personality disorder patients: a double-blind, placebo-controlled pilot study. *Journal of Clinical Psychiatry* **62**, 849–854.

Zanarini MC, Frankenburg FR (2003). Omega-3 fatty acid treatment of women with borderline personality disorder: a double-blind, placebo-controlled pilot study. *American Journal of Psychiatry* **160**, 167–169.

Zanarini MC, Frankenburg FR, Hennen J *et al.* (2004*a*). Axis I comorbidity of borderline personality disorder: description of six-year course and prediction to time-to-remission. *American Journal of Psychiatry* **161**, 2108–2114.

Zanarini MC, Frankenburg FR, Parachini EA (2004*b*). A preliminary, randomized trial of fluoxetine, olanzapine, and the olanzapine–fluoxetine combination in women with borderline personality disorder. *Journal of Clinical Psychiatry* **7**, 903–907.

Zanarini MC, Frankenburg FR, Vujanovic AA *et al.* (2004*c*). Axis II comorbidity of borderline personality disorder: description of six-year course and prediction to time-to-remission. *Acta Psychiatrica Scandinavica* **110**, 416–420.

Zanarini MC, Gunderson JG, Frankenburg FR, Chauncey DL (1990). Discriminating borderline personality disorder from other axis II disorders. *American Journal of Psychiatry* **147**, 161–167.

Ziegenhorn AA, Roepke S, Schommer NC *et al.* (2009). Clonidine improves hyperarousal in borderline personality disorder with or without comorbid post-traumatic stress disorder: a randomized, double-blind, placebo-controlled trial. *Journal of Clinical Psychopharmacology* **29**, 170–173.

Index

Printed in the United States
By Bookmasters